Mosby's

RADIATION THERAPY

Study Guide and Exam Review

LEIA LEVY, MAdEd, RT(T)
Program Director
Radiation Therapy Program
Swedish American Health System
Rockford, Illinois

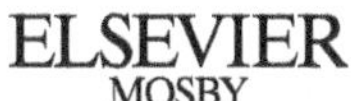

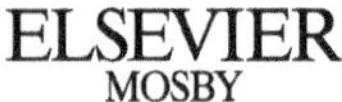

3251 Riverport Lane
St. Louis, Missouri 63043

MOSBY'S RADIATION THERAPY STUDY GUIDE AND EXAM REVIEW

ISBN: 978-0-323-06934-2

Notices

Knowledge and best practice in this field are constantly changing. As new research and experience broaden our understanding, changes in research methods, professional practices, or medical treatment may become necessary.

Practitioners and researchers must always rely on their own experience and knowledge in evaluating and using any information, methods, compounds, or experiments described herein. In using such information or methods they should be mindful of their own safety and the safety of others, including parties for whom they have a professional responsibility.

With respect to any drug or pharmaceutical products identified, readers are advised to check the most current information provided (i) on procedures featured or (ii) by the manufacturer of each product to be administered, to verify the recommended dose or formula, the method and duration of administration, and contraindications. It is the responsibility of practitioners, relying on their own experience and knowledge of their patients, to make diagnoses, to determine dosages and the best treatment for each individual patient, and to take all appropriate safety precautions.

To the fullest extent of the law, neither the Publisher nor the authors, contributors, or editors, assume any liability for any injury and/or damage to persons or property as a matter of products liability, negligence or otherwise, or from any use or operation of any methods, products, instructions, or ideas contained in the material herein.

ISBN: 978-0-323-06934-2

Acquisitions Editor: Jeanne Olson
Developmental Editor: Luke Held
Publishing Services Manager: Julie Eddy
Senior Project Manager: Andrea Campbell
Design Direction: Karen Pauls

Printed in the United States of America

Last digit is the print number: 13 12 11 10

To my husband, Rick, for your support and encouragement,
and my children, Reia and Malcolm,
for your understanding during those long hours at the computer.
To my parents, for your encouragement and cultivation of my faith.

To every radiation therapy student who has passion and determination
to make a difference in the lives of every patient encountered.

Contributors and Reviewers

CONTRIBUTORS

Beverly K. Coker, MA, RT(R)(T)

Program Chair/Assistant Professor for Radiation Therapy
Baptist College of Health Sciences
Memphis, Tennessee

Elva Marie Dawson, MSEd, RT(T)

Clinical Coordinator
Radiation Therapy Program
Swedish American Health System
Rockford, Illinois

Mike Hosto, RT(T), CMD

Medical Dosimetrist
Swedish American Hospital
Rockford, Illinois

Robert P. Laureckas, MS, PhD (ABD)

PhD Candidate
Department of Medical Radiation Physics
Rosalind Franklin University of Medicine and Science
North Chicago, Illinois
Medical Physicist, Radiation Oncology
Advocate Christ Medical Center
Oak Lawn, Illinois

Contributed questions to Exam Review on the Evolve site

Jayme Leavy, RN, MSN, ANP-BC, OCN

Adult Nurse Practitioner
Rockford, Illinois

Christine C. Zielinski, BA, MSEd

Director, Academic Resource Center
University of St. Francis
Joliet, Illinois

REVIEWERS

Robert D. Adams, EdD, CMD, RT(R)(T)

Assistant Professor
UNC School of Medicine, Department of Radiation Oncology
Chapel Hill, North Carolina

Stacy L. Anderson, MS, RT(T), CMD

Associate Professor and Interim Chair
University of Oklahoma Health Sciences Center
Department of Medical Imaging and Radiation Sciences
College of Allied Health
Oklahoma City, Oklahoma

Lisa Bartenhagen, MS, RT(R)(T)

Program Director
University of Nebraska Medical Center
Omaha, Nebraska

Beverly K. Coker, MA, RT(R)(T)

Program Chair, Radiation Therapy
Baptist College of Health Sciences
Memphis, Tennessee

Annette M. Coleman, MA, RT(T)

Product Manager Radiation Oncology Charting and Imaging
IMPAC Medical Systems
Sunnyvale, California

Patricia A. Davis, BS, RT(R)

Acting Program Director
University of Virginia Health System Program of Radiography
Charlottesville, Virginia

Stephanie Eatmon, EdD, RT(R)(T), FASRT

Program Director
California State University, Long Beach
Long Beach, California

Kathryn E. Frye-Oakley, MS, RT(R)(T)

Associate Professor/Educational Program Director
Weber State University
Ogden, Utah

Ahmad Hammoud, BS, RT(T), CMD

Supervisor, Dosimetry Services
Karmanos Cancer Hospital
Detroit, Michigan

Jana L. Koth, BS, RT(R)(T)

Clinical Education Coordinator
University of Nebraska Medical Center
Omaha, Nebraska

Deborah A. Kuban, MD, FACR, FASTRO

Board Certified Radiation Oncology, 1986
M.D. Anderson Cancer Center
Houston, Texas

Ronnie Lozano, MSRS, RT(T)

Program Chair and Associate Professor
Radiation Therapy Program
Texas State University
San Marcos, Texas

Shirlee E. Maihoff, MEd, RT(T)

Associate Professor, Retired - Currently as Consultant
University of Alabama at Birmingham
Birmingham, Alabama

Sandy L. Piehl, RT(R)(T), MPA

Program Director, School of Radiation Therapy
Northwestern Memorial Hospital
Chicago, Illinois

Judith Mae Schneider, MS, RT(R)(T)

Master of Science Degree in Education
Clinical Coordinator/Assistant Clinical Professor
Indiana University
IUPUI
School of Medicine
Radiation Therapy Program
Indianapolis, Indiana

Zachary D. Smith, AAS, BS, MBA

Director - Radiation Therapy
Baton Rouge General, Pennington Cancer Center
Baton Rouge, Louisiana

Megan Trad, MSRS, RT(T)

Assistant Professor
Texas State University
San Marcos, Texas

Amy Carson VonKadich, MEd, RT(T)

Program Director, Radiation Therapy
New Hampshire Technical Institute
Concord, New Hampshire

Paul E. Wallner, DO, FACR, FAOCR, FASTRO

Radiology (AOBR), Therapeutic Radiology (ABR)
Senior Vice President, 21st Century Oncology, Inc.
Fort Myers, Florida
Adjunct Professor, NYU School of Medicine, Dept of Radiation Oncology
New York, New York

Tracy B. White, MS, RT(R)(T)

Program Director, Associate Professor
Arkansas State University
Jonesboro, Arkansas

Preface

Content and Organization

Mosby's Radiation Therapy Study Guide and Exam Review is intended to be a comprehensive study guide and review of radiation therapy curriculum content and the traditional core competencies for the radiation therapist. The guide is divided by subject area. The first eight chapters are subject-concentrated so that students may use them to reinforce notes following lecture or to prepare for subject-related examinations. The final chapter is intended to show readers how curriculum content is actually applied in clinical situations and should allow students to see how all curriculum content areas are used in everyday practice.

Each chapter contains the following material:

- **Focus questions**, which should give students a glimpse into the highlights of the subject matter. Students and faculty may use focus questions as a means of testing knowledge in the subject area *before* reading through the chapter.
- **Review material**, which is presented using bulleted high-point phrases and detailed illustrations, including drawings, diagrams, radiographic images, and tables, when appropriate.
- **Reference textbooks for suggested reading**, which are texts that are available and used by many programs in radiation therapy, radiation oncology, oncology nursing, and medical physics. The hope is that the user will have access to at least one text on the list to explore theories and find illustrations and justification for the published correct answers.
- **Review exercises**, which are designed to engage the student in active review of the material. There are fill-in-the-blank, complete-the-table, true/false correctives, matching, puzzles, diagramming, labeling, and other active-learning exercises among traditional multiple choice–type questions.

ANCILLARIES

The study guide is also available for purchase in electronic format for convenience of use in any setting where the internet is available. Faculty with access to the electronic study guide may use focus questions or end-of-chapter activities during class time for content review.

Online Mock Examinations

To supplement the study guide, online mock examinations are available through Elsevier's Evolve website at http://evolve.elsevier.com/Levy/radiationtherapy/. The online mock examinations feature a bank of more than 1000 multiple-choice questions in topic areas relating to the core competencies for the radiation therapist. The exam questions may be used for study or exam preparation.

Study Mode. In study mode, students can choose to view questions from all topic areas or select specific area(s) in which they would like to concentrate. During study mode, the user will be provided immediate feedback after answering each question.

Exam Mode. When a student elects to take a mock examination, they will be administered a 200-question test, with questions randomly selected from the question bank. The random selection of questions will provide the student with access to multiple comprehensive examination opportunities while minimizing the chances of seeing repeat questions. At the end of the mock examination, the student and/or faculty will be able to review results and become cognizant of areas needing further study or areas of relative proficiency.

Because some radiation therapy programs require program exit examinations, the mock examinations accompanying the study guide will provide programs with an exit examination tool and insight into content area strengths and weaknesses per cohort, across cohorts, or for individual students. These examinations may also be used periodically by students and faculty as developmental assessments. For example, a student or program may begin taking mock examinations by the mid-point of the curriculum and then take examinations periodically thereafter, to assess improved and increased understanding of content.

How to Use

The maximum benefits of this study guide and online examinations can be realized when student and faculty implement use starting at the beginning of the academic program. By using the guide from the beginning, content areas may be reinforced gradually. The table of contents is expanded such that students and faculty can selectively review material as curriculum content delivery order prescribed by individual programs. By the end of an academic program, students may use previously completed activities to help prepare for comprehensive exit examinations and also to prepare for certifying examinations.

Acknowledgments

I would like to thank all of the radiation therapy professionals who contributed to this project. To Elva Dawson, radiation therapist and clinical coordinator, for being so willing to commit to helping with this project during a very demanding period in your professional and family life. To Robert Laureckas, medical physicist, for committing to helping with this project while working on your doctoral degree and meeting the demands of a full-time physicist. Mike Hosto, dosimetrist, for being courageous in committing to a project such as this that required you to step into an area you had reservations about. To Jayme Leavy, oncology nurse educator, for not hesitating in committing to helping with this project in the midst of developing new nurse competencies, assisting in pharmaceutical promotions, and completing the graduate nurse practitioner program. To Beverly Coker, radiation therapist and program director, for committing to helping with this project in the midst of the most demanding program director duties and personal challenges.

To Christine Zielinski, I am so grateful for our meeting. Your contribution is invaluable. Your daily work impacts so many; so much more now that you have given your talent to this work. You never know exactly how one encounter can blossom.

Very special thanks to Luke Held, Developmental Editor, for your guidance, patience, and flexibility. Thanks for reviewing drafts of this work, and for your honesty and most helpful feedback. Thanks also to Jeanne Olson, Publisher, and Andrea Campbell, Senior Project Manager, as well as to the other Elsevier staff members who contributed to the publication of this project.

Contents

Mosby's

RADIATION THERAPY

Study Guide and Exam Review

CHAPTER

1

Developing Good Study Habits in the Health Professions

Christine Zielinski

FOCUS QUESTIONS

- What are some ways to strengthen study skills in reading, note-taking, and critical thinking?
- How can creating a personalized study plan based on your strengths, course requirements, and objectives, improve retention of important material?.
- How does effectively preparing for examinations both enhance performance and save time?
- What are some successful strategies for taking tests?

Expectations for a student in the health professions are challenging. You need to understand and retain a growing base of complex information. Additionally, the knowledge and skills must last throughout your lifetime. Now is the time to take charge of your success. Good strategies for taking notes and reading difficult material provide an essential start to assimilating the information. Efficient individualized study plans provide the platform for deep comprehension. Finally, effective test preparation and test taking approaches allow you to recall and demonstrate your knowledge of the material. This chapter offers tools and ideas to create the conditions for your success.

DEVELOPING SKILLS FOR UNDERSTANDING

Class lectures, activities, clinical discussions, and written text and journals provide the essential information for your health field. Two skills that are crucial to gathering and understanding the information are reliable note taking and effective reading skills. These abilities not only capture the material needed to learn, but supply the basis for comprehension.

Compose Valuable Class Notes

Class notes are your collection of facts, figures, formulas, and advice. Learning the vast amount of facts depends on your creation and use of these comments. How can students effectively capture all the important information of lectures? The most useful note taking proceeds through three phases: before, during, and after the class.

Preview Lesson. Taking lecture notes is only part of a thorough note-taking process. Good notes actually begin before you even step into the classroom. A targeted focus aids identification of the most important ideas to put in the notes. To gain this focus, read or preview the topic to be covered for the day and review previous notes. Write down any questions that result from this preview. By all means, come prepared to class.

Record Notes. In the classroom, effective note taking begins with effective listening, not just writing down every word you hear. The most valuable notes result from selective recording in your own words. The focus gained from previewing puts you in the moment and better able to recognize verbal clues and main ideas (Box 1-1). Tape recorders are helpful if the amount of information or speed of delivery make the accurate recording of all the necessary information challenging. New pen voice recorders write and function as ordinary pens but also capture voices through digital recording. Some offer an option to download the information to a computer. Good and useful notes should include:

- Terms, definitions, and main ideas including theories, explanations, and processes
- Threads of comments from class discussion and questions
- Answers to your preview questions

Note Formats. The note-taking technique used depends on your personal choice and the type of information presented. A standard outline of main ideas with bullet points provides sound organization and a logical approach to note taking. PowerPoint slide presentations

BOX 1-1 Key Verbal Clues

Important Points	Cause And Effect	Comparisons	Exceptions	Processes
most important above all remember that a key idea most significant pay attention to the main point for example to illustrate for instance specifically	because due to consequently reason result cause effect outcome findings therefore consequently	similar different equal related in contrast on the other hand advantages disadvantages contrary to types characteristics	however although but nevertheless though except excluding apart	steps numbers (1,2,3. . .) stages first, second,. . . phase cycle procedure method

accompany many lectures now. These lectures often provide the basic outline, but expect that you add more information, such as explanations and examples, to fully understand and remember the details.

Using the format of a rough paragraph or sentences is helpful when the information is not easily organized or easy to follow. Combine ideas that are related into the same paragraph to keep thoughts organized. The writing can be rough and incomplete, but use complete sentences for important points such as quotes or definitions.

The Cornell system of notes created by Walter Pauk provides a technique that can also be used to review material (Figure 1-1). This method divides each note page into three parts. To create this format, draw a line from the top to almost the bottom of the page, about 2 inches from the left side of the page. Next, draw a line across the page, about 2 inches from the bottom. Write your notes in the largest (right side) portion of the paper. After class, use the left column to review and insert the key terms and main concepts. The bottom section is the summary area. Here, write the most critical points in your own words. This last step will reinforce your comprehension.

Visual strategies can be inserted into any note-taking format. The best part is you do not need to be an artist to use them. Use charts to demonstrate hierarchies or comparisons. Tables and maps help organize information. Flow charts assist in procedures. Draw pictures with labels for concepts and processes. Go ahead, be creative. Make it meaningful to you.

	Sept. 8
2 types of cells	Germ cells, responsible for sexual reproduction
	Somatic cells, perform all other body functions
4 possible results	• radiation may pass through w/o change
when radiation hits	• may temporarily damage cell
cells	• may damage cell & no repair takes place
	• may kill cell
lymphocytes	Most radio sensitive cells
& radiation	type of white blood cell in the vertebrate immune system
	play an important and integral role in the body's defenses
	Die immediately after radiation damage and before they
	complete cell division. This is unusual, most other cells
	divide a few times before they die
What are the kinds	three major types of lymphocyte are T cells, B cells and
of lymphocytes?	natural killer (NK) cells

Summary: Radiation can have different effects on cells. Not all cells are automatically killed by radiation. Lymphocytes are most sensitive to radiation and die immediately. 3 types of these cells are T cells, B cells and natural killer (NK) cells.

FIGURE 1-1 Cornell notes.

Make Notes Meaningful. No matter what format you choose, special measures make the notes more meaningful and effective. Start by dating all notes and numbering pages. This habit allows for an easier search for specific information as you go back to review. Use abbreviations and graphic symbols, such as arrows or stars, to write quickly or provide visual signals (Table 1-1). Be consistent and careful in your approach so that the abbreviations and shorthand you use are fully understood when you return to your notes. Avoid short forms that may be confused for more than one word, such as *comm.* which might be community, committee, or a variety of other words.

The note-taking format should also provide opportunities for adding information later. Place question marks along the way where you do not understand the matter or would like more clarification. Leave holes in your notes or keep the opposite page blank to provide the opportunity to go back and add additional ideas from your text or review.

After the lecture, one more set of steps await; review, rewrite, and reflect. Retention of information drops dramatically after the first 24 hours so it is important to revisit notes within the first day, while the information is still fresh and remembered. Take this time to complete incomplete notes and organize the material. Compare notes with other students and with the material in the text. Visual indicators aid in the organization. Use color codes to highlight terms, major concepts, theories, and processes, but limit colors to three or four to maximize effectiveness and limit confusion. Some students find typing or rewriting their notes provides good reinforcement. Reciting your lessons into a voice recorder fosters clarification as you must think through your notes. As you study and complete your notations, notice where questions or confusion still remain and mark these concerns.

"*I don't have time!!*" you say. Actually, using this system can make your time more efficient. Effective organization makes it easier to have all the correct material to study in a good format. Reciting and reflecting allow the material to be committed to memory sooner, so that only reviews are needed instead of cramming. Regular reviews help you retain more material for longer periods of time, making studying for examinations easier.

Read to Remember

Text and journal assignments present challenges in reading for many students. Reading in the health arts sometimes feels overwhelming with the breath of content and difficulty of concepts. Active reading techniques make reading meaningful and result in improved comprehension, memory, and analysis of concepts. As with any project, however, the work is easier with a plan. Start by creating a strategy of how much you will read and when you will complete each section in order to read all of the necessary material. Set reasonable expectations, choose a good setting, and make sure you do not fall behind your schedule.

Engage in Reading. You gain the most from reading when actively engaged in the process. Reading is meant to provide essential information and make you think and analyze the information. One of the most effective approaches to reading for comprehension was developed over 60 years ago by Francis Robinson. *SQ3R* is an acronym for "Survey, Question, Read, Recite, Review".

Knowing in advance the purpose and main ideas of the content provides a focus just as previewing provided focus for note taking. To *survey*, scan the information to be read and identify the main topics and questions. Look at titles, headings, and bold notations to give you the general idea of what you are about to read. Read introductions, abstracts, and summaries. Make note of terminology, graphics, and charts.

As you search over the material, notice any *question* that comes to mind. Write down these inquiries or indicate a question mark near the corresponding spot in the text. As you proceed to reading, keep these questions in mind and search for their answers.

To *read* effectively requires active involvement. Annotate the text to make it your own. Highlight the important terms

TABLE 1-1 Abbreviations and Symbols

Standard Abbreviations		Letters and Numbers (text talk)	
&	and	b4	before
/	divided by	b/c	because
<	less than	2	to, too
>	greater than	w	with
@	at	w/o	without
?	question	**First Syllables or Beginning of Words**	
=	equals	diff	difference
c/o	care of	ex	example
eg	for example	biol	biology
→	results in	ind	individual
≈	about	**Shortened Words**	
Δ	change	prblm	problem
∴	therefore	estmt	estimate

and concepts, or jot notes in the margins to explain difficult ideas in your own words. To isolate the key information and avoid confusion, read a section first, think about the important elements, and then highlight, underline, or make notations. Read the assignment in chunks and over small short periods of time instead of marathon reading sessions. Attention wanes and comprehension lessens during extreme reading periods. A large assignment or difficult reading does require extra work and concentration, so take frequent breaks and do not expect to master things on your first reading. Instead, try reading aloud and reading the material more than one time. E-readers with speech capability and text-to-speech software or shareware may also aid reading comprehension.

The final SQ3R stages of *recite* and *review* allow a reader to understand, analyze, and remember what is read. A deeper understanding can be achieved by "talking to the author" about what you have learned. After reading a section or chapter, find the essential details, explanations and examples, and talk about them. Make sure you address cause and effect, arguments, and assumptions to help you analytically evaluate the material. With any applications, discuss their goals and the related information, actions or procedures.

Come back once again to the text to reinforce your comprehension. When lectures are not clear, go back to your textbook and search for the section that provides clarification. Locate where the reading connects to lectures and insert this information into the blank pages or holes left open in your notes. The end of chapter summaries and questions should be part of your routine review. Study time is your opportunity to pull material together in creative ways by making terminology lists or flash cards, generating questions and summaries, or developing applications related to your experiences. Above all, find the answers to the questions you generated in your scan of the reading material.

Ideas for ESL Students. Textbooks in health arts can be challenging for any student. For students whose native language is other than English, reading can provide additional obstacles. The techniques of SQ3R can serve all students well, but if scanning and reading as described in the previous approach is not sufficient to comprehend the complex ideas, try this method.

- Read an entire section quickly to get your mind connected to the information.
- Then read the piece again, but slowly, to pick out more detail.
- Concentrate on understanding the main ideas in the text, and searching for key information, not by trying to understand or translate every word you read.
- Continue using markings and notes within the book.

Other helpful techniques are:

- Outline each chapter
- Start with the conclusion since it holds the essence of the chapter
- Try reading aloud

When you come to vocabulary or ideas you do not understand, employ strategies to help clarify the information. Writing has no one's body language to offer clues, but the text itself may provide hints. For words you do not know, read the sentences before and after the word since they often give suggestions to the meaning of the word. Sometimes another book may offer explanations in ways that help understanding. Create your own personal dictionary or a journal with your questions. A dictionary should be used only to look up key words that you must understand to get the point.

Fellow students can also help to improve your reading comprehension. Create a community of friends to review and discuss the readings. Such groups also provide chances to practice listening and pronunciation skills. Groups are especially helpful with learning to understand idioms such as "at arm's length" or "labor of love." Above all, other students offer support and encouragement.

LEARNING STYLES

Use Your Learning Style

Learning styles are the ways that learners perceive, interact, and respond to new knowledge. People take in, process, and work with information in different ways. No one manner is superior; they are just different. When you understand your learning style, you can build on it to make studying more efficient.

Identify Your Learning Style

Your learning style is a combination of four categories: visual/verbal; sensory/intuitive; active/reflective; and sequential/global. Everyone finds themselves in each of the eight areas at some time, but people gravitate to or favor only some modes. These favorites define your learning style. To determine your preferred style, answer the following four questions.

- How do you prefer to take in new information? Visually with pictures or diagrams, or verbally with words?
- How do you prefer to perceive information? Through your senses and facts, or through thoughts and concepts?
- How do you like to process new information? By engaging in activity or discussion, or through introspection?
- How do you come to understand information? By taking logical measured steps, or seeing the "big picture"?

Apply Your Learning Style

Particular study techniques build on each strength or comfort area. The learning activities in your preferred style will make learning more comfortable and efficient. Combine methods from each of the four categories. For instance, if you are a reflective, sensory, visual, linear learner, study in a quiet place drawing color-coded diagrams and outlines. Table 1-2 contains additional information on learning styles and ways to help yourself. Do you use techniques that place you in your preferred learning mode, or are your study strategies unrelated to your style? Are they simply habit?

The health professions expect flexibility in approaches to understanding and providing knowledge. Effective professionals in the health professions need to strengthen their skills in each learning type and not limit themselves to only one mode. Practicing the activities in areas outside of your preferred style develops new skills and broadens your comfort zone for learning.

LEARNING TECHNIQUES AND AIDS

Make Connections

Knowledge in the health fields must also go beyond the specific context to a generalized and unified understanding for the practical settings. This type of comprehension only comes from manipulating the material and information to find the connections. Graphic organizers help review and organize the material from your notes and text. Visual aids emphasize important relationships, compress large amounts of information, or focus on the essential material. A deeper understanding results from prioritizing, inferring, analyzing, problem solving, and evaluating the information.

Mind and Concept Maps

Concept or mind maps, developed by Tony Buzan, turn abstract ideas into a visual diagram of related ideas (Figure 1-2). This method quickly shows processes and relationships through creating a web of ideas. Maps go from general to specific facts. The construction uses a main topic and then focuses on the subordinate ideas. Only key words and phrases are used to make the connections that illustrate the relationships.

- Start with the main topic; draw a circle or box around it.
- Go back to the concepts and find the key ideas that come from your main topic.
- Draw a line from the topic to the idea.
- Write down facts that pertain to the idea, on lines stemming from it.
- Continue the process as needed.
- Use color, arrows, stars, and symbols, and create links.

Matrixes

Critical thinking and analysis is central to all health professions. A versatile and effective analytical tool is a matrix. A comparison matrix shows the in-depth relationship between two or more complex groups of information in a concise and quick way (Figure 1-3). Such a chart is flexible in its composition and allows for categorization, comparison, or decision making. The development of the matrix allows you to see the bigger picture and can also be used for review.

To create a matrix:

- First identify the basic elements of the concepts involved.
- Place the concepts to be analyzed in the block chart, along the side.
- Brainstorm the features of each concept, or in the case of decision making, decide on the alternatives.
- Include the features of comparison or alternatives across the top of the matrix.
- Fill in the table with the specifics for each block of comparison or the effect of each option to complete the process.

Other Visual Aids

Other types of critical thinking may involve processes or setting priorities. Visual aids are helpful here too. Processes or action steps fit well into a flow chart (Figure 1-4). For procedures with repetitive steps, a cycle diagram can be employed. Priorities, such as the Maslow's hierarchy, can be visualized through a pyramid or ladder (Figure 1-5). The fishbone technique displays the important elements of a topic at one glance (Figure 1-6).

Create a Personalized Study Plan

Just like a journey, learning success starts with planning, and any plan starts with knowing where you are and where you want to go. An effective plan works with specific goals and optimizes your time and physical surroundings.

Design the Right Environment. A focus for your study time offers the best results for all your efforts. A good atmosphere and goals based on your strengths and weaknesses provide this direction. Success happens when you know where to study, what to study, and how to stay on track.

TABLE 1-2 Strategies for Learning Styles

Active	Reflective
• Study in a group in which members take turns explaining and discussing	• Study in a quiet place
• Think of practical uses of the material	• Stop during reading to think about the material
• Walk and talk	• Do not just memorize, but make it meaningful
• Act out	• Write short summaries
• Use flash cards	• Jot your thoughts down, then share
• Teach it	
Sensory	**Intuitive**
• Seek how ideas and concepts apply in practice	• Think of concepts and theories that link facts together
• Brainstorm and look for specific examples	• Read test questions carefully and thoroughly before answering
• Make connections between theories and the real world	• Look for systems and patterns
• Draw diagrams	• Analyze the material
• Fill in details	
• Establish "rules and procedures" for yourself	
Visual	**Verbal**
• Add diagrams to your notes—use timelines, graphs, symbols, flow charts	• Talk about what you learn
• Organize your notes to see main points and then supporting facts	• Work in a study group
• Have your notes show connections	• Read your book aloud
• Color code	• Rewrite your notes
• Outline and organize material to study	• Outline chapters
	• Highlight only man points/words
Sequential	**Global**
• If your professor jumps around a lot, spend time with someone who can fill in the gaps; see a tutor	• Realize that until you "see the whole picture" you must be patient
• Rewrite class notes to follow a logical pattern that you can understand	• Before reading, preview a chapter and write questions in margins
• Outline material	• Working on one subject in depth at a time makes more sense for you
• Write out steps for procedures	• Look for the objectives of the class, the chapters
	• Start at the end—look at the summaries, chapter questions

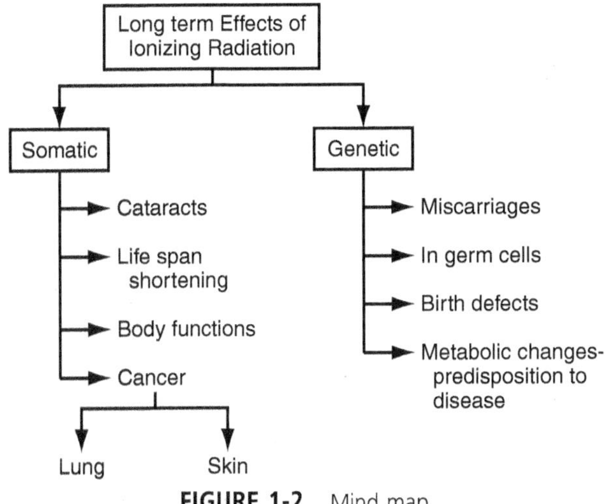

FIGURE 1-2 Mind map.

Build a Good Setting. The place and time to study can make a huge difference in learning effectiveness. Once again, start with knowing how you learn best. Do you need an absolutely quiet environment or a little background noise? Do you study well in a comfy chair or would you fall asleep in that seat? And lighting—do you prefer bright or dim? Even the time of day plays a role. When are you at your best and most alert? When are there fewer demands on you and your time? Now the trick is to find the closest fit to your preferred setting. The best spot may be your room in the early morning, a table or a sofa in the evening or a corner in the library in the afternoon. Claim a space for study and make it your own.

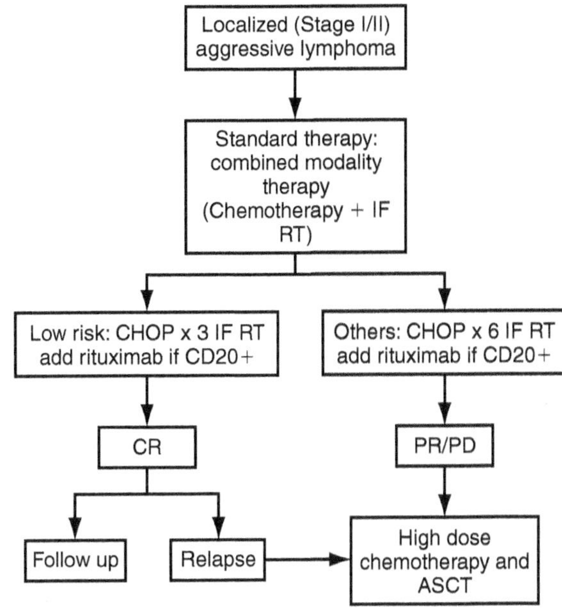

FIGURE 1-4 Flow chart.

This spot should be your routine place to study. Since this place has a purpose, make sure you have the tools to

Emergency	Symptoms	Causes	Response
Hypoglycemia	• Nervousness • Sweating • Intense hunger • Trembling • Weakness • Palpitations • Often have trouble speaking or concentrating	• Imbalance of insulin, especially in a diabetic • Prolonged fasting • Some drug interactions	• 10–15g of glucose or carbohydrate • Glucogon if needed
Hyperglycemia	• Increased thirst • Headaches • Blurred vision • Frequent urination • Difficulty concentrating • Weight loss • Blood glucose >180 mg/dL • High levels of ketones in the urine • Dry or flushed skin • Fruity odor on breath	• Diabetes • Skipping insulin for diabetics • Eating too many carbohydrates • Infection • Increased stress • Illness	• Drink lots of fluids • Electrolyte replacement • Insulin therapy

FIGURE 1-3 Matrix.

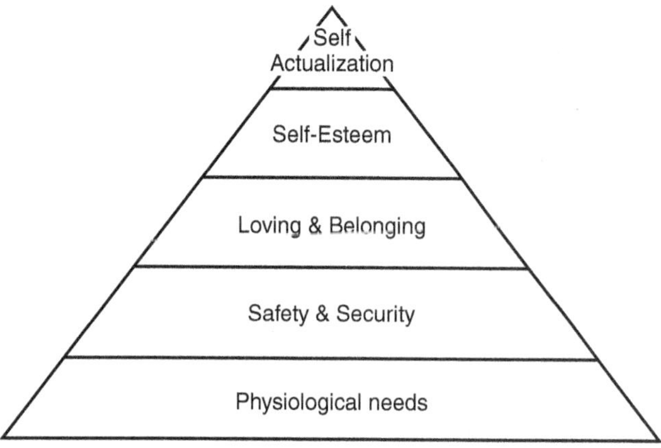

FIGURE 1-5 Pyramid visual aid.

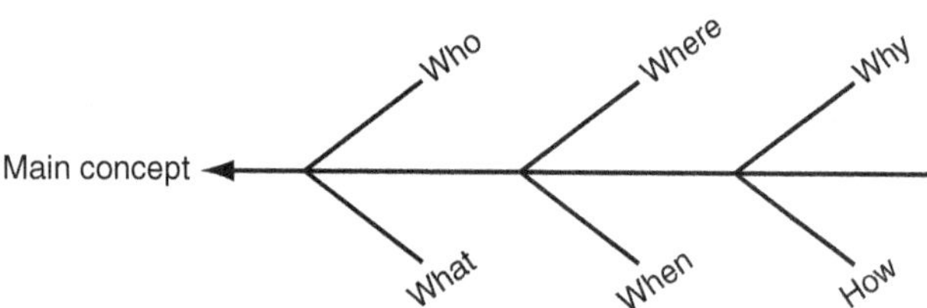

FIGURE 1-6 Fishbone graphic aid.

accomplish what you need to do. Make sure a computer is available, with paper and books in easy reach. Have index cards, highlighters, and other supplies handy as well. And remember to keep a calendar nearby.

A word of caution: distracters make some spots undesirable for deep and serious learning. Student unions, cafeterias, and other high traffic areas can tempt a person's attention. Though many people now multitask, focus becomes divided as a result, and lack of focus results in missed knowledge. So turn off televisions and cell phones, and avoid e-mail, texting, and other communications during your study periods. Let voice mail work for you and establish a reputation with others that your designated time is not to be disrupted. If you study in your room, think of hanging a "do not disturb" sign on the door. Study where and when you will be alert, attentive, and with limited distractions.

Assess Strengths and Weaknesses. Knowing your strengths and weaknesses in your course material will direct the emphasis for your study time. Reviewing your notes and reading on a regular basis not only provide early and consistent feedback for yourself, but actually shortens the overall time you need to assimilate the information. Reviews that are days apart require you to backtrack and relearn material instead of just reviewing it.

One way to assess your understanding is to examine your notes and reading. Identify the concepts, terms, processes, and procedures that are important and sort between those that you fully understand and those that may cause some confusion. Which areas are strong and which need some work? Look, where appropriate, to make comparisons, find relationships, perform applications, offer implications, or create correct evaluations.

Other sources also provide feedback of your comprehension and abilities. Look at questions that accompany the chapters in the books. Some texts also have additional supplemental resources online or a companion CD. Your quizzes and tests are also an essential piece of the puzzle in identifying concepts that still require some work to master. Analyze the items that you missed, trying to discover why you got the answer incorrect. Such discoveries will provide information on what and how to study.

Establish Goals for Studying. Each study session will accomplish more when you set a specific objective for your time. In fact, establishing a *goal* is the secret to making a study plan (Box 1-2). The four elements to a good and effective study plan include creating a specific *goal*, identifying *obstacles*, selecting the methods for *action*, and assessing what you *learned*.

From your analysis of your personal course strengths and weaknesses, or from the upcoming expectations of your classes, decide on the purpose of your time. What do you want to accomplish in the session at hand? Be as specific as you can. Avoid setting your purpose as "studying the chapter." Instead, list what those words mean to you, such as "to define the terms and major concepts within Chapter 3," or "to re-create the process for radiation therapy treatment for breast cancer." With a specific target, you will be able to establish a better plan to achieve it.

Also, identify the challenges that may exist in accomplishing your goal. Consider what must be done to overcome or compensate for these difficulties. With this information in mind, decide on what methods you will use to reach your goal. "Looking over your notes and highlighting" is not a plan nor is it sufficient to comprehend and remember the complex information you need as a health provider. Combine reading, comprehension, and memory techniques in ways that make sense for the material and for your learning needs. Think of the actions you will take to integrate the information and reach your goal.

Finally, decide on how you will know if you achieved your main purpose in studying. How will you know if you need to change your methods or apply more time to reaching your goal? You may quiz yourself or review notes again. Other methods include writing summaries or creating lists or diagrams. Find a means that is appropriate for the goal, the information, and your learning style.

BOX 1-2 Making a Study Plan

Steps for a Study Plan
Goal—Make it specific
Obstacles—Identify potential problems
Action—Apply effective methods
Learned—Confirm what you learned

USING TIME EFFECTIVELY

Make the Best Use of Time

Making the most of your study time allows for learning as much as you can, as well as you can. Time, however, cannot be managed; it is a given unchanging commodity. Therefore, you need to manage yourself. Effective management is dependent on setting priorities that should include time to read, review, and study. By general rule of thumb, these tasks should require about 2 hours of study for every class hour. Time management techniques are critical for academic success.

Find the Time to Study

Yet, how often we wonder where the time has gone. Each day we are given the same number of hours, but at times they seem to disappear. Our lives are conducted under the impression that we effectively use each set of minutes. To really understand how your time is spent, take a few minutes to complete a weekly time tracker (Box 1-3).

Write the number of hours you spend per week in each category. Take a look at your total number of hours. How does it compare to 168? That is how many hours are in 1 week. If you are trying to squeeze more hours in, something needs to be trimmed. Find the spots where you can save time to use for the areas that are most important. On the other hand, if you have fewer hours than the 168 total, you might be squandering time without realizing it. If time has disappeared, time wasters may be to blame.

Everyone has time wasters, ways we misuse our time and realize no accomplishments. Hours in front of the television or computer, talking on the phone, sleeping, or daydreaming can all rob us of valuable time to accomplish our necessary goals. Any of these activities is not bad in itself, but extended time that inhibits productivity can be a barrier to your aspirations. Note what activities tend to result in your wasted time.

Time wasters often take hold when we procrastinate. Tasks that are difficult, boring, or disliked are among the first to be ignored. A few simple rules help conquer procrastination.

- Do first the tasks and work that is difficult or unpleasant. Attacking the hard material early allows peak energy to be applied and lowers the likelihood of avoidance.
- Break the job into smaller parts and attempt to do only one part. Eating one bite of an elephant is less overwhelming than staring at the entire animal.
- Agree to an effort for a designated period of time. Deciding to work for 15 minutes is very easy and often once you start, you will continue for much longer. Even if you only work at your task for 15 minutes, that is 15 more than zero.
- Schedule the chore into your calendar, making a commitment to it.
- Promise to reward yourself when the job is complete, whether it is a tasty delight or a special television show or movie.
- Work in your prime time, rest in off peak hours.

People also learn best during their own peak time. That time is usually during daylight hours, but not always. Discover your best time, when you are most alert and able to deal with complex thoughts or problems, whether early in the morning before the world gets busy, late in the evening after all are in bed, or a time in between. For maximum effectiveness, schedule as much your study time as possible during that period. Box 1-4 contains additional study tips for parents.

BOX 1-3 Weekly Time Tracker

List the average number of hours per week that you spend doing each of the following activities:

_________ Sleeping
_________ Eating
_________ Personal grooming/care
_________ Working at your place of work
_________ Work you bring home from your job
_________ Family obligations—includes caring for others and chores
_________ Cooking and cleaning
_________ Shopping
_________ Television
_________ Reading for pleasure or personal interest
_________ College classes
_________ Computer/e-mail/games
_________ Traveling/transportation
_________ Organizations—clubs, church, meetings
_________ Volunteer work
_________ Exercising/sports
_________ Entertainment
_________ Talking on phone/texting
_________ Other
_________ Homework and studying
_________ TOTAL

Use Time Management Tools

A big trick to taking charge of your time is to make things less urgent. When tasks become routine and expected, anxiety lessens. Three time management tools help accomplish this mission. These tools assist with long-term goals, weekly work, short-term tasks, and even large projects.

Calendars. A calendar or academic planner will help display at a glance what needs to be accomplished

BOX 1-4 Ideas for Parents

Study after children are in bed or while they are at school
Share babysitting coops; take turns finding quiet time
Include very small children in study time by reciting your notes to them
Preschoolers might enjoy role-playing study cases
Find activities, games, or projects, to keep them occupied
Older children can share the same time to do their homework
Do not be afraid to ask for help
Look for waiting time, the small periods while waiting for a doctor's appointment or for the dryer to finish its cycle. Use the small time periods to

- Review notes or flashcards
- To preview a chapter
- Study terminology
- Listen to the material (e.g., tape-recorded lectures or podcasts)

during a month or semester (Figure 1-7). A good approach to planning begins with the syllabus from each course. In your calendar, include all the tests and major assignments from each course. To these dates, add the important times from your personal activities, such as doctors' appointments, weddings, birthdays, and other major commitments. One additional step to complete the plan requires the academic calendar from your school. Check for important academic dates to be added. Important times include withdraw dates, days of finals, and deadlines for other important academic requirements.

One of the biggest benefits to using this type of plan is a limit to surprises. Frequent use of the calendar will keep you sensitive to what is coming ahead. This awareness allows you to plan ahead and avoid last minute rushes to complete work. Knowing that there is a doctor's appointment the day before a paper deadline allows you to choose, which days earlier in the week or month are available to work on the project. A good way to use this method is to work backwards. See when a project or examination is scheduled. Decide on the steps needed to accomplish the homework or study for the test. Now select the days to schedule each step in the process. Make sure you allow some "wiggle" room in case the unexpected happens. The resulting calendar is your timetable to accomplish your goals.

November						
Sun	Mon	Tue	Wed	Thu	Fri	Sat
	1 **Start Paper**	2	3 **Study Calc Prob**	4	5 **Dr. Appt.**	6
7	8	9 **Revise Paper**	10	11 **Study Calc Prob**	12	13 **Study Calc Memorize**
14 **Dad's birthday**	15 **Study Calc Prob**	16 **Do Final Draft of Paper**	17 **Final Study for Calc**	18 **Calc Test!! Review Final Draft**	19 **Paper Due****	20
21 **Study Psych Organize**	22 **Study Psych Organize**	23	24 **Study Psych Memorize**	25	26	27
28	29 **Final time to Study Psych**	30 **Psych Test!!**				

FIGURE 1-7 Calendar planning.

Schedules. Finding the time you need throughout the week or day becomes easier with a weekly schedule. Create a daily schedule with times from early morning until you sleep. With the same approach used in the calendar, insert all your regular weekly obligations starting with classes and jobs. With the open times, identify opportunities to study, aiming to reach the time commitment of 2 hours per hour of class time. Avoid a large-scale study session. Long hours result in fatigue and poor retention. Instead, look for openings between classes or other commitments, and leave some holes in your schedule to offer some flexibility for the unexpected. Figure 1-8 provides a sample schedule and one for you to complete for your personal goals.

To-Do List. For days that are filled to the brim, a to-do list keeps you focused and helps remind you of the essential assignments (Figure 1-9). If there are more tasks than time, set priorities so the most important or necessary will get accomplished. One of the best pleasures is to mark off each job done.

STUDY WITH AND WITHOUT A GROUP

Learning does not have to be a lonely experience. Advantages are realized in both solitary and group study modes. Well-defined and structured groups add efficiency and depth of comprehension to the learning experience.

Advantages of Each Approach

Your individualized study plan targets the material and study methods that meet your specific needs. Memorization, review of facts and processes, and self-testing are served well by this approach. This arena is where comprehension begins. Health care, however, requires higher order thinking: application, analysis, and evaluation. Some individual learning techniques help with this type of thinking, but some views or alternatives may be missed.

Working with others assists with the ability to see multiple perspectives, leading to deeper thinking. The

Personal Weekly Time Schedule

	Sunday	Monday	Tuesday	Wednesday	Thursday	Friday	Saturday
6:00							
7:00							
8:00							
9:00							
10:00							
11:00							
12:00							
1:00							
2:00							
3:00							
4:00							
5:00							
6:00							
7:00							
8:00							
9:00							
10:00							
11:00							
12:00							

A

FIGURE 1-8 Weekly time schedule. **A**, Blank;

Continued

Personal Weekly Time Schedule

	Sunday	Monday	Tuesday	Wednesday	Thursday	Friday	Saturday
6:00							
7:00							
8:00	Study	Study			Study		
9:00		Class	Study	Class	Study	Class	Work
10:00		Study	Class	Study	Class	Study group	Work
11:00		Study		Study		Study group	Work
12:00							Work
1:00	Work	Class		Class	Class	Class	Work
2:00	Work	Study	Lab	Study		Study	
3:00	Work					Study	Study
4:00							Study
5:00				Work	Work		
6:00		Work	Study	Work	Work		
7:00		Work	Study	Work	Work		
8:00	Study	Work		Work	Work		
9:00	Study	Work	Study				
10:00							
11:00							
12:00							

B

FIGURE 1-8, Cont'd **B** completed sample.

My Daily to Do List

- Complete reading of chapter 2
- Take draft of paper to writing center
- Create flash cards for Prof. Smith's class
- √ Confirm date of next study group meeting
- Do laundry, at least essentials
- Exercise at fitness center

FIGURE 1-9 Daily to-do list.

diverse offerings of ideas and solutions reinforce important concepts while making more efficient use of time and energy. The group setting also provides a venue where mistakes and questions are acceptable. Study partners even help to increase motivation and provide some social life in the busy life of a student. The power of the group, however, can also be weakened or counterproductive. Working with others can, at times, be distracting, resulting in less productive time instead of more.

Tips for Effective Group Study

To make the best use of teamwork, a few guidelines are valuable. Just refer to the simple questions of who, what, and how. Start by inviting two or three classmates who have similar goals and will challenge you to do your best. Each member should expect to be a full participant, taking turns in leading the group. A comparison of how each person studies or prepares for examinations will show who does what best. If the group members have different approaches, you will reap the benefits from the diversity.

Next, establish the expectations. Determine a regular schedule with leadership rotation and how each person will be accountable. Discuss what will keep you on track and what the team will do if you hit an obstacle.

A specific goal for each session such as to test preparation or a chapter review provides focus for the gathering. Talk about the ways the group will work together to achieve the goal. The members might pool and review notes, teach each other a difficult concept, or create questions or flashcards. Use the group to develop memory devices and study materials. Teamwork is helpful to clarify notes or quiz each other. Distance does not have to hurt you; the group can even text questions back and forth to quiz each other. Be creative in your learning.

BOX 1-5 Mnemonic Examples

Mole: signs of trouble: **ABCDE**
Asymmetry
Border irregular
Color irregular
Diameter usually >0.5 cm
Elevation irregular
Head CT scan: evaluation checklist "**B**lood **C**an **B**e **V**ery **B**ad"
Blood
Cistern
Brain
Ventricles
Bone
Supine vs. prone body position
Supine is on your **spine**.
Therefore, prone is the "other" one.
Tumors that metastasize to skin: BLOCK
Breast
Lung
Ovary
Colon
Kidney

PREPARE EFFECTIVELY FOR TESTS

As examinations grow closer, it is time to step up your study tactics. A good and thorough strategy for your examination will not only prepare you but also minimize your stress level. The most important keys to successful preparation are an early start to avoid cramming, use of reinforcement tools, question prediction, continuous practice, and physical and mental preparation.

Reinforce Memory

The mind, at times, needs signposts to help recall all the stored information. Memory tools are ways to train your brain to associate important information with images or codes that form meaningful organization. Several techniques reinforce your memory and supply your mind with critical thinking skills. Tools and templates help you organize, connect concepts, and strengthen recall. All memory systems are most effective when they are meaningful and memorable. The more practice with these techniques, the more effective they become. The critical elements and ideas, however, also require you to overlearn.

Memory Aids.

Association. Associations are an excellent way to remember. Some of the easier memory devices are mnemonic tools. A simple approach is to take the first letter of a series of terms and create an acronym, a representative word, or sentence. For instance, the main sites for distant metastases in lung cancer might be classified as: ***BLAB***: ***B***one, ***L***iver, ***A***drenals, ***B***rain; Box 1-5 lists other examples. Play with your choices to discover one that is meaningful to you. Mnemonics for the medical field are also found in books and on the web.

Imagery. Personalize your memory tools with stories containing strong mental images or familiar journeys. A technique that works well for the health field is to create an anecdote inserting all the details to be remembered. Code information vividly, based on familiar items, or with a sense of humor to increase the likelihood of remembering the facts. Make the story's characters more memorable by creating backgrounds related to your personal life or so unique to be unforgettable. Perhaps your patient is a professional clown. Imagine the patient, picturing how they look, feel, and even what they say, as you rehearse your tale.

Another method of story and association involves a familiar setting from your everyday life, such as your bedroom. Mentally picture the room and locations around the room. Imagine that each item to be remembered sits at a particular spot in the room. To remember the *radiations in the electromagnetic spectrum*, your fantasy could envision the room's window (*visible light*), then see the floor register (*heat*), followed by the table next to your bed (*radio*), your bed (*microwave*), and so forth. More ideas are available on websites like mindtools.com.

Flash Cards and Study Sheets. Writing, paired with repetition, also provides good avenues for recall. Traditional flash cards have been used for years because they work. Write a word or key information on one side and an explanation on the reverse side, then carry them with you and review in those available small time slots. This technique easily turns into a system of concept cards. Put a concept's key word(s) on the one side of the card with an image, mnemonic, or other memory device, and main points on the reverse side. Use the cards to make flow charts and mind maps to rehearse the connections between concepts.

Sometimes the vast amount of information makes using cards impractical. Creating summary sheets can yield a similar result (Figure 1-10). On a sheet of paper, create a column about 2 inches from the left side of the page. Use the left margin as you would the front of the flash card and write key terms. Write details, definitions, or summary in the right side. Just fold back the column to review and quiz yourself.

radio sensitivity of	1 type of cell
cancer cells	2 phase of cell life
depends on	3 division rate of cell
	4 degree of differentiation
record radiation	absorbed energy per unit mass
dose as	
One Gray	100 rad
1cGy	1 rad
Simulator	Machine that simulates the treatment machine & its
	movement and positioning
blocks	shielding devices made of lead or high density
	alloys minimize radiation exposure to nearby
	normal tissues

FIGURE 1-10 Summary sheet.

Anticipate Questions

An effective way to process information and prepare for examinations is to anticipate the material you could expect on the test. To accomplish this task, it helps to think like a teacher and predict questions that may be asked.

Identify Key Theories, Processes, and Procedures. The syllabus often identifies key theories, processes, formulas, and procedures and is the first clue to what tests will emphasize. This document also lists the important objectives of the course. With these goals in mind, review your sources to detect the principal facts.

- In your book, flag key terms and concepts. Go back to the questions you generated when you previewed readings. Reexamine the end of chapter summaries and questions.
- From lecture notes, pay attention to items emphasized by repetition, placed on the board, or given in handouts. What are the questions the instructor posed in class? Save and view past quizzes, tests, and assignments. Discussion with fellow students will also reveal new perspectives.

Identify the Common Situations. Common situations are more likely to be tested. Detect the most ordinary problems and tasks. Find the who, what, where, and when to situations and problems. Within those situations, however, anticipate unexpected circumstances and how they affect the situation.

Create Examination Items

Once you establish the important and most likely material, continue the teacher role and develop your own pretest. To create questions, go back to the questions you had in previewing your readings or reviewing your notes. Information and concepts can be quizzed by creating your own scenarios. Develop problems around an imaginary patient or about a particular process. This method is a good exercise for group study, pulling talents of the entire team together.

Practice, Practice, Practice

With practice questions identified, remember that rehearsals are not limited to the arts. The best preparation for performing on assessments is frequent practice of similar questions and problems.

Practice Random and Various Types of Questions. Though many test items may be multiple choice, practice a variety of question types to be prepared for other kinds of questions and to stimulate your critical thinking. Practice questions from texts, supplementary material, and other students.

- Multiple choice examinations require a review of nearly everything.
- Story or scenario questions require theory and practice combined together.
- Short answer and matching short items test your memorization of key definitions and theories, and expect that you have "overlearned" the information.

You may want to take advantage of clues within questions, but do not count on them. Good test items leave few if any clues. No matter what type of question, watch for qualifiers such as *all, some, never, always*, and negatives that indicate an answer that is opposite of the given situation such as *except, not,* or *but.* Do not hesitate to underline or circle important information within the question. For specific strategies for each item type, see the "Tackle the Questions" section later in this chapter.

Seek Patterns in Thinking

Though each test item is unique, patterns exist among the questions and concepts. Determine these patterns by dissecting recurring question structures. First, step back from the particulars of the question to see the broad idea or concept of each question. Discover how each item is similar to others, the causes, effects, and theories behind the answers. Then examine the logic in questions and situations to uncover recurring situations. Often there is a particular theory that is repeatedly part of understanding the items. Once you begin to see how concepts are tested, you can recognize the type of question and the needed approach (Box 1-6).

Learn From Your Previous Performance

Each test and assignment is an opportunity to learn. A test analysis shows your strengths and where you need improvement (Figure 1-11). Investigate why you were not successful. If you were careless in reading the question thoroughly, try to read more slowly. Possibly you were surprised by a question so you may want to look at the concepts missed in your studying. If you did not study a particular point, your notes may need to be more detailed. Did you think into the question too much and make unjustifiable assumptions? Such analysis allows you to make changes in your study approach and improve on future examinations.

BOX 1-6 Steps for Critical Analysis

Identify Essential Information
Facts
Evidence
Inferences based on evidence
Assumptions

Evaluate Evidence
From the information you identified, use logical thinking and reasoning skills to
- Classify; determine cause and effect; solve problems
- See parts and wholes; compare and contrast; seek patterns and analogies
- Anticipate next steps; predict; draw conclusions
- Assess values; judge; determine a rationale for support

Avoid Fuzzy Thinking
Unwarranted assumptions
Overgeneralization
Failure to see subtle differences
Oversimplification
Hasty conclusions

Manage Life Stress

Stress and a college student's life seem to be intertwined. The demands on the days of a student in the health professions only heighten anxiety levels. At the same time, tension interferes with successful studying. Manage stress and keep it in control with a creative approach to setting your priorities and activities.

Reducing Stressors. Stress is reduced as you take control of your life, so step number one is to side step unnecessary sources of stress. To begin, recognize and assess the stressors in your life; consider aspects of work, school, and family. The commitments you make should be realistic, so it is OK to say "no." Decide what can go for now. What can you do without and what can you do differently? Flexibility with your schedule or setting new priorities offers noticeable relief. A less than perfectly made bed is better than an unsuccessful test. Slow your pace by doing one important thing at a time and only multitask the less important duties. Above all, eliminating procrastination of important obligations will bring more relief than anything else.

Plan ahead wherever possible and prepare for surprises. They will happen. A plan "B" for all important events reduces the anxiety that comes with sudden situations. Consider what you will do if your car breaks down, if your computer printer spits out blank pages, if the babysitter gets sick. Remember to think about the happy events too. Arrange for the evening of your birthday or anniversary, and the weekend of your son's soccer tournament.

Develop a Support Network. Companions can also assist in managing the stressors of life. Friends, relatives, neighbors, and fellow students can act as your personal cheerleaders. Those who understand your goals and the work demanded can offer encouragement to lift your spirits. Students who share the work and obligations of your academic life will comprehend the challenges and support your goals. Identify your supporters and network with the students who share your experiences.

Positive Exercises. Stress relief methods start with good positive self-talk and thinking. Keep a journal to help your thoughts pour out onto paper. Writing your feelings down is one way to defuse them. Write everything on your mind, all the feelings in your heart, good and bad. Complete the exercise by responding to your thoughts with new positive and empowering statements that reaffirm your abilities. Remind yourself "I can do this" or "don't sweat the small stuff."

Recreation and participation in activities you enjoy also provide means for coping with pressure (Box 1-7).

Test Analysis for ______________________ Exam on __________ (date)

Reason	Q#	Q#	Q#	Q#	Q#	Q#	Q#
Test Taking Skills							
Did not read question thoroughly							
Did not choose the "best" answer							
Did not notice qualifiers							
Did not check grammar flow							
Answered too quickly							
Changed from right answer							
Did not consider ALL possibilities							
Did not include ALL essential information							
Used assumptions							
Did not address all points of the question							
Effective Studying							
Did not understand what was asked							
Did not study material well enough							
Could not recall information							
Could not find a way to remember this							
Only remembered part of it							
Did not spend enough time on concept							
Did not see the relationship involved							
Comprehension							
Unable to make an inference							
Unable to make a comparison							
Unable to use different wording							
Unable to summarize							
Unable to use or apply the concept							
Unable to make an analogy							
Unable to make a prediction							
Unable to put material together in a new way							
Comprehensive Studying							
Did not have material in notes							
Had not read this material							
Had not considered this important							
Skipped this & did not return to it							
Left it blank							
Anxiety							
Ran out of time							
Got nervous/anxious							
Went blank/froze up							
Was distracted by environment							
Lost concentration							
Other:							

FIGURE 1-11 Test analysis.

BOX 1-7 Stress Relievers

30 Ways to Reduce Stress

1. Take a walk
2. Watch a movie
3. Read a book
4. Jog
5. Pet a dog or cat
6. Whistle
7. Fly a kite
8. Ride a bike
9. Go for a swim
10. Have a long iced tea
11. Plant some flowers
12. Pick some flowers
13. Do a puzzle
14. Play a game
15. Dance
16. Listen to music
17. Take a nap
18. Call a friend
19. Tell jokes
20. Take a bubble bath
21. Paint your nails
22. Hit a ball
23. Tickle a baby
24. Sing a song
25. Feed the birds
26. Go on a picnic
27. Stroll in the woods
28. Watch a ball game
29. Light a candle
30. Smile

Many pursuits fulfill this need: nature, music, movies, or reading. A sense of humor inserted into any situation releases tensions too.

Exercise not only improves your physical health, but reduces stress by releasing endorphins, adrenaline, serotonin, and dopamine—chemicals that give you a sense of well-being. Any form of exercise, even something as simple as walking, can release tensions and produce a relaxed feeling. Find a method that works for you and fits your personal life. More relaxation ideas are found later in this chapter in the "Cope with Test Anxiety" section.

Be Physically Prepared

Your life may be busier than ever, but now is the time to really take care of yourself. "Mom" does know best about eating, sleeping, and other self-care advice. Your mind cannot function at its best without your body feeling at its best.

Eating to Help Your Memory. Stress can diminish certain mineral or vitamin supplies and attack your ability to learn and remember. Stress also establishes a drive to reach for foods that are detrimental to your body and learning. Cravings for sugar, donuts, and chocolate candy bars seem to be a quick solution to nutrition on the run while you study and prepare for examinations. However, sugar will leave your brain muddled. While that fast energy gets you through the remaining stretch of study time, your body pays for the simple solution with a roller coaster ride for your blood sugar. Just when you need all the cells of your brain the most, your brain does not have all the fuel it needs. Look at your food environment. Surround yourself with healthy carbohydrates and protein. Do not skip meals; instead, eat to feed your brain.

Sleeping Guidelines. Sleep-deprived bodies and minds also have trouble functioning at their peak. College students often feel they must make a choice between sleep and academics. But sleep is an essential part of academic success, despite the fact that students pride themselves in marathon all night study sessions. After studying late into the night, the next morning you wake up feeling tired and miserable, not the way you want to start an important day. Lack of sleep results in lower concentration and memory, and higher levels of stress. Sleep allows your brain to be reenergized and tackle new ideas and solutions.

To get good sleep, follow a few simple guidelines. Avoid caffeine and stimulants before you go to bed. Caffeine is not only found in coffee, but it is also in some soft and energy drinks, tea, and chocolate. Complete tasks and homework at least an hour before sleep so your mind will slow down and not worry. During the day, find ways to relax or reduce stress with exercise or walks.

Attack the Examination

The first part of understanding any examination is to know the expectations of the test; what it covers, how it will be administered, its format, and its scoring policies. Creating a plan to take the test and manage anxiety puts you in control. The more you know about what the test will be like, the better you can prepare for the examination and the less nervous you will be. These steps are especially important in preparing for your certification examination.

Know the Test Procedures. Well before your examination, investigate and learn about the procedures, design, and timing of the examination. This type of preparation will eliminate surprises and give you a sense of security.

Understand the Expectations. Read all you can about the examination, its format, and content. Start with how the test is delivered. ARRT examinations are administered on computers. Tutorials, offered before the examination, provide some familiarity and comfort for using this format. The types of questions, the allowed time, the number of items, and how the examination will be scored give important information for your preparation. ARRT employs scaled scores on a range from 1 to 99 with a scaled score of 75 to pass. Scaled scores are not the same as percentage, but take into account the difficulty of a particular test form.

Identification of the concepts and material covered in the examination supplies the blueprint for your study plan. ARRT examinations are related to practice. Knowledge and skills from anatomy and physiology to technical skills will be included in the certification test. Questions will also examine exhibits and unusual circumstances. Consult the ARRT website for more information and current details. This knowledge will allow you to develop a study plan and test taking strategy.

Know the Testing Situation. The testing situation and procedures may cause undue anxiety if you are not prepared to deal with the requirements in the necessary timeframe. It is important to familiarize yourself with all the policies, procedures, and deadlines. Identify the test center and learn their procedures and expectations, especially for scheduling or cancelling an appointment. Find out what information you need to register and schedule an examination appointment, and what you need to bring to the test. Check on the current fees and their deadline. Early investigation and preparation will ease your process and avoid disappointments.

Understand the Types of Questions. Four types of questions are used in certification examinations (Box 1-8). Success on examinations depends on understanding how to approach each item type. While some test items require a simple recognition of facts and basic concepts, others require deeper thinking and understanding. Comprehending how and why things are done and applying principles to clinical practice will be tested. Keep in mind that new items of any type may be inserted as a try out. These questions are not identified as pilot questions, but are unscored.

Question Types.

Multiple Choice Questions. ARRT examinations use multiple choice questions (MCQs) as one of the main types of questions. Two formats for these items are questions and incomplete statements. These problems are also known as *selected-response* items because an answer is chosen from several provided. Incorrect responses or distractors are often based on elements from a related concept or a common misconception. MCQs test simple facts, but are also sophisticated enough to assess evaluation and application.

Situation-Judgment Items. The certification examination may contain one or more situation-judgment items (SJTs). A written scenario describes a problem and is followed by a list of possible solutions. The item is answered by selecting *two* answers, one that is the most desirable answer to the problem and the other the least desirable solution. SJTs test the ability to deal with multiple steps or decisions as in the case of providing radiation therapy to a patient over time. Note that this type of question takes more time to read and answer than standard multiple choice questions.

Sorted Lists. Another question type provides a list of items in random order. The task asks the items be placed into a designated order, creating a sorted list. On the computerized examination, the mouse is used to drag each item into its correct order. Processes and information where order or placement are important are candidates for sorted lists.

BOX 1-8 Question Samples

Multiple Choice

The primary concern in radiation to the gonads is to prevent:

a. Somatic effects
b. Chronic effects
c. Genetic effects
d. Erythema Answer: c

Situation Judgment Item

Mary, a 78-year-old patient is accompanied by her neighbor, Nancy, for her appointment. Her neighbor agreed to drive her today because Mary's daughter, who usually accompanies the patient, is ill. As you transport the patient in a wheelchair, Mary asks to see her chart. She just wants to "check it out." In this situation, which is the most appropriate and least appropriate response?

Most Least

A. Mary is frail and has poor eyesight, so hand the chart to her friend, Nancy.
B. Since you are in the hall among many people, suggest that Mary waits until you are in a room with some privacy.
C. Hand the chart to Mary; she has a right to know as a patient.
D. Stop walking, offer to read any information Mary wants to know.
Answer: Most: B; Least: A

Sorted List

Place the following list in order from shoulder to wrist:

- Carpal
- Humerus
- Radius
- Phalanges
- Metacarpal bone

Humerus
Radius

Hot Spot

Place an X on the location of the thymus in Figure 1-12.

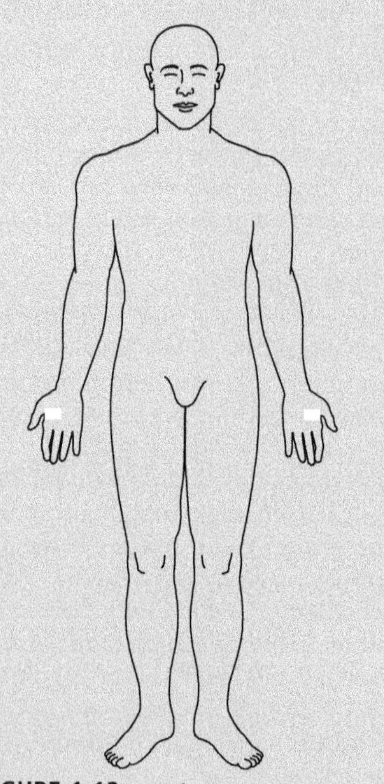

FIGURE 1-12 Surface anatomy model.

Hot Spot Items. Radiologic science is filled with radiographs, CT scans, sonograms, and other images. Medical images and illustrations are represented in "Hot Spot" items. Among the questions, you may be asked about structure such as anatomy or functions as in physiology, positioning, or equipment. This item will require the move of the mouse cursor to indicate the location of a specific feature.

Tackle the Questions. To tackle the test, start by selecting the best spot in the room for you and make yourself as comfortable as you can. Have a watch so you can budget your time. If you fear that you might forget some essential knowledge, dump that information down at the beginning of the examination, writing down facts, formulas, or diagrams that you might then retrieve throughout the test. ARRT will provide a white-board to use. Read directions carefully, survey the assessment, and make a mental plan of attack. Start at the beginning, middle, or end, doing first the questions that come quickly or easy to you.

The key to correctly answering the questions is to identify what the item is really asking and what the options are. A systematic strategy provides steps to analyze each question stem and the choices.

Reading the Question Carefully. Careful reading of each test item involves scrutiny of the question. To start, classify the question within a larger context; are you being asked about proper positioning, a treatment option, proper communication, or other category. Isolate the facts and decide what additional knowledge is implied by the given information. Identify the relevant processes and procedures associated with the question. Avoid assumptions; answers should be only based on given details. If you are thinking, "perhaps...," you may be assuming. Speculation will lead you down incorrect paths.

Rank the Options. A few strategies after you have carefully read and thought about the question help distinguish correct choices. Before reading the options, consider how you might respond to the question. Distractor responses are placed there to distract and will often do their job if you read them before considering a response. Treating each alternative as a true or false statement helps to eliminate obvious incorrect responses. The remaining choices require incorporating theories, processes, and logic to establish priorities and make your final decision.

Some questions will have only one correct answer. However, judgment is tested by questions that seek the "best answer." Some responses may only be partially true, or not the highest priority, best method, or best action. When the answers are narrowed down, consider the following to set priorities and select an answer among the remaining items.

- The underlying principle or theory that is involved in the overall question
- Any indications or contraindications for a procedure
- The steps or priorities within a process or procedure, and their purpose
- Where the test item lies within a process, and the next step to be executed
- The type of equipment and instrumentation required and how it works

Changing Answers and Guessing. Too often students do not have faith in their own knowledge and ability. As a result, they second guess themselves and change answers on tests. Some students find that this strategy has harmed them, yet others find it beneficial. How do you know when to change your answer? One simple test is to reflect on your self-talk. If you are debating between answers, you may find that your first choice or your "gut" choice is correct more often. If you notice that you have misread the question or response, or missed a detail on first reading, your new answer may be more likely to be the accurate one.

When there is no penalty for guessing on an examination, use your critical thinking to eliminate choices and make a good guess among remaining choices based on theory. Answer the sure things first. On your second round through the test, use your critical thinking. Save your guesses for the third time around. Do not leave unanswered questions. Remember that an unanswered question is definitely wrong.

Cope with Test Anxiety

Anxiety indicates the importance we place on an event. A certain amount of apprehension is normal and can even be helpful going into a testing situation. If anxiety interferes with your ability to study or take a test despite the following or other techniques, seek assistance from a professional counselor. There are, however, steps you can use before and during the examination to minimize your anxious feelings and keep them under control.

Relaxation Exercises. Relaxation can be enhanced through imagery and exercises. Progressive relaxation, based on muscle physiology, employs a process of tension awareness and muscle relaxation. The method starts as you lie comfortably and focus your attention on your feet and toes. Create tension in these muscles for a few seconds, and then allow the muscles to relax. Now, concentrate on your legs and do the same. Slowly move up your body repeating this process. Include your back, diaphragm, neck, shoulders, hands and arms, and face and forehead; each time be aware of the tense feelings and commanding your body to relax. Soon your mood will follow.

Another method paints a mental vacation. Close your eyes and imagine yourself in a beautiful and peaceful place. Use your senses to imagine how it feels, what it smells like, what you see and hear. Envision each aspect of the scene and make this your special place. Practice taking this imaginary trip and place yourself there when life becomes stressed.

Breathing Techniques. When people are anxious, their breathing gets shallow and rapid. The pattern feeds the anxiety. Belly breathing helps before and during the examination. Concentrate on breathing in and out as air enters and exits your lungs. Inhale deeply beginning in the abdomen instead of the chest. Push your stomach out so the air has somewhere to go. Inhale through your nose and exhale though your mouth. Repeat the steps a few times until you are relaxed.

Other breathing techniques combine exercise and meditation such as yoga, *tai chi,* and *qi gong*. You may need some training at first to learn them, but you can do all of these techniques at home. Books and videos are also available for instruction.

Methods During the Examination. Anxiety is often caused by a perceived knowledge level that does not match the anticipated challenge. To counter this discrepancy, your knowledge level needs to be as strong as possible. All your studying and test preparation are the best way to beat any test anxiety.

At the time of the test, before you begin, start with a deep cleansing breath. Tell your shoulders and arms to relax. Drop your head forward and slowly roll it left and right to release the last tensions. Then focus on the task at hand, one question at a time. Keep a positive stream of self-talk; reminding yourself that you can do this, you will be successful.

If your mind seems to go blank, do not panic—it will only steer you downward. Instead, slow down, talk positively to yourself, and slowly continue to read each question until you feel comfortable to answer one. It may seem like a long time, but it will actually be shorter than you imagine and you will be able to continue with the examination. Most importantly, remember that you have done all the work you needed to prepare for the examination; now believe in yourself.

BIBLIOGRAPHY

Barnet S, Bedau H: *Critical thinking reading and writing: a brief guide to argument*, ed 6, Boston, 2007, Bedford/St. Martin's.

Carter C, Bishop J, Kravits SL: *Keys to success*, ed 5, Upper Saddle River NJ, 2009, Pearson Education.

Ellis D: *Becoming a master student*, ed 12, Boston, 2007, Houghton Mifflin.

Felder RM, Brent R: Understanding student differences, *Journal of Engineering Education* 94(1):57–72, 2005. Available at: http://www4.ncsu.edu/unity/lockers/users/f/felder/public/Papers/Understanding_Differences.pdf.

Gardner JN, Jewler AJ, Barefoot BO: *Your college experience: strategies for success*, ed 8, Boston, 2008, Wadsworth.

Gurley LT, Callaway WJ: *Introduction to radiologic technology*, ed 6, St. Louis MO, 2006, Mosby.

Jenkins C: *Skills for success: developing effective study strategies*, Belmont CA, 2005, Wadsworth.

Langhorne M, Fulton J, Otto SE: *Oncology nursing*, ed 5, St. Louis MO, 2007, Mosby.

Mindtools (website): Available at: http://www.mindtools.com. Accessed April 12, 2009.

Nist SL, Diehl W: *Developing textbook thinking*, ed 5, Belmont CA, 2001, Wadsworth.

Pauk W, Owens RJO: *How to study in college*, ed 9, Boston, 2007, Wadsworth.

Rogan L: Tips for Developing English Reading Skills, Ezine Articles (website). Available at: http://EzineArticles.com/?expert=Lesley_Rogan. Accessed April 13, 2009.

Saia DA: *Lange Q&A: radiography examination*, ed 7, New York, 2008, McGraw Hill.

Staley C: *Focus on college success*, Boston, 2009, Wadsworth.

The American Registry of Radiologic Technologists (website): Available at: http://www.arrt.org. Accessed May 2, 2009.

REVIEW EXERCISES

1. Name at least two things to do before class to gain more out of what is presented in the classroom.

2. Identify the parts of a study goal represented by the acronym *GOAL*.

3. Cell phones can cause distractions during study sessions. List one way that this disruption may be limited while studying.

4. In selecting the correct answer to a multiple choice test item, what factors should be considered to establish priorities among the responses?

Multiple choice items may have more than one correct response

5. To remember how to spell the word "arithmetic," Charlene uses the phrase "A rat in Tom's house might eat Tom's ice cream." This memory technique is an example of:

   a. A peg system
   b. Mnemonics
   c. Chaining
   d. Visualization

6. Sara's goal is "to get a good grade in my chemistry course." Select the additional elements that can improve this goal and increase the likelihood of success?

a. List the dates for examinations and assignments.
b. Set a deadline for the goal.
c. Write the course number.
d. State the target grade Sara wants to earn.
e. List steps Sara needs to accomplish a good grade.

7. Which of the following has a positive effect on memory and learning?

a. At least 7 hours of sleep daily
b. Study sessions at least 5 hours long
c. Caffeine drinks to allow longer study sessions
d. A well-balanced diet that includes fruits and vegetables
e. Multitask while studying

8. There are steps to take before reading or taking notes and after you have completed these tasks. Create a matrix that compares the strategies to use before and after reading or note taking.

9. Michael keeps putting off his research paper, a long and difficult assignment. Give Michael your best advice to stop his procrastination.

10. Marie learns best when she can talk through things. She prefers to actively work through new information step by step to understand how to apply new concepts. Name the four elements of her learning style and offer her at least two suggestions for ways to use her style in studying and comprehending new material.

11. Jose is trying to balance a part-time job and his studies. He has a presentation due in 6 weeks, two examinations within that time, and his child's first birthday. Give three suggestions to Jose that will help him manage his time and successfully complete his obligations. Be specific.

12. How many stress management techniques can you find in the following puzzle?
Look horizontally, vertically, diagonally, and backwards.

N	O	P	L	E	N	T	S	A	A	M	U	S	R	E	F
A	D	E	E	A	T	R	I	G	H	T	H	M	E	D	I
N	I	K	X	T	N	D	F	Y	D	H	K	I	P	T	E
B	D	F	E	S	A	E	O	B	O	L	V	L	C	A	H
W	E	P	R	N	L	D	U	E	N	G	A	E	A	L	T
N	E	H	C	L	K	Q	O	G	O	Y	A	X	N	P	E
E	P	E	I	K	F	P	K	G	M	E	D	T	D	N	R
T	B	V	S	W	I	M	I	W	F	L	G	N	L	I	B
W	R	S	E	T	P	R	I	O	R	I	T	I	E	S	D
O	E	H	X	W	L	Z	S	R	E	A	D	J	S	H	K
R	A	D	N	J	A	G	X	I	A	Y	B	Z	H	U	G
K	T	L	S	I	N	L	P	K	N	F	P	R	D	M	E
S	H	D	E	D	A	H	K	E	O	G	E	A	J	O	G
F	I	N	D	C	H	E	E	R	L	E	A	D	E	R	S
J	N	E	H	O	E	N	H	G	R	E	X	E	I	W	U
A	G	F	I	M	A	G	E	R	Y	A	L	V	N	F	Q
P	N	K	M	E	D	I	T	A	T	I	O	N	I	I	Y

CHAPTER

2

An Overview of Cancer and Management Modalities

Leia Levy

FOCUS QUESTIONS

- What are some epidemiologic factors associated with cancer?
- What is carcinogenesis?
- What are some etiologic factors associated with cancer?
- How might you differentiate, compare, and contrast benign and malignant tumor cell populations?
- What are the various roles in cancer management served by surgery, chemotherapy, and radiation therapy?
- Describe the basic principles of surgical oncology.
- Describe the basic principles of chemotherapy.
- What are some examples of biologic response modifiers?
- Describe the basic principles of radiation therapy.
- Compare and contrast various staging and grading systems.
- Define morbidity and mortality.
- Which types of cancers show the highest mortality and incidence rates in the United States?

DEFINITIONS AND TERMINOLOGY

- *Oncology* is the study of a large variety of diseases that behave in a similar way with lethal potential; it is the study of neoplastic disease.
- A *tumor* is a neoplasm composed of cells with abnormal proliferation capacity.
- Tumors may be classified as *benign* or *malignant.*
- Malignant tumors are referred to as *cancers.*
- Hippocrates, a Greek physician who lived in the fourth century bce, was the first to identify a group of diseases that appeared to manifest as a central mass with extensions similar to the anatomy of a crab. He named the disease "karkinos," the Greek word meaning crab (Figure 2-1). Today we accept the crab as the symbol for the zodiac sign Cancer.
- Hippocrates and physicians who followed him also observed that this disease had the tendency to spread to distant locations in the body. The means by which the disease spread was not completely understood at the time.
- It is understood now that cancer has the ability to spread through three main routes: local extension, lymphatics, and blood.
- When cancer has spread outside of the original location to distant locations in the body, the phenomenon is known as *metastasis.*
- The study of cancer as it is distributed in a given population is known as *epidemiology.* Epidemiologic studies help reveal patterns of *incidence.* Populations may be divided by race, gender, common social habits, occupation, geographical location, age, religion, or marital status, among others.
- The study of cancer causes and risk factors is known as *etiology.* Etiologic factors include smoking, asbestos exposure, arsenic exposure, ultraviolet radiation, and nickel compounds, among many others.
- Epidemiologic and etiologic studies have resulted in recommendations for cancer screenings by agencies such as the American Cancer Society.
- Continued study and research means that screening recommendations may change over time.

CARCINOGENESIS

- Cancer causing agents are known as *carcinogens.* The multistage process that occurs following exposure to a carcinogen leading to malignancy is termed *carcinogenesis.*
- Development of a tumor likely requires two or more mutations in the stem cells of the tissue of origin, but expression of the mutation as a tumor depends on how the cell population proliferates and a number of host factors.

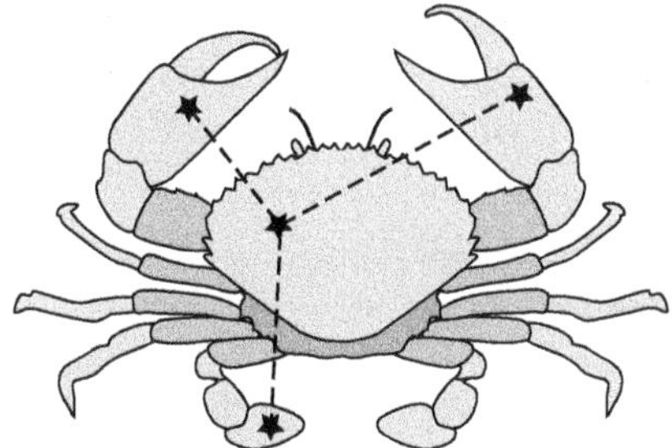

FIGURE 2-1 Sketch of the crab.

- Carcinogens may be categorized as chemical factors, physical factors, viral agents, or genetic factors.
- There are known chemicals that increase the likelihood of developing a cancer, such as soot, tar, nickel compounds, asbestos, arsenic, and benzene.
- Some viruses have been proven to cause transformation of normal cells by attaching to the cells' DNA or RNA, therefore leading to multiplied mutations, eventually forming a tumor (Figure 2-2).
- All mammalian cells contain genes known as *proto-oncogenes, oncogenes,* and *antioncogenes* (tumor suppressor genes).
- Proto-oncogenes are responsible for controlling cellular proliferation.
- Proto-oncogenes can be transformed into oncogenes when activated by the presence of certain viruses or chemical agents.
- When oncogenes cannot be combated by antioncogenes, or negated and eliminated by the body's other immune system components, the oncogenes can take control of proliferation and manifest as a malignancy.
- Ionizing radiation is an example of an extensively studied carcinogen. Cigarette smoke is another.
- Being exposed to a carcinogen does not guarantee the manifestation of a cancer; hyperplasia, metaplasia, or anaplasia may be the result of carcinogen exposure.
- Whether a cancerous condition manifests is influenced by many things including immune status, inherited and intrinsic factors that increase the risk for developing cancer, and the total time over which exposure has occurred.
- Most cancers are not inherited. Those cancers attributable to extrinsic factors are classified as sporadic. Inherited cancers are classified as familial. Familial cancers are a result of a genetic translocation, loss of chromosomes, or amplification of genes causing genetic instability.
- Sporadic cancers typically are caused by multiple outside factors. These cancers are likely due to a change in cell genes following multiple encounters with a carcinogenic agent.
- Familial cancers show up in families who share a common environment and/or genetic abnormality that is passed down through generations. The mother's side tends to be most influential. Familial cancers tend to have an early age of onset; tumors may be multifocal/bilateral, multiple family members are often affected and each family member has a high risk of multiple primary cancers in their lifetime.

DETECTION AND DIAGNOSIS

- Taking a medical history is the initial step toward the diagnoses of cancer.
- The medical history should include documentation of:

1. Chief complaint and main symptoms
2. Details of known or present illnesses

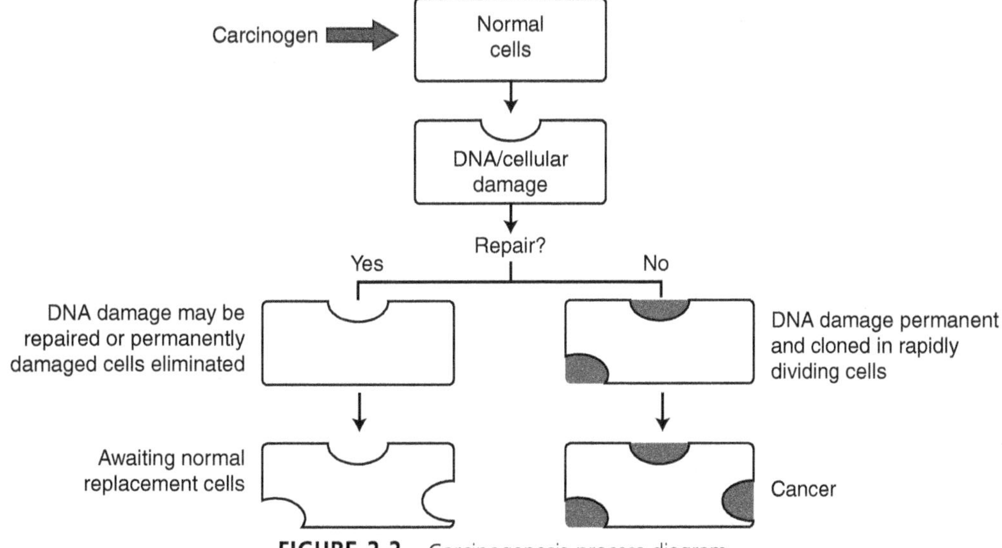

FIGURE 2-2 Carcinogenesis process diagram.

3. Review of all body systems
4. Past medical history
5. Social history
6. Family history
7. Work history
   - Reliance on early symptom reporting is the foundation of cancer detection and subsequent management.
   - Physical examination is also critical in diagnosing cancer.
   - The examiner should check the status of the skin, lymph nodes, oral cavity, breast, testis, perineum, and central nervous system.

The American Cancer Society publishes 7 Warning Signs of Cancer signified by the acronym CAUTION.

C change in bowel habits
A a sore that will not heal
U unusual bleeding or discharge
T thickening or lump
I indigestion or difficulty swallowing
O obvious change in a wart or mole
N nagging, persistent cough

- The next critical step toward accurate diagnosis is to obtain a cell sample.
- A *biopsy* is the removal of tissue or cells for microscopic evaluation.
- There are several types of biopsy procedures including:
  1. Collection of body secretions such as sputum or urine
  2. Scraping or curettage of tissue surfaces
  3. Aspiration of fluid as from the chest, abdomen, fluid-filled mass, or other body cavity with a small bore needle (fine needle aspiration [FNA])
  4. Core needle sampling in which a larger bore needle can actually "punch-out" a bit of tissue from a mass
  5. Dermal punch is similar to core needle; however, a special instrument is used to remove a plug of tissue.
  6. Scalpel incision or excision; incision refers to cutting into a mass whereas excision refers to the total removal of a mass with a margin of gross normal tissue
  7. Direct biopsy or endoscopy uses special flexible, fiber optic instruments directed into a body lumen with an instrument on the end for tissue sampling.
  8. Open surgery is a formal surgical procedure performed under general anesthesia that allows the surgical oncologist to visualize the tumor and surrounding tissues leading to an opportunity to perform a total excision of the tumor and any areas appearing positive for disease.

- To help determine the proper management strategy and to give caregivers an idea about the prognosis of the patient, tumors may be classified and sorted by:
  a. Biologic behavior—benign versus malignant, slow-growing versus aggressive
  b. Anatomic site—breast, prostate, pancreas
  c. Tissue origin—epithelial, connective, reticulo-endothelial
  d. Differentiation—how well the cells can carry out the normal functions of cells of this origin; how well the cells exhibit normal physical characteristics; also known as the tumor grade
  e. Stage—the extent of disease; whether there is only local involvement or involvement of distant tissues (metastasis)
- Cancerous tumors originating in epithelial tissues are referred to as *carcinomas*.
- Epithelial tissues line, cover, or are glandular. Cell types that form epithelial tissues include basal cells, squamous cells, and transitional cells.

  ADENO + CARCINOMA = adenocarcinoma; cancerous tumor of glandular epithelium.
- Cancerous tumors originating in connective tissues are referred to as *sarcomas*.
- Connective or mesenchymal tissues provide our bodies with support, and comprise our blood tissues. Cell types that form these tissues are osseous, muscular, fatty, cartilaginous, and vascular.

  OSTEO + SARCOMA = osteosarcoma; cancerous tumor of the bone
- The suffix -OMA may be combined with other root words to indicate benign growths in various tissues.

  LIP + OMA = lipoma; benign tumor of fatty tissue
- There are exceptions to the root + suffix rule such as:

  LYMPHOMA = malignancy originating in the lymphatic system
  LEUKEMIA = malignancy originating in the blood, specifically the white blood cells
  GLIOMA = malignancy originating in the central nervous system
- There are many organizations responsible for staging system recommendations.
- The American Joint Committee for Cancer Staging (AJCC), the International Union Against Cancer (IUCC), the Pediatric Oncology Group (POG), the World Health Organization (WHO), the International Federation of Gynecology and Obstetrics (FIGO) are a few organizations with well-known recommendations for certain cancers.

- The stage of disease may be assessed clinically or pathologically.
- Clinical staging requires the use of the practitioner's senses.

What is seen, felt, or heard on physical examination can provide enough information for clinical staging.

- Pathologic staging requires the use of imaging and histologic study.

Imaging studies such as CT, MRI, or PET and tissue sampling provides information for pathologic staging.

- The most widely used and internationally accepted staging system is the TNM system.
- The TNM system describes the *tumor*'s size, circumference, depth of invasion, or mobility status. The involvement of lymph *nodes*, their size and mobility are also evaluated. Finally, the presence of distant *metastasis* is assessed as well.
- Each category may be assigned a numerical value. Typically the values are 0 to 4. Once each category has been assigned a value, then multiple combinations may be placed in stage groups indicated by Roman numerals.

Stage Grouping Sample

Stage I	Stage II	Stage III	Stage IV
T1 N0 M0	T2 N1 M0	T3 N2 M0	T4 N3 M1

- Whenever the value "X" is assigned to one of the categories, that indicates that the status could not be accessed and has to be documented as "status unknown."

MANAGEMENT MODALITIES

- The three main cancer management modalities include surgery, chemotherapy, and radiation therapy.
- Immunotherapy is another cancer management modality; while not used as widely as the main three, its use may become more prevalent as we continue studying the mechanisms for carcinogenesis, remission, and recurrent disease.
- The specialized areas of medical practice that apply these modalities are known as surgical oncology, medical oncology, and radiation oncology.

Surgery

- Surgery is a local approach used to diagnose or aid in disease staging, palliate symptoms, curatively manage, or as an adjunct (complementary) to other cancer management modalities.
- Surgery may also be used following cancer therapy for rehabilitation, restoring of normal organ function, or cosmetic restoration.
- Surgical diagnosis is achieved through tissue sampling. Some biopsies may be performed in the surgical suite with the aid of specialized imaging modes such as ultrasound or fluoroscopy.
- Nonoperative staging is desired and essential before a curative surgical procedure is planned; however, surgical lymph node dissections have been helpful in staging certain cancers, such as breast cancer and those of the head/neck region.
- Historically, surgical staging laparoscopies were performed for systemic cancers such as lymphoma; today, the advances in medical imaging have made invasive procedures such as this unnecessary.
- Surgery may be used to debulk or decrease the size of a tumor before other management modalities are attempted.
- Large tumors may be difficult to totally excise when they may be invading neighboring tissue, wrapped around a neighboring organ, or in an anatomic region where it may be difficult to excise without compromising the quality of the postsurgical life for the patient.
- Surgical treatment is optimally used as curative therapy, where the goal is for the patient to be pronounced cancer-free or in remission after surgery.
- Cancers that are easily cured with surgery are small and localized with no evidence of distant metastasis.
- The role of surgery may also be prophylactic; an example may be a bilateral mastectomy for a patient with diagnosed breast cancer in one breast, who is at an increased risk for developing cancer in the opposite breast.
- The surgical oncologist has to be knowledgeable of all cancer types, patterns of spread, various staging and grading systems, and be proficient in surgical technique suitable for cancer detection and/or eradication of disease.
- Since surgery is a local approach, the anticipated side effects are local.
- Once a patient has been determined as a suitable candidate for surgery, he or she should be educated on possible postsurgical complications such as pain, swelling, infections, limited or altered function, lengthy rehabilitation, or recovery and cosmetic consequences.

Chemotherapy

- Chemotherapy is the use of anticancer drugs (cytotoxic drugs) or hormonal agents to cure, palliate, maintain remission, or as a prophylactic measure.
- Chemotherapy is prescribed and supervised by a medical oncologist.

- Chemotherapy may also be used as an adjunct to other cancer management modalities.
- In most cases, chemotherapy is administered intravenously or orally. Its use is a systemic approach to managing cancer.
- There are a few cytotoxic drugs that may be applied topically or administered locally.
- The effectiveness of cytotoxic drug therapy is influenced by: the tumor cell burden, the growth rate of the tumor, the vascular supply, the patterns of cell division, and the concentration of the drug made available to malignant cells.
- Cytotoxic drugs may be grouped into two broad categories: Phase-specific and non–phase-specific.
- Phase-specific drugs are most effective during certain stages of cell division. In order for these drugs to work, the tumor cells must be dividing. As cell division occurs, in many malignant populations every 4 to 6 hours, it is desirable that phase specific drugs be available during multiple cell dividing cycles. The longer the drug is in the system, the better chance for death of malignant cells. These drugs are the ones you may observe being administered over a long period of time (i.e., a few days of continuous infusion).
- Non–phase-specific drugs are effective at any stage of cell division and may be effective on tumor cell populations that are no longer dividing, or are sparsely dividing. These drugs are the ones you may observe administered as a bolus injection or taken orally.
- Further, cytotoxic drugs may be divided into classes such as follows (Figure 2-3):

  Alkylating agents
  Antitumor antibiotics
  Antimetabolites
  Plant alkaloids
  Nitrosoureas

- Although hormonal agents and biologic response modifiers (BRMs) in the management of cancer are also administered under the care of a medical oncologist, these agents have a different action than the cytotoxic groups.
- The cytotoxics are intended to act as a poison to malignant cells.
- Hormones are administered to counteract the body's response to the presence of certain types of cancers.
- Biologic response modifiers are administered to induce or enhance the body's natural response to the presence of disease or physiologic imbalance.

Examples: Certain breast cancers nurtured by the presence of estrogen may be stunted by the administration of an antiestrogen, such as tamoxifen.

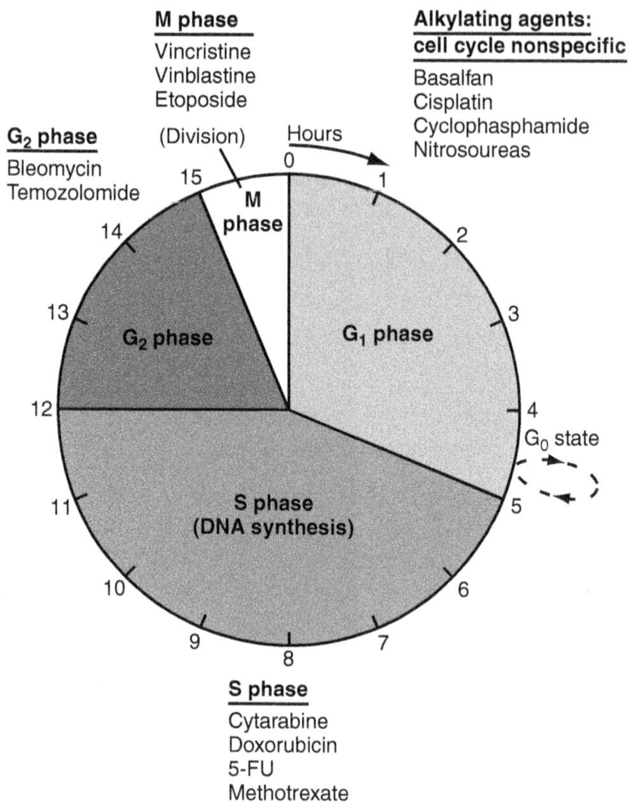

FIGURE 2-3 Cell cycle and cytotoxic targets of common antineoplastic agents.

Central Nervous system cancers may cause increased swelling in the cranium. An antiinflammatory, such as dexamethasone, could decrease swelling.

Monoclonal antibodies may be harvested from cancer infected animals and given to the cancer patient to induce an antigen-antibody complex reaction so that the patient may fight the disease.

- Some chemotherapy agents sensitize the cancerous tissues to other cancer therapy such as radiation. They are called *radiosensitizers.*
- Some chemical agents protect the normal tissues from other therapy such as radiation. They are called *radioprotectors.*
- Radiosensitizers and radioprotectors have limited duration, so it is important to administer radiation in a timely manner after these drugs are administered.
- Single drugs may be administered, but most often drugs are used in combination to improve effectiveness.
- Past *clinical trials,* the known biologic behavior of the cancer, its vascular supply and spread pattern strongly influence the use of chemotherapy as a management strategy.
- In instances where there is no evidence of systemic disease, but there is a strong possibility of systemic disease in the future, as past case studies have proven, the prophylactic use of chemotherapy is warranted.

- When chemotherapy is administered systemically, the side effects manifest systemically.
- Cytotoxic drugs are not only toxic to malignant cells but to normal cells as well. The number of surviving cells decreases as the cycles of therapy progress, but regrowth may start if therapy is prematurely stopped (Figure 2-4).
- Administerers and handlers of chemotherapy agent containers should take care not to expose skin or eyes to drugs.
- Some common side effects across chemotherapy cytotoxic agent classes are: myelosuppression, nausea, vomiting, alopecia, skin rashes, diarrhea, renal disease, and cardiomyopathy.
- All chemotherapy agents do not have the same side effects.

Radiation Therapy

- Radiation therapy, like surgery, is a local approach to cancer management.
- Radiation may be used to cure, palliate, maintain remission, or for prophylaxis.
- The effectiveness of radiation is similar to that of chemotherapy and is influenced by: the tumor cell burden, the sensitivity of both the cancerous and normal tissues to radiation, the cumulative dose given, the type of radiation applied, and the patterns of cell division and the vascular supply.
- The law of Bergonie and Tribondeau describes the most radiosensitive cells as ones that rapidly divide, divide often, have a long mitotic future, and are undifferentiated.

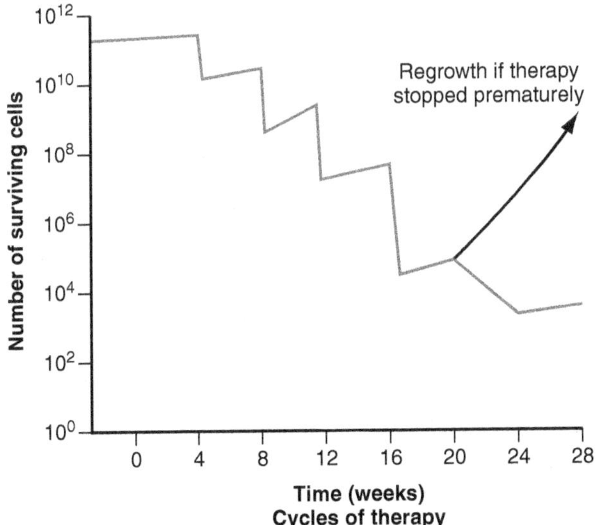

FIGURE 2-4 Cell survival curve for cytotoxic chemotherapy administration.

- Tumors with a larger cell burden tend to have necrotic, slow-dividing cells at the core. Necrotic, slow-dividing cells have decreased radiosensitivity.
- Reaching lethal doses for the tumor while sparing normal tissue from damaging doses is challenging.
- The *therapeutic ratio* is a measure of potential success with radiation (Figure 2-5).

$$\text{Therapeutic ratio} = \frac{\text{Normal Tissue Tolerance Dose(NTTD)}}{\text{Tumor Lethal Dose(TLD)}}$$

- When the ratio is 1.0 or greater, the potential for success is favorable.
- Strategies such as fractionation and complex treatment planning assist in making a favorable therapeutic ratio easier to achieve.
- Certain types of radiation are more lethal to tissues than others.
- When conditions are conducive, adequate doses of radiation can lead to cell death in the local area targeted.
- When tumors are localized and confined, radiation can be focused over the tumor and local areas of anticipated cancer spread, with the expectation of complete eradication of disease.
- In instances where the tumor is large and there is proven distant metastasis, radiation may also be administered to shrink the tumor to relieve symptoms due to compression or obstruction.
- Radiation therapy may also be used as an adjunct to surgery and or chemotherapy to "sterilize" any areas of possible disease spread.
- Radiation therapy is a local approach, so side effects remain local.
- Patients undergoing radiation therapy must be made aware of anticipated side effects as indicated by the region irradiated.
- Radiation side effects may include: hair loss in the area, local redness and swelling, nausea and vomiting when irradiating the abdomen and possibly diarrhea when irradiating the bowel.
- The radiation oncologist must be knowledgeable of the various cancer types, their sensitivities/resistance to radiation, proven dose and fractionation protocols, tolerance doses of normal tissues, and the biologic behavior of certain types of cancers and their spread patterns.
- Some radiation oncologists may specialize in certain age-related cancers or certain cancers of anatomic regions.

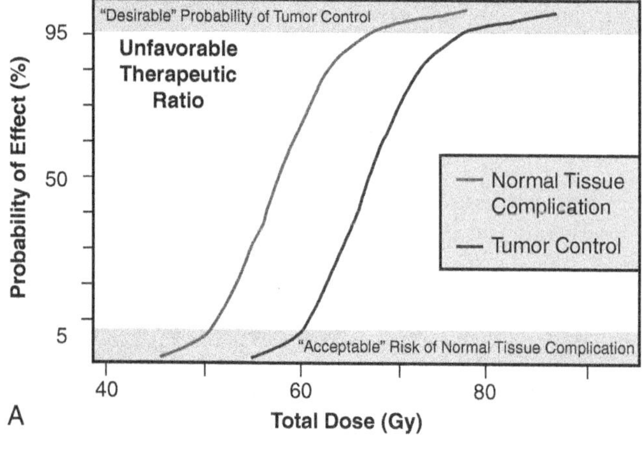

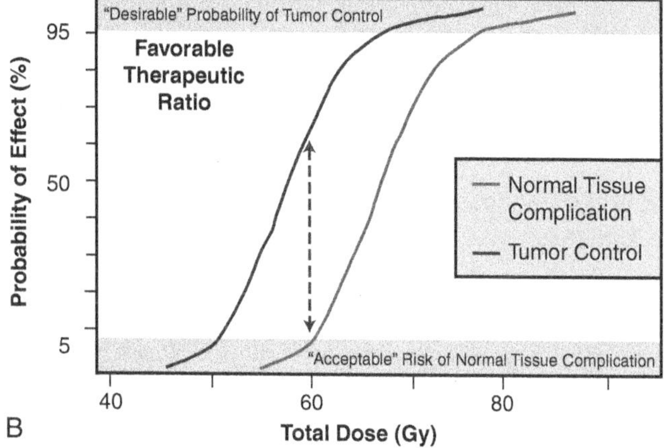

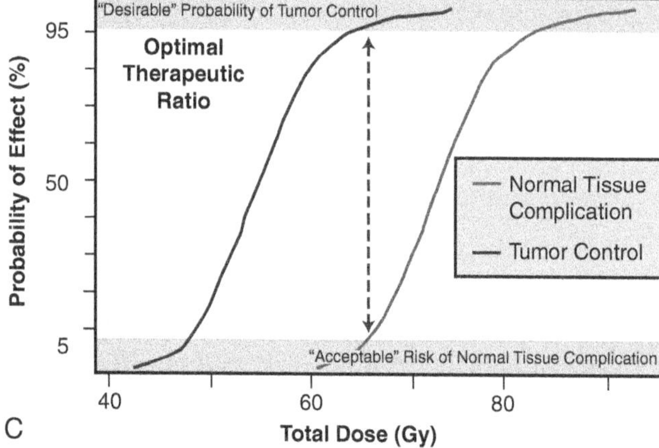

FIGURE 2-5 Therapeutic ratio diagrams. **A**, Poor therapeutic ratio; **B**, Good therapeutic ratio; **C**, Optimal therapeutic ratio.

Immunotherapy

- Immunotherapy, or the use of biologic response modifiers (BRM), is a systemic approach like chemotherapy.
- BRMs include proteins, such as interferon, capable of attacking cancer cells, monoclonal antibodies, vaccines, and natural killer B and T cells.
- The goal of immunotherapy is to use the body's natural defense mechanisms to control malignancy.
- It has been substantiated that certain cancers occur as a result of the body's inability to naturally defend itself against disease. At some point, the body may loose its ability to differentiate between self and nonself and allows malignant, nonself cells to thrive and eventually take control of the host.
- Immunotherapy is often reserved for use in the end stages of malignancy, as much more research needs to occur while the main three modalities continue to perfect their effectiveness against the majority of cancers.
- Interferon is a protein that is naturally produced by the body, but when it seems production has failed, it may be produced technologically and administered to the cancer patient. T and B cells may be donated by compatible donors, and monoclonal antibodies are lymphocyte clones produced in animals such as mice.
- Before any drug therapy is initiated, the medical oncologist must consider the biology of the disease, the pharmacology of the drug(s), the effectiveness of drugs as proven in clinical trials, and the clinical condition of the patient.
- Moreover, the medical oncologist must be a knowledgeable internist so that he is familiar with signs of possible complications and side effects that may occur in any body system.

MANAGEMENT MODALITY OVERVIEW

- Cancer management modalities are often used together to improve the potential for remission, limit side effects, and to improve patient prognosis.
- When modalities are used complementary to each other, the supporting modality is known as *adjuvant* therapy. The modality intended to initiate remission is known as the *neoadjuvant* therapy.
- The determination whether to use modalities at the same time or one after the other has to be justified by clinical trials and outcomes recorded in tumor registries.
- When modalities are used together, one after another, the term *concomitant* may be used.
- When modalities are used together at the same time, the term *concurrent* may be used.
- The surgical oncologist, medical oncologist, and radiation oncologist have to work together closely to design the optimal treatment plan for every patient.
- The management goals must be clearly defined, all alternatives must be presented and all expected side effects and expected outcomes should be disclosed to the patient so that they may make the ultimate decision regarding the management of their disease.

BIBLIOGRAPHY

Bomford CK, Kunkle IH: *Walter and Miller's textbook of radiotherapy*, ed 6, London, 2003, Churchill Livingstone/Elsevier.
Gunderson LL, Tepper JE: *Clinical radiation oncology*, ed 2, Philadelphia, 2007, Churchill Livingstone/Elsevier.
Lenhard R, Gansler T, Osteen R. *Clinical oncology*, ed 8, American Cancer Society, 2001.
Washington CM, Leaver D: *Principles and practice of radiation therapy*, ed 3, St. Louis, 2010, Mosby.

REVIEW EXERCISES

1. Use the table to compare and contrast benign and malignant tumor cell populations.

Benign Tumors	Malignant Tumors

2. List current cancer-screening recommendations from the American Cancer Society for men and women.

3. List and describe five different methods of tissue sampling/biopsy.

4. The following group of terms is associated with cancer management. Circle the term in each group that does not belong among the others.

Group 1
Basal cell Squamous cell Adenocarcinoma Glioma

Group 2
Cytotoxic drugs Antitumor drugs Chemotherapy drugs Antiemetics

Group 3
Methotrexate 5-flourouracil Purinethol Tamoxifen

5. Define prophylactic cancer management.

6. Match the terms and descriptions.

____ **Adenocarcinoma**	A. Malignant tumor occurring in striated muscle
____ **Myeloma**	B. Malignant tumor occurring in bone
____ **Leukemia**	C. Malignant tumor originating in the central nervous system
____ **Osteosarcoma**	D. Abnormal proliferation occurring in the bone marrow
____ **Rhabdomyosarcoma**	E. Malignant tumor of glandular epithelium
____ **Glioma**	F. Abnormal proliferation occurring in the bone marrow, especially the white blood cells

7. Unscramble the letters to reveal general oncology or pathology terms.

G O C N E C N E

S C A R I E S N E C O N G I

Y B I S P O

O T M R U

T N D I N O F E R F E T A I I

S S S A T E M I T A

8. Complete the chemotherapy table.

Phase-specific Cytotoxic Drugs	Phase Nonspecific Cytotoxic Drugs
	Effective on nondividing cells
One such class would be antimetabolites	
	Examples are: nitrogen mustard, Cytoxan
Toxicities include: myelosuppression, anorexia, nausea	

9. Compare and contrast hyperplasia, metaplasia, and anaplasia.

10. Mortality rates are based on the number of persons per________ population.

a. 1,000,000
b. 1000
c. 100,000
d. 50

11. Any substance or agent that produces or incites cancer is called:

a. Carcinosis
b. Carcinogen
c. Mutant
d. Carcinoid

12. The seven warning signs of cancer include all of the following except:

a. Thickening or lump
b. Nagging cough
c. Pain
d. Change in bowel habits

13. The TNM staging system evaluates:

a. The size and extent of the tumor
b. Whether the primary tumor has metastasized
c. The grade of the tumor
d. a, b
e. a, b, c

14. Malignant neoplasms that originate in lymphoreticular tissues are called:

a. Sarcomas
b. Lymphosarcomas
c. Lymphomas
d. Lymphoreticulomas

15. When more than one cancer modality is used simultaneously, it is known as:

a. Concurrent therapy
b. Concomitant therapy
c. Systemic therapy
d. Immunotherapy

16. The class of cytotoxic agents that has the potential to burn the skin of the administerer is:

a. Alkylating agents
b. Antimetabolites
c. Plant alkaloids
d. Hormones

17. The cancer warning sign most likely indicating colon/rectal cancer would be:

a. Pain
b. A sore that will not heal
c. A change in a wart or mole
d. Change in bowel habits

18. Which of the following cytotoxic drugs may produce heart failure?

a. Methotrexate
b. Actinomycin-D
c. Adriamycin
d. Bleomycin

19. A tumor classified as T3, N2, M0 is likely a stage:

a. I
b. II
c. III
d. IV
e. V

20. The tissue of a malignant carcinoma is:

a. Epithelial
b. Cartilaginous
c. Skeletal
d. Neural

21. The method used to establish definite malignancy is:

a. Radiologic imaging
b. Hematologic study
c. Histopathologic screening
d. Clinical staging

22. A cancerous tumor composed of glandular tissue would be called a/n:

a. Neurilimoma
b. Adenocarcinoma
c. Epithelioma
d. Chondrosarcoma

23. A malignant tumor of striated muscle would be called a/n:

a. Leiomyoma
b. Fibrosarcoma
c. Epithelioma
d. Rhabdomyosarcoma

24. A surgical procedure in which an incision is made through the abdominal wall to examine lymph nodes and establish the extent of disease is called a/n:

   a. Incisional biopsy
   b. Laparoscopy
   c. Mastectomy
   d. Radical excision

For questions 25 to 30, circle the word(s) that would correctly complete the sentence.

25. The highest incidence of malignancy for adult males in the United States occurs in the (prostate, liver, colon). The highest incidence of malignancy for adult females in the United States occurs in the (liver, breast, colon).

26. The process by which tumors are induced by certain chemical or physical agents is called (carcinosis, carcinogenesis, carcinitis).

27. (Hair loss, weight loss, myelosuppression) is the most common side effect associated with cytotoxic drugs.

28. Most cancers are (sporadic, familial).

29. The removal of cells by scraping is called (FNA, total excision, curettage).

30. The (stage, grade, histology) of a tumor is an evaluation of the degree of cellular differentiation.

31. According to Bergonie and Tribondeau, factors that may influence the sensitivity of a group of cells to ionizing radiation are:

   1. Mitotic activity
   2. Time of cell division
   3. Cellular differentiation
   4. Length of mitotic activity

      a. 1, 2
      b. 2, 3
      c. 1, 3, 4
      d. 1, 2, 3 and 4

32. Cancer management modalities such as radiation and chemotherapy work by interfering with or modifying DNA synthesis. This synthesis occurs in the____ phase of cell division.

   a. S
   b. M
   c. G0
   d. G1

33. Mr. Jones and Mr. Smith have larynx tumors. Mr. Jones' tumor is classified as T2 and Mr. Smith's as T4. What difference(s) would you expect to see in these tumors?

34. Palliation is:

   a. To treat for cure
   b. Treatment for the relief of symptoms
   c. The skin color indicative of low oxygen flow
   d. Treatment to prevent the manifestation of disease

The following are true/false corrective statements. If the statement is true, place a T on the line. If the statement is false, place an F on the line and correct the statement so that it becomes true without changing the intent of the statement.

35. ______ One of the characteristics of benign tumors is that they are never fatal.

36. ______ A patient being treated with radiation to the abdomen will experience epilation of the scalp.

37. ______ The term for transmission of disease from one original site to one or more sites elsewhere in the body is metastasis.

38. ______ Oncogenes are also known as tumor-suppressor genes.

39. ______ In general, children have the highest incidence of cancer.

40. ______ Surgery is never used prophylactically.

41. Which of the following is not a possible side effect of cytotoxic drugs?

a. Nausea
b. Cardiac toxicity
c. Myelosuppression
d. Alopecia
e. None of the above

42. Factors considered in chemotherapy drug selection include which of the following?

1. Histology
2. Tumor location
3. Rate of drug absorption
4. Tumor resistance to the drug(s)

a. 1, 2
b. 1, 3
c. 2, 3, 4
d. 1, 2, 3, 4

43. The oldest cancer management modality is:

a. Chemotherapy
b. Radiation therapy
c. Surgery
d. Immunotherapy

44. All of the following are characteristic of malignant tumors except:

a. Blood vessel invasion
b. Rapid growth
c. Encapsulation
d. Metastatic

45. One unique characteristic of substitute ureas is:

a. They may burn the skin on contact
b. They can cross the blood-brain barrier
c. They are the most expensive class
d. They are exclusively used for metastatic disease

46. The cancer warning sign most likely indicating breast cancer would be:

a. Pain
b. A sore that will not heal
c. A lump or thickening
d. Change in bowel habits

47. The incidence of cancer in a given area may be affected by:

a. Race
b. Environmental exposures
c. Cultural practices
d. All of the above

48. An imaging technique used to detect lung cancer would be:

a. Ultrasound
b. Routine radiography
c. Lymphangiography
d. Venography

49. A tumor marker for the detection of germ cell tumors is:

a. PSA
b. CEA
c. PAP
d. Beta HCG

50. The American Cancer Society recommends____ for men beginning at the age of 45.

a. Annual PAP smear
b. Manual testicular examination
c. Colonoscopy
d. Annual chest x-ray

51. Mr. Anthony and Mrs. Anthony are chronic smokers. Mr. Anthony smokes 1 pack per day and has been for the past 5 years. Mrs. Anthony smokes 1 pack per day and has been for the past 25 years. Who probably has the greatest risk for the development of lung cancer? Explain your answer.

52. If Mrs. Anthony successfully quits smoking next week and Mr. Anthony quits 10 years later. Who has the greatest risk for the development of lung cancer? Explain your answer.

53. Briefly describe the following curative surgical procedures:

Prostatectomy—

Radical mastectomy—

Modified radical mastectomy—

Exenteration—

54. Prophylactic therapy is intended to:

a. Relieve pain
b. Heal or stall ulceration, fungation, or fracture
c. Improve the quality of life
d. Sterilize areas of microscopic disease

55. Curative therapy is intended to:

a. Relieve pain
b. Heal or stall ulceration, fungation, or fracture
c. Totally eradicate disease
d. Counteract the presence of hormones

Think About It

56. If the administration of cytotoxic drugs poisons both malignant and healthy cells, how are we able to continue using this modality to treat cancer and return the cancer patient to a healthy state?

57. Systemic chemotherapy and local radiation similarly rely on adequate vascular supply. What is the significance of vasculature and the effectiveness of both therapy modalities?

58. Cure rates for early stage carcinoma of the cervix, glottic larynx, and basal cell carcinoma of the skin are the same whether radiation *or* surgery is used for management. If this is so, why would radiation therapy become the treatment of choice for most?

59. We generally report survival rates in 5-year increments. Breast cancer survival rates are reported at a different time interval. What is the time interval? Explain why this is appropriate.

60. Regardless of the reported successes of the widely used management modalities for cancer, we still see disease recurrence and mortality. List a few possible reasons for treatment failures.

61. Most cytotoxic chemotherapy drugs cannot cross the blood-brain barrier. Explain how certain cytotoxic chemotherapy drug(s) or combinations, unable to cross the barrier, are effectively used in the management of central nervous system malignancies today.

62. Fractionation of radiation doses allow for:

a. Repair of normal tissue
b. Decrease in the oxygen concentration of the cells
c. Efficient use of high voltage equipment
d. Depletion of circulating blood cells

63. Which of the following treatment modalities, if used alone, would best treat a patient with metastatic disease?

a. Surgery
b. Radiation therapy
c. Chemotherapy
d. Hormone therapy

64. Hippocrates is credited with:

a. The first use of cytotoxic drugs
b. Establishing cell sensitivity theory
c. Writing radiation therapy protocols
d. Identifying the disease we know as cancer

65. The youngest modality used in the treatment of cancer is:

a. Surgery
b. Radiation therapy
c. Chemotherapy
d. Blood letting

66. Effective cancer management should involve interactive communications between:

a. Surgical oncology
b. Medical oncology
c. Radiation oncology
d. b and c
e. All of the above

67. The following is true regarding excisional biopsy:

a. Involves the removal of a portion of the tumor
b. Generally appropriate for cure in relatively small tumors
c. Provides a definitive diagnosis
d. b and c
e. a, b, c

68. Possible routes for cytotoxic drug administration are:

a. Intravenous
b. Topical
c. Enteral
d. a, c
e. a, b, c

69. Actinomycin D is a/an:

a. Alkylating agent
b. Antitumor antibiotic
c. Antiemetic
d. Hormonal agent

70. The ____of a tumor is an evaluation of the degree of differentiation.

a. Grade
b. Stage
c. Extent
d. Histology

71. Generally, a lesion classified as T1, N0, M0 is likely a stage____

a. IV
b. III
c. II
d. I

72. Which of the following is not recognized as a carcinogen:

a. Ionizing radiation
b. Asbestos
c. Ultraviolet light
d. Crude oil

73. A patient receiving radiation therapy to the brain is expected to experience:

a. Epilation
b. Diarrhea
c. Dysuria
d. Dysphagia

74. A likely symptom of testicular cancer is:

a. Change in bowel habits
b. A sore that will not heal
c. Nagging cough
d. Painless lump

75. The most widely used staging system is known as the____ system:

a. Therapeutic ratio
b. TNM
c. BRM
d. ABDE

CHAPTER

3

Radiation Therapy Physics

Leia Levy

FOCUS QUESTIONS

- How does radiation interact with matter?
- Where does radiation exist in the universe?
- What are the characteristics of electromagnetic radiation?
- How does an x-ray photon differ from a microwave photon?
- What are the influences on types of radiation interactions?
- Distinguish electron interactions from photon interactions.
- What happens during radioactive decay?
- What is radioactivity?
- Are photon interactions different from particulate radiation interactions?
- Can we predict the interaction of radiation with the atom?
- How are x-rays produced?
- How do x-rays and naturally occurring radiations differ?
- What is the importance of understanding radiation interactions with matter for the radiation therapist?

ATOMIC PHYSICS

- Radiation physics is the study of radiation interactions with matter.
- All matter in its smallest form is composed of atoms.
- There are several models for the composition of the atom.
- Bohr's model is used often and demonstrates a centralized nucleus, containing neutrons and protons, and electrons orbiting the nucleus at various levels around it in "shells" (Figure 3-1).
- Bohr's theory states that most of the atom's mass is in the nucleus where there are neutrons, protons, and nucleons.
- The mass of atoms are expressed in terms of atomic mass units (amu) or atomic weight; 1 amu = 1.66×10^{-27} kg.
- The mass in grams numerically equal to the atomic weight is the gram atomic weight.
- According to Avogadro's law, every gram atomic weight of an element contains the same number of atoms.
- The number of atoms per gram is given by Avogadro's number/atomic weight; Avogadro's number is accepted as 6.0228×10^{23}.
- Atoms are represented by the formula $_{Z}X^{A}$.
- The X is the chemical symbol, Z is the atomic number (the number of protons or electrons), A is the atomic mass (the sum of protons and neutrons).
- Neutrons have no charge and protons have a positive charge; nucleons have the ability to transition between positive and neutral charge; the nucleus is positively charged.
- Both neutrons and protons have a substantial mass as compared with orbiting electrons; protons are about 1800 times more massive than electrons and neutrons are slightly heavier than protons.
- The orbiting electrons have virtually no mass but may be stripped from the atom to go on to interact with other atoms or particles. The mass, charge, and LET of some key particles is provided in Table 3-1.
- With electrons orbiting carrying a negative charge, they are bound to the atom by the attraction of their negative charges to positive charges in the nucleus; this attraction is known as electrostatic force.
- The closer the electrons are to the nucleus, the more tightly bound they are to the nucleus.
- Atoms have a maximum number of required electrons in each shell.

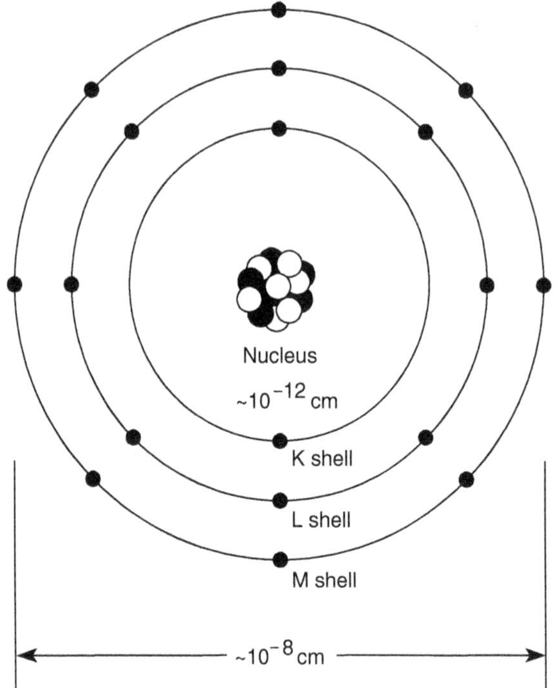

FIGURE 3-1 Bohr's model of the atom.

TABLE 3-1 Particles with Mass, Charge and LET

	Mass (kilograms)	LET(KeV/ micrometer)	Charge
Cobalt gamma	0	0.2	0
250 kV x-rays	0	2.0	0
Beta	0.000548	0.2-2.0	−1, +1
Protons	1.67×10^{-27}	0.5-4.7	+1
Neutrons	1.68×10^{-27}	75	0
Alpha particles	6.65×10^{-27}	166	+2

- $2n^2$ is the formula used to find the maximum number of electrons in a shell. N represents the shell number or quantum number. Each shell, beginning with the inner shell is assigned a letter, K, L, M, N or quantum number 1, 2, 3, 4 and so on.
- The stability of the atoms in an element is determined by a balance of positive and negative charges and evenly paired electrons.
- An atom is electrically neutral or said to be in its ground state when it has as many positive charges as negative charges and has evenly paired electrons.
- An encounter with radiation can manipulate any of the atom's components.
- Electrons can be stripped from the atom and interact with other atoms or positively charged particles.
- Neutrons may also be stripped from the atom but will not interact with electrons due to its neutral charge, but may interact with other particles.
- Protons can be stripped and will likely interact with electrons or neutrons.
- Any encounter that would cause an electron to be raised to a higher electron shell or made to vibrate in place, would lead to an energy emission known as excitation (Figure 3-2).
- Any interaction with the atom that would cause an electron to be totally removed from the atom is known as ionization (Figure 3-3).

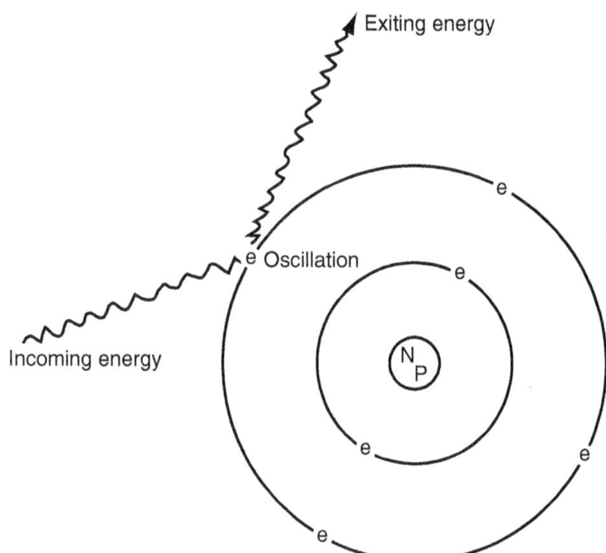

FIGURE 3-2 Excitation occurs when an electron is raised to a higher shell or made to vibrate.

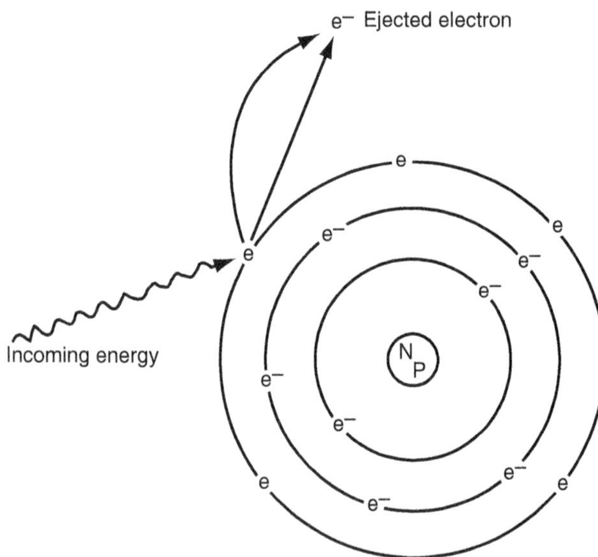

FIGURE 3-3 Ionization occurs when an electron is ejected from the atom.

- Once an atom is ionized, it is no longer stable. Rather, it has charge. If an atom captures an electron then it is called a negative ion. If it loses an electron, then it is called a positive ion.
- Great energy has to be expended to raise electrons to a higher shell. The closer the electrons are to the nucleus, the stronger the binding energy, or electrostatic force.
- As electrons are held tight to the nucleus by energy and have energy at rest in the shell, any change in the status of an otherwise resting electron causes an energy loss or redistribution of energy.
- If the incoming or interacting energy of an atomic particle, or energy bundle, has at least 124 electron volts of energy and a wavelength shorter than 10^{-6} cm, it has the greatest potential to be ionizing.
- Energy ranges commonly used in radiation therapy are 200 keV-50 MeV.
- The kilo electron volt (keV) is 10^3 electron volts or 1000 electron volts.
- The mega electron volt (MeV) is 10^6 or 1,000,000 electron volts.

ELECTROMAGNETIC SPECTRUM

- Ionizing radiation is in the family of electromagnetic radiation.
- All radiation in the electromagnetic spectrum are photons, or bundles of energy, that travel in straight lines, have velocity as the speed of light, and have wavelength and frequency.
- Radiation in the electromagnetic spectrum includes visible light, heat, radio, microwaves, ultraviolet rays, gamma rays, and x-rays (Figure 3-4).
- These photons are called electromagnetic because they exhibit similar characteristics as electric and magnetic

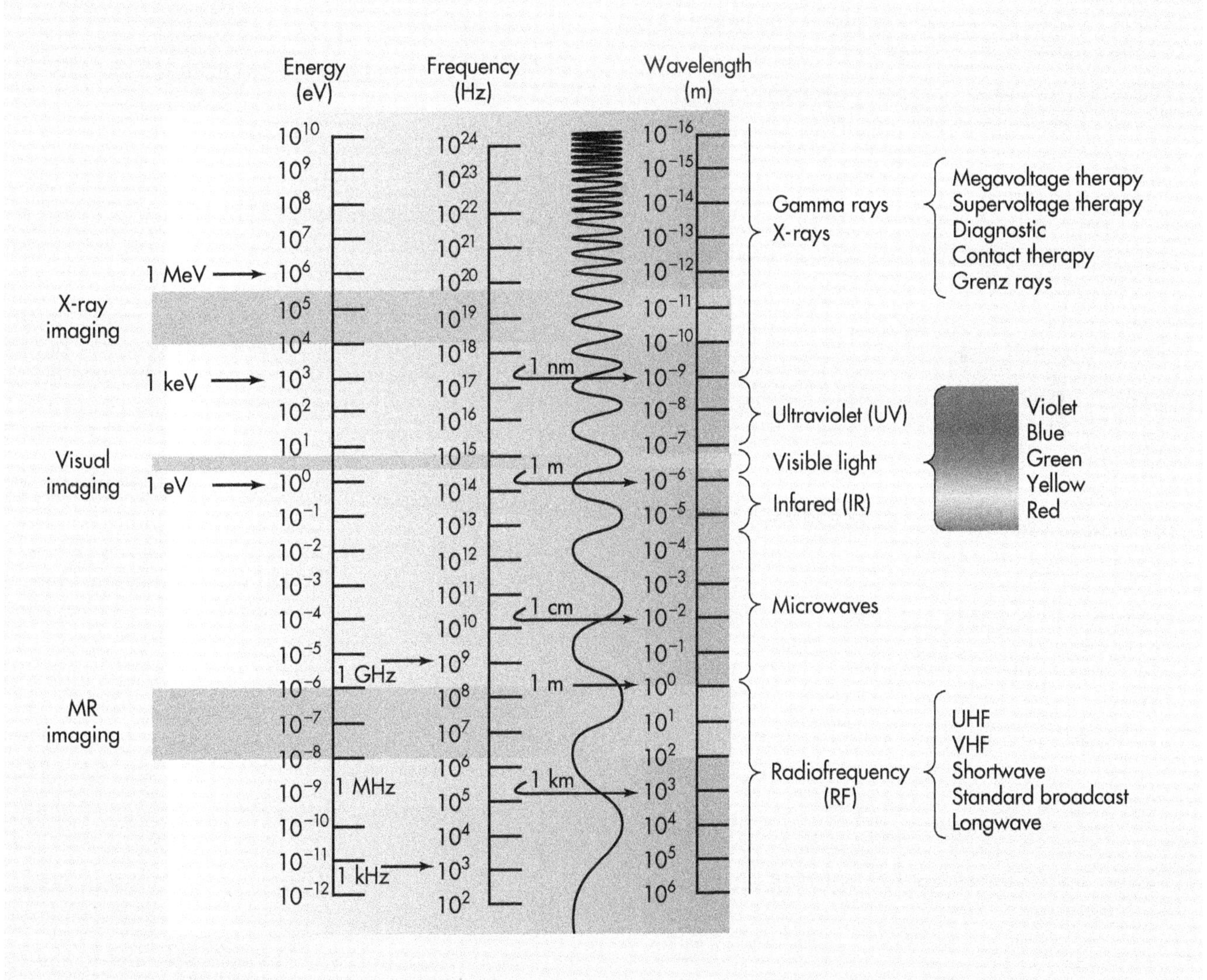

FIGURE 3-4 The electromagnetic spectrum.

fields (oscillating wave patterns, frequency, wavelength, energy, and velocity).

- Frequency is measured in cycles per second using the unit Hertz.
- Wavelength is measured in meters using the unit Angstrom.
- Energy is measured in joules or expressed in electron volts (eV).
- Radiation in the electromagnetic spectrum used in radiation therapy includes gamma and x-radiation; x-rays and gamma rays are found at the upper end of the spectrum with short wavelengths, high frequency, and high energies.
- X-rays and gamma rays are ionizing.
- X-rays and gamma rays only differ by where they originate.
- Gamma rays are a result of natural nuclear decay; x-rays have to be created and are a result of interaction or deceleration of electrons with the atoms of a target material.
- Positrons (positively charged electrons), electrons, protons, neutrons, alpha particles, and pi mesons are examples of other radiation known as particulates.
- Particulates may also be ionizing; electrons, protons, neutrons, and alpha particles may be used in radiation therapy.
- Positrons only exist in motion and are used in imaging, such as PET scanning.
- Particulates with high mass are more directly ionizing than gamma rays, x-rays, and low mass electrons.
- Wavelength, frequency, and the speed of light are related according to the formula:

$$C = \lambda \upsilon$$

where C = speed of light, λ = wavelength, υ = frequency

- The speed of light is constant at 3×10^{10} cm/sec in vacuum or 3×10^{8} m/sec.
- The kinetic energy of an electromagnetic radiation is related to wavelength according to the formula:

$$E(KeV) = \frac{12.4}{\lambda}$$

- Kinetic energy is related to frequency according to the formula:

$$E = h\upsilon$$

where h = Plank's constant(6.626×10^{-34} joules/second)

PARTICLE INTERACTIONS AND X-RAY PRODUCTION

- The physical characteristics of heavy particles such as protons, neutrons, alpha particles (2 neutrons + 2 protons), or deuterons (1 neutron + 1 proton) allow them to penetrate and deposit energy at short range.
- The heavy particles have a high linear energy transfer (LET).
- The energy deposit increases to a maximum and produces a more dense ionization near the end of its path. The dense ionization region is called a Bragg peak (Figure 3-5).
- The rate of energy loss by a charged particle is proportional to the square of the particle charge.
- Electrons are commonly used charged particles in radiation therapy. Electrons have a low mass and distribute energy in a finite range in an absorber. The electron's low mass allows it to have a low LET and therefore does not show the same distribution pattern as Bragg's peak.
- There are two types of electron interactions with matter. They are:
  1. Collision (elastic and inelastic)
  2. Radiative
- Collision interactions involve electrons interacting with orbiting electrons in matter and transferring momentum and energy.
- An elastic collision involves the incoming electron coming to rest, giving all of its energy to the particle encountered; an inelastic collision involves the incoming electron only giving a portion of its energy to the encountered particle.
- Excitation and ionization are examples of collision interactions.
- When a bit of energy is given to an orbiting electron, the electron may vibrate; when large amounts of energy are transferred, the energy state of the encountered electron changes.
- An encountered electron may be relocated to a higher shell level in the atom; this vacancy may be filled with another orbiting electron. Any energy loss may exit the atom in the form of a photon.
- Orbiting electrons have a resting energy and a binding energy.
- The binding energy of an inner shell electron is large; the binding energy of an outer shell electron is small.
- The potential energy difference between where the relocated orbiting electron used to be and where it ends will be the resulting energy of the exiting photon.

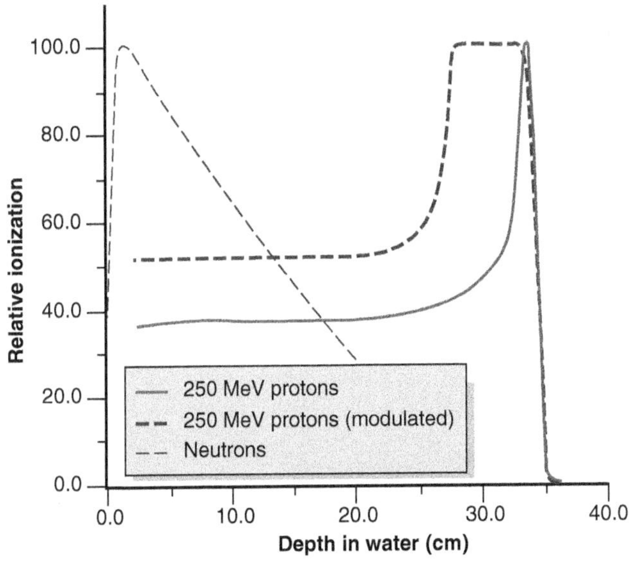

FIGURE 3-5 Examples of Bragg peaks.

- The exiting photon is in the form of characteristic x-rays (Figure 3-6).
- If the electron encountering the atom does not interact with an orbiting electron but is drawn to the positive charge in the nucleus, its velocity is slowed and its direction changes.
- The change in velocity causes a loss in the kinetic energy of the incoming electron; the energy loss exits the atom in the form of bremsstrahlung radiation (Figure 3-7).
- When x-rays are produced, both characteristic and bremsstrahlung radiation are emitted from the target atoms.
- X-ray production requires: a high voltage source, cathode, anode, glass envelope, and vacuum (Figure 3-8).

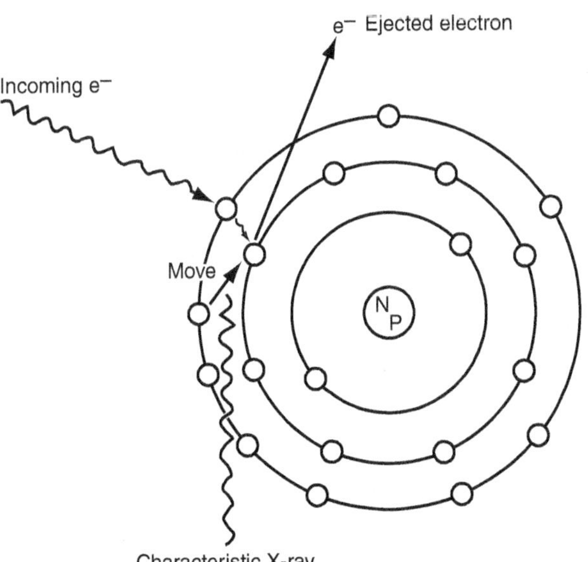

FIGURE 3-6 Characteristic x-ray production.

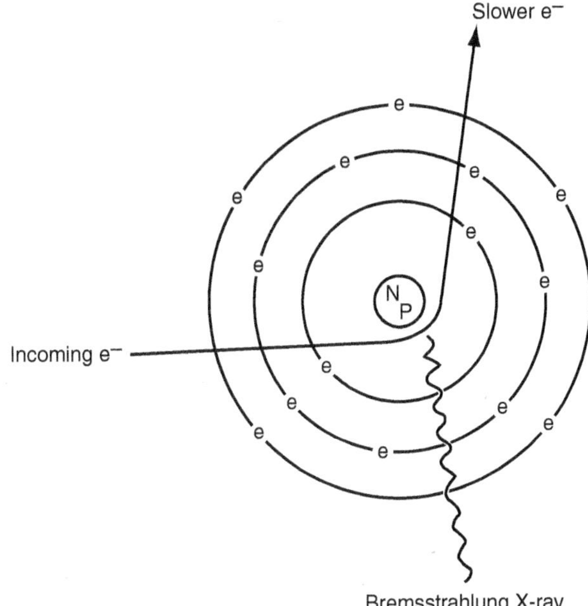

FIGURE 3-7 Bremsstrahlung x-ray production.

- The deceleration of electrons as they encounter the atoms of the target cause both x-ray and heat emission.
- In diagnostic tubes about 99% of the electron energy is converted to heat, while only 1% is converted to x-ray.
- During megavoltage x-ray production, a higher proportion of electron energy is converted to photons.
- The proportion is influenced by the atomic number of the target and maximum energy of the electrons in MeV.
- The following equation may be used to figure the converted energy to photons:

  $F = 3.5 \times 10^{-4}$ (Z) (E)
  F = fraction of the incident electron energy converted to photons
  Z = atomic number of the target
  E = maximum energy of electrons in MeV

PHOTON INTERACTIONS

- There are five major types of photon interactions with matter. They are:

  a. Photodisintegration
  b. Coherent scattering (Rayleigh scattering)
  c. Photoelectric effect
  d. Compton effect
  e. Pair production

- Photodisintegration occurs when high-energy photons interact with the nucleus; this leads to the emission of one or more nucleons or neutrons; energies greater than 10 MeV have the greatest probability.
- Coherent scattering occurs when the photon bundle passes near an orbiting electron and sets it into

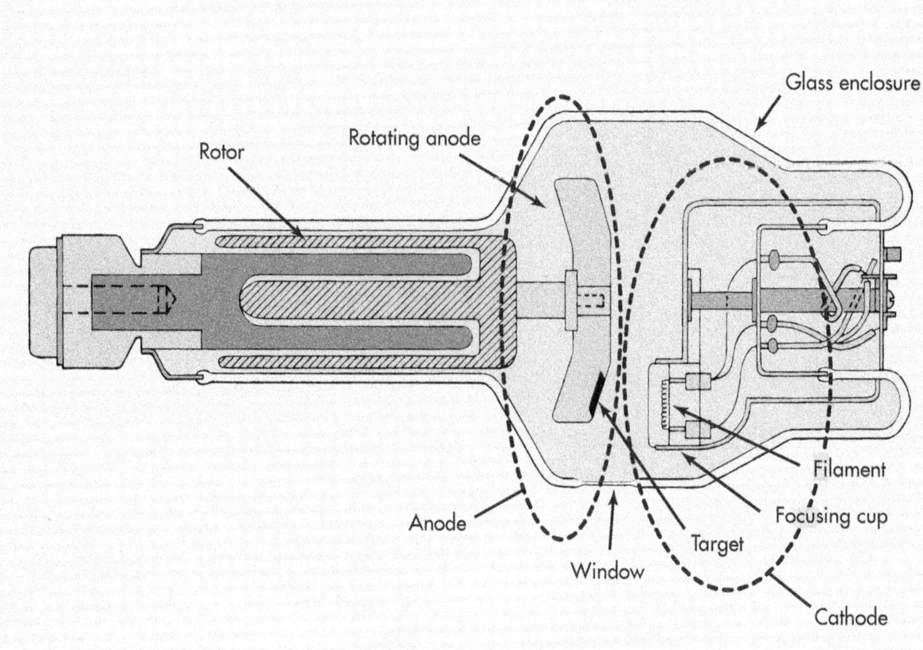

FIGURE 3-8 The basic x-ray tube.

motion; no energy is absorbed by the atom, just redirected; this is probable in high atomic number materials and low energy beams less than 10 KeV.

- Photoelectric effect occurs when a photon ejects one of the orbiting electrons. The entire energy of the photon is first absorbed by the atom and then transferred to the atomic electron. This happens in the innermost shells. The ejected electron is called a photo-electron. When vacancy occurs, another electron drops in to fill the space and energy emitted is in the form of characteristic x-rays or Auger electrons. The higher the energy, the greater the probability of this type of interaction.
- Compton effect occurs when a photon interacts with an electron as though it were a free electron. This happens in the outer shells. The encountered electron receives some energy from the photon and is emitted at an angle from the atom. The photon, with reduced energy, is also scattered at an angle. There could be a direct hit where the electron will move out and forward and the photon will travel backward. The higher the energy, the smaller the probability of this type of interaction. The Compton effect is independent of atomic number of the material.
- Pair production occurs when the photon energy is greater than 1.02 MeV. The photon interacts with the electromagnetic field of the nucleus and gives up all its energy in the process of creating a pair of particles consisting of an electron and positron. The particles are emitted in the forward direction; probability of this type of interaction increases with atomic number.

RADIATION INTENSITY AND BEAM QUALITY

- *Intensity* is defined as the amount of energy present per unit of time per unit of area perpendicular to the beam direction.
- Beam quality refers to the energy of the beam expressed in electron volts, or the absorbing potential or penetrating power of the beam expressed in half value layers (HVL) of material.
- Intensity of the beam is reduced by two effects: beam divergence and attenuation.
- Beam divergence is an expression of the scattering of photons away from the original point source.
- An area at a certain distance from the source (distance 1) would have an amount of photons passing through it (intensity 1). At a greater distance (distance 2), the same amount of photons would be scattered apart further and result in a less intense beam (intensity 2) (Figure 3-9).
- The ***inverse square law*** governs the principle of divergence and demonstrates that the intensity of the beam is inversely proportional to the square of the distance from the original point source:

$$I_1(D_1)^2 = I_2(D_2)^2$$

- Beam ***attenuation*** is the removal of energy from the beam.
- When a photon or particulate beam passes through matter, some energy is removed from the beam as a result of

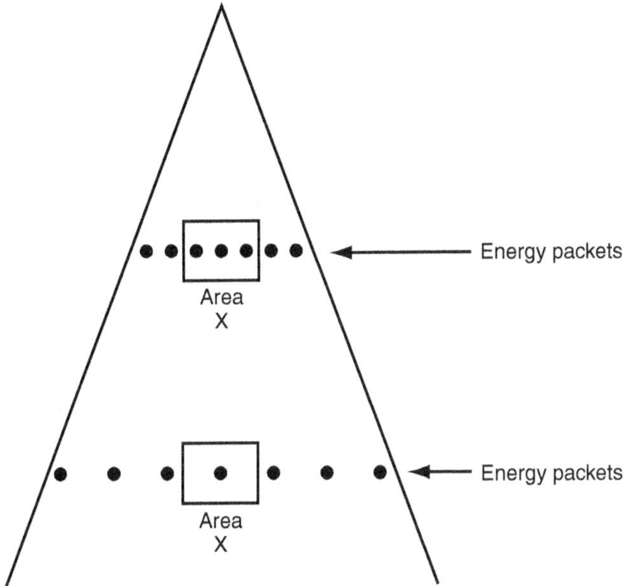

FIGURE 3-9 Illustration of beam divergence.

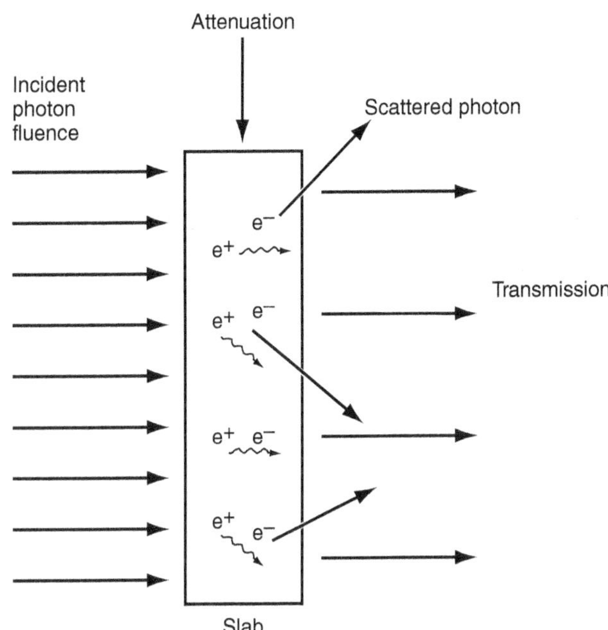

FIGURE 3-10 Photon fluence, attenuation, and transmission illustration.

absorption and scattering; the energy that is removed or absorbed by the material is said to be attenuated.

- The number of photons passing perpendicular through an area of 1 m square may be referred to as photon fluence.
- The energy passing perpendicularly through an area of 1 square meter would be called energy fluence.
- Some photons or particles are unaffected by the attenuator and pass through; the photons or particles passing through are referred to as ***transmission.***

$$\text{Transmission} = \frac{I}{I_0}$$

Io = original intensity
I = final intensity

- Some photons are totally absorbed; some may be partially absorbed and exit the material with reduced energy and changed direction.
- Photons that are totally or partially absorbed in tissue contribute to the absorbed dose. Figure 3-10 illustrates attenuation, fluence, and transmission.
- Refer to Figure 3-10 and consider the following:

If N_0 is the number of photons incident on a slab of material (photon fluence) and it encounters a thickness of material (t) to absorb some energy, the following mathematical equation could help us solve for the number of photons transmitted.

$$N = N_0 e^{-\mu t}$$

μ = linear attenuation coefficient

- The energy attenuated or transmitted is influenced by the incident beam energy and the type of material it passes through.
- The amount of material that would reduce the incident photon fluence to half its original value would be called its half value thickness (HVT) or HVL.
- The HVT and linear attenuation coefficient are related by the formula:

$$\mu = \frac{\ln 2}{\text{HVT}}$$

μ = linear attenuation coefficient

- As the material thickness increases, the intensity of the attenuated beam decreases.
- If we use a photon source with only one energy, the attenuation of the beam follows the relationship:

$$I = Ioe^{(-\mu t)}$$

- The meaning of the equation is that each millimeter of thickness added to an absorber reduces the beam intensity by a constant percent.
- In low energy x-ray tubes, filters may be used as absorbers to harden the beam.
- Beam hardening refers to the phenomenon where the effective energy of the beam increases as it passes through the filter: the filter absorbs the low energy rays and allows the higher energy rays to be transmitted. Since the hardened beam has more high energy rays, then the amount of material needed to decrease the original intensity by subsequent increments of 50% actually decreases due to beam hardening.
- 2 HVLs is not exactly HVL(2), due to beam hardening.
- HVT or HVL can be used to express the beam quality in lower energy beams.

- HVL is also used in the design of beam shielding blocks; the acceptable transmission of shielding blocks is approximately 3% or 5 HVLs of material.
- HVL is not used to specify beam energy for high energy photon or electron beams. Rather, an equivalent energy is used to characterize high energy beams used in radiation therapy.
- In radiation therapy, the beam energy is expressed in eV (KeV for imaging and MeV for therapy).
- The energy specified refers to the maximum energy in the spectrum of energies exiting.

RADIOACTIVITY AND NUCLEAR TRANSFORMATION

- Atoms represented by the formula $_{Z}X^{A}$ are called nuclides. When elementary particles of the stable atom are manipulated, they become unstable elements grouped by radionuclide families of isotopes, isotones, isobars, or isomers (Table 3-2).
- Radioactivity was discovered by Henri Becquerel in 1896 while exploring the naturally irradiative element, uranium.
- At around the same time, similar irradiative characteristics were found in radium by Marie and Pierre Curie.
- Radioactive decay, or disintegration, is a phenomenon in which radiation is emitted by the nucleus in the form of particles or electromagnetic radiation as an unstable element attempts to become stable again.
- On the periodic table of elements, the elements with atomic numbers higher than 82 tend to be unstable and are at some point attempting to become stable; as they are emitting particles or electromagnetic radiation, we refer to them as radioactive.
- Disintegrations are a statistical phenomenon and occur exponentially; 1 disintegration per second = 1 dps.

TABLE 3-2 Radionuclide Families

Isotopes	Same number of protons but different number of neutrons
Isotones	Same number of neutrons but different number of protons
Isobars	Same number of nucleons but different number of protons
Isomers	Same number of protons and neutrons except in a different nuclear state

- The mathematics of radioactive decay is based on the fact that the number of atoms disintegrating per unit of time is proportional to the number of radioactive atoms present. There is constant proportionality known as the decay constant.
- The symbol for the decay constant is λ and may be found by the equation:

$$\lambda = \frac{\ln 2}{T½} \text{ or } \frac{0.693}{T½}$$

- T ½ is the half-life; this is the time required for the number of radioactive atoms to decay to half the initial value.
- T_a is the mean or average life; this is the average lifetime for the decay of radioactive atoms.

$$T_a = 1.44(T½) \text{ or } \frac{T½}{0.693}$$

- In theory, the time it takes for all atoms to decay is infinite.
- Activity refers to the rate of decay or the strength of radioactive material. The traditional unit for activity is the Curie (Ci). The international unit is the Becquerel (Bq).
- Important equations to remember related to nuclear transformations are:

$N = No\ e^{-\lambda t}$ N = number of atoms No = initial number of atoms

$A = Ao\ e^{-\lambda t}$ A = activity Ao = initial activity

$1\ \text{dps} = 2.7 \times 10^{-11}$ Ci = 1Bq

$1\ \text{Ci} = 3.7 \times 10^{10}$ dps

- Radioactive nuclides undergo successive transformations in which the original nuclide—known as the parent (X)—give rise to a radioactive product nuclide known as the daughter (Y).
- Naturally occurring radioactive materials are grouped into three decay series: uranium series, actinium series, and thorium series.
- If the half-life of the parent (X) is longer than that of the daughter (Y), then after a certain time, a condition of equilibrium occurs where the activity of the parent and daughter become constant.
- Nuclear transformations manifest as:

  a. Alpha decay
  b. Beta decay (negative and positive)
  c. Electron capture
  d. Internal conversion

- Alpha decay occurs with very high atomic number nuclides where two protons and two neutrons are emitted; an example would be in the decay of radium-226.

- Beta negative decay occurs when there is an excessive number of neutrons or high neutron to proton ratio; the element tends to emit negative electrons; the decay of phosphorus-32 is an example.
- Beta positive decay occurs when there is a deficit of neutrons and is usually accompanied by the emission of gamma rays; sodium-22 decay is an example.
- Electron capture occurs when one of the orbital electrons is captured by the nucleus, transforming a proton into a neutron or neutrino. The neutrino would be ejected from the nucleus and carry away excess energy. The captured electron leaves an empty space in an electron shell, which in turn will be filled by another orbiting electron causing a release of energy known as characteristic x-rays.
- The characteristic x-ray may kick an outer shell electron out of the atom as it is expelled; such an electron is referred to as an Auger electron.
- Internal conversion occurs with the emission of gamma rays from the nucleus. In most transformations, the daughter nucleus loses energy immediately in the form of gamma radiation. Orbiting electrons may bombard the nucleus and receive some energy from the nucleus. The energized electron may subsequently be ejected from the atom and travel away with an energy equal to the difference between the energy lost by the nucleus and the binding energy that held the electron.
- Other interactions include fission and fusion; these interactions are a result of producing radioactive materials.
- Fission is a result of bombarding certain high atomic number nuclides with heavy neutrons; the nucleus splits into nuclei of a lower atomic number.
- Fusion can be considered the reverse of fission; low mass nuclei are combined to produce one nucleus.

SUGGESTED READINGS

Bomford CK, Kunkle IH: *Walter and Miller's textbook of radiotherapy*, ed 6, London, 2003, Churchill Livingstone.

Bushong SC: *Radiologic science for technologists*, ed 9, St Louis, 2008, Mosby.

Kahn FM: *The physics of radiation therapy*, ed 4, Philadelphia, 2010, Lippincott Williams & Wilkins.

Podgorsak EB: *Radiation physics for medical physicists*, Berlin, 2006, Springer.

Stanton R, Stinson D: *Applied physics for radiation oncology*, ed 2, Madison, 2009, Medical Physics Publishing.

Washington CM, Leaver D: *Principles and practice of radiation therapy*, ed 3, St Louis, 2010, Mosby.

REVIEW EXERCISES

1. 1 mCi is equivalent to:

a. 3.7×10^{10} disintegrations/min
b. 2.22×10^{12} disintegrations/min
c. 3.7×10^{4} disintegrations/sec
d. 3.7×10^{-2} disintegrations/sec

2. The half-life of iridium 192 is 74 days. The decay constant is:

a. 3.7 days^{-1}
b. 37 days^{-1}
c. 106.6 days^{-1}
d. 0.0094 days^{-1}
e. 0.027 days^{-1}

3. What are the differences between the electron and proton?

4. Types of nuclear decay include all of the following except:

a. Alpha decay
b. Neutron decay
c. Beta decay
d. Internal conversion

5. During x-ray production, the resulting x-ray beam comes from electrons colliding with the target causing interactions such as:

a. Characteristic radiation
b. Bremstrahlung radiation
c. Auger electrons
d. All of the above

6. The positive side of the basic x-ray tube is known as the:

a. Anode
b. Cathode
c. Filament
d. Vacuum

7. A radioactive source has an initial activity of 60 mCi. Its half-life is 8 days. What is the remaining activity after 10 days?

a. 30 mCi
b. 40 mCi
c. 25 mCi
d. 20 mCi

8. The average life of the source above is:

a. 16 days
b. 0.086 days
c. 12.3 days
d. 11.5 days

9. The ratio of x-ray to heat during x-ray production is:

a. Constant at 99% heat and 1% x-ray
b. Constant at 90% heat and 10% x-ray
c. Variable depending on the maximum energy of electrons traversing the tube
d. Variable depending on the strength of the target

10. The radioactive decay of a radioisotope is characterized by its:

a. Secular equilibrium
b. Decay constant
c. Fraction decay rate
d. Transient equilibrium

11. An elastic collision is one in which:

a. The incoming electron gives all of its energy to the electron it encounters
b. The incoming electron shares its energy with the electron it encounters
c. The incoming electron is captured by the nucleus
d. The incoming electron takes the place of an ejected electron

12. The energy of an electromagnetic radiation is inversely proportional to its:

a. Frequency
b. Mass
c. Speed
d. Wavelength

13. If a 50 keV electron collides with an inner shell electron with a binding energy of 25 keV, the resulting photoelectron will have an energy of:

a. 25 keV
b. 75 keV
c. 100 keV
d. 150 keV

14. The energy of an electromagnetic radiation is directly proportional to its:

a. Frequency
b. Wavelength
c. Velocity
d. a and b

15. Complete the table:

Photon Interactions	Electron Interactions

16. The decay of cobalt-60 to stable lead is an example of _______ decay.

a. alpha
b. beta negative
c. beta positive
d. fusion

17. Regarding isotopes; isotopes of an element have the same number of ______________ but a different numbers of neutrons.

18. Complete the table:

	Mass (kilograms)	Rest Energy	Charge
Electrons			
Positrons			
Protons			
Neutrons			
Alpha particles			

19. Match the following:

Isotopes _______	A. Ir^{192} Ir^{192m}
Isobars _______	B. $_{27}Fe^{59}$ $_{27}Fe^{58}$
Isotones _______	C. $_{28}Ni^{60}$ $_{31}Ga^{60}$
Isomers _______	D. $_{11}Na^{22}$ $_{10}Ne^{21}$

20. A photon of 25 Å has a kinetic energy of _______KeV.

21. If the decay constant of a particular isotope is 45 sec^{-1}, the half-life is________.

22. If the half-life of cobalt-60 is 5.26 years, the average life is________.

23. If using a tungsten target, the fraction of 4 MeV electrons converted to photons is ____.

24. Which has the highest photon energy?

a. Radio waves
b. Ultraviolet light
c. Microwaves
d. Infrared

25. Circle the correct word(s).

The probability of a photoelectric interaction (increases/decreases) with increasing energy and (increases/decreases) with the atomic number of the medium.

26. The majority of the mass of the atom is derived from:

a. Protons and electrons in the nucleus
b. Protons and neutrons in the nucleus
c. Protons, neutrons, and electrons in the nucleus
d. Alpha, beta, and gamma radiation emitted

27. A neutral atom that loses an electron by ionization is called a:

a. Negative atom
b. Positive atom
c. Negative ion
d. Positive ion

28. After alpha decay, the daughter nuclide will have an atomic mass number _____ amu lower than the parent.

a. 1
b. 2
c. 4
d. 6

29. A certain atom has binding energies of 70 eV in the L shell and 10 eV in the M shell. During an M shell to L shell transition, the photon emitted will have an energy of:

a. 80 eV
b. 60 eV
c. 35 eV
d. 5 eV

30. What type of nuclear decay is realized when:

a. $_{88}Ra^{226}$ decays to $_{86}Rn^{222}$ _______
b. $_{11}Na^{22}$ decays to $_{10}Ne^{22}$ _______

31. An atom is neutral if the number of its electrons is equal to its:

a. Protons
b. Nucleons
c. Atomic weight
d. None of the above

32. What is the threshold energy for pair production:

a. 0.511 MeV
b. 1.53 MeV
c. 9.81 MeV
d. 1.02 MeV

33. Solve for λ in hours^{-1}
A = 5 mCi
Ao = 18 mCi
t = 50 hours

34. Solve for Ao
A = 10 mCi
T ½ = 8 hours
t = 22 hours

35. The System International unit for activity is the:

a. Becquerel
b. Curie
c. Hertz
d. Roentgen

36. To interact by photoelectric effect, the interacting photon must have energy:

a. Less than the binding energy of the orbiting electron
b. Equal to or greater than the binding energy of the orbiting electron
c. Of any level
d. Of at least 1 MeV

37. The photons produced during the orbital transitions of electrons from a higher to lower energy are called:

a. Characteristic radiation
b. Corpuscular radiation

c. Gamma radiation
d. Vacancy radiation

38. An electron with the lowest binding energy is most likely located in the:

a. K shell
b. L shell
c. M shell
d. All binding energies are the same

39. Two or more chemicals with the same chemical formula, but having different nuclear states are known as:

a. Isomers
b. Isotopes
c. Isobars
d. Isotones

40. Which is not true of the electromagnetic spectrum? They all have the same:

a. Velocity
b. Energy
c. Mass
d. Charge

41. Radon has a half-life of 3.83 days. Its average life is:

a. 3.83 days
b. 4.4 days
c. 5.5 days
d. 6.6 days

42. Carbon-14 and nitrogen-14 are:

a. Isotones
b. Isotopes
c. Isobars
d. Isomers

43. How many disintegrations per minute (dpm) are there in 1 Ci?

a. 3.7×10^{10} dpm
b. 29.7×10^{18} dpm
c. 3.14×10^{21} dpm
d. 2.2×10^{12} dpm

44. How many electrons are there in 1 g of tissue?

a. 3×10^{10}
b. 3×10^{23}
c. 6.02×10^{23}
d. None of the above

45. On January 1, we receive 80 mCi of an isotope with a half-life of 8 days. The activity remaining on January 25 would be:

a. 8 mCi
b. 10 mCi
c. 20 mCi
d. 40 mCi

46. The fraction of cobalt-60 atoms remaining after 10 years is approximately:

a. 1/3
b. 1/8
c. ½
d. ¼

47. The wavelengths of x-rays are measured in:

a. millimeters
b. centimeters
c. Roentgens
d. Angstroms

48. The relationship between mass and energy is given by Einstein's equation: $E = mc^2$
The C stands for:

a. Energy
b. Mass
c. Velocity of light
d. 3×10^8 cm/second

49. The photoelectric process is essentially an interaction between a photon and:

a. A free electron
b. The nucleus
c. A bound electron
d. All of the above

50. As the wavelength of light is decreased, its speed is:

a. Increased linearly
b. Decreased linearly
c. Unchanged
d. Increased exponentially

51. The frequency of radiation with a wavelength of 5×10^{-7} meters is:

a. 6×10^{14} Hz
b. 1.66×10^{15} Hz
c. 6×10^{-15} Hz
d. 1.66×10^{-15} Hz
e. 3×10^8 Hz

52. A radionuclide decays at the rate of 20% per hour. Its half-life is approximately:

a. 2 hours
b. 2.5 hours
c. 3 hours
d. 3.5 hours
e. 4 hours

53. Bragg peak is:

a. An ionization maximum near the end of the range of a heavy charged particle
b. A maximum in the curve of activity and time for a parent and daughter radionuclide in equilibrium
c. A maximum concentration of Compton interactions
d. The maximum activity of an isotope

54. Different isotopes of the same element will have equal numbers of ________.

a. Electrons
b. Protons and electrons
c. Neutrons
d. Electrons and neutrons
e. Protons and neutrons

55. A radioactive source has a half-life of 6 hours and an activity of 10 mCi at noon on Monday. The activity at noon on Tuesday will be ________ mCi.

a. 9.375
b. 6.25
c. 2.5
d. 0.625
e. 0.31

56. The half-life of a radionuclide is:

a. Influenced by temperature and pressure
b. Directly proportional to the decay constant
c. Less than the average life
d. Usually shorter for beta negative than beta positive emitters

57. In the formula $A = Ao\ e^{-\lambda t}$, λ is ________.

a. The number of atoms decaying per unit of time
b. The fraction of atoms decaying per unit of time
c. The fraction of atoms decaying in time
d. The linear attenuation coefficient

58. When a very long-lived radionuclide decays to a short-lived daughter, it is known as ____ equilibrium.

a. thermal
b. secular
c. transient
d. temporary

59. Which of the following is not a type of ionizing radiation?

a. 2 MHz ultrasound
b. Cobalt gamma rays
c. Strontium beta
d. 15 MV x-rays.

60. An electron, proton, and alpha particle each have 20 MeV kinetic energy. Which of the following is true?

a. The alpha particle travels at almost light speed
b. The alpha particle has the least total energy
c. The proton has the highest total energy
d. The electron travels at almost light speed

61. The mass of an electron is:

a. The same as a proton
b. Half that of a proton
c. The same as a neutron
d. Much smaller than that of a neutron

62. Ionization implies:

a. An excited state of the atom
b. The production of x-rays
c. The removal of an electron from the atom
d. A neutral state of the atom

63. A deuteron is the nucleus of an isotope of H^2. Which of the following is true?

a. It has a mass number of 2
b. It has an atomic number of 2
c. It has a positive charge of 2
d. It has an energy of 2 MeV

64. When a radionuclide decays, radiation is emitted from the:

a. Outer shell electrons
b. Inner shell electrons
c. The nucleus
d. All of the above

65. The probability that a photon interacts with a material is:

a. Dependent on its density
b. Proportional to the total attenuation coefficient

c. Inversely proportional to the number of protons in the atom
d. All of the above

66. The rate of energy loss by a charged particle is:

a. Proportional to the particle charge
b. Proportional to the square of the particle charge
c. Independent of charge
d. None of the above

67. Heavy particles lose most of their energy:

a. Immediately as they enter the medium
b. In the middle of their range
c. Near the end of their range
d. Equally throughout their range

68. Bragg peak is not observed in electrons because of their:

a. High speed
b. Negative charge
c. Small mass
d. Short half-life

69. Excitation produced by electron beams occurs in the:

a. Nucleus of the atom
b. Neutrons of the atom
c. Orbital electrons of the atom
d. Protons of the atom

70. In the production of bremsstrahlung, the electron:

a. Ejects a cloud of electrons
b. Slows down and loses some of its energy as an x-ray photon
c. Produces a heavy particle
d. Ejects an electron from the atom

Write the letter A for alpha particle, B for beta particle, P for proton, or N for neutron on the line with the appropriate description.

71. ____Has the largest mass

72. ____Has the highest LET

73. ____Particulate radiation that possesses no charge

74. ____Produced during natural radioactive decay

75. ____Can carry either a positive or negative charge

76. ____Helium nucleus

77. ____Hydrogen nucleus

78. ____The greatest internal hazard

79. ____Cannot ionize directly; interacts only with the nucleus

80. ____May be referred to as an electron or positron

Write the letter Q for quantity, H for quality, or B for both to show which is affected by altering the following in the x-ray tube.

81. ____Time of exposure

82. ____Tube current

83. ____Target material

84. ____Distance

85. ____Filtration

86. ____kVp

87. ____Generator type

88. The term x-ray refers to a part of the electromagnetic spectrum having an energy of :

a. More than 1 million electron volts
b. Less than 1 electron volt
c. Between 1 and 100 electron volts
d. Between 100 and 1 million electron volts

89. Which of the following types of radiation has a positive electrical charge?

a. Alpha
b. Beta
c. Delta
d. Gamma

90. Radiation can be described as energy:

a. In transit
b. Destroyed
c. Recovered
d. In the form of heat

91. I^{131} and I^{125} have different:

a. Chemical properties
b. Z values
c. Numbers of protons
d. Numbers of neutrons
e. K shell binding energies

92. If the distance from a radiation source is decreased by half, the intensity is:

a. Increased by half
b. Increased by four times
c. Decreased by half
d. Decreased by a quarter

93. 10^6 photons from a source are incident on a 1.5 cm thick lead plate. The HVL of the beam in lead is 1.1 cm. The number of photons transmitted through the lead plate would be:

94. 10^8 photons from a source are incident on a water tank 0.2 meters thick. The linear attenuation coefficient of this beam in water is 11.55 m^{-1}. The number of photons transmitted through this 0.2 meters of water would be:

95. What is the HVL of the source encountering the water in the previous problem?

CHAPTER

4

Radiation Biology

Leia Levy and Elva Marie Dawson

FOCUS QUESTIONS

- What physical factors affect tissue response to radiation?
- What biologic factors affect tissue response to radiation?
- What aspects of tissue response are demonstrated with the dose-response curve?
- What aspects of tissue response are demonstrated with the cell-survival curve?
- What are the principles of target theory?
- What aspects of radiation biology may be applied to radiation safety practices?
- What are the primary acute and late whole body radiation responses?
- What are the differences between somatic and genetic effects?
- In what ways may we manipulate tissue response to radiation?
- What are the tolerance doses of certain tissues to fractionated radiation?

RADIATION BIOLOGY OVERVIEW

- Radiation exposure to living tissue may cause direct or indirect effects.
- Direct effects would be consequences of events directly causing the disabling of cellular function.
- Indirect effects would be consequences of a series of events ultimately leading to the disabling of cellular function.
- The response of living tissue to radiation exposure can be examined on various levels: atomic, molecular, cellular, and systemic.
- Responses may be observed within a short time frame (acute) or after a long time period following exposure (latent).
- Specific tissue responses are influenced by multiple factors such as:
  1. Total dose
  2. Radiation type
  3. Cellular sensitivity to radiation
  4. Volume of tissue irradiated
  5. Protraction (period of time over which total dose is absorbed)
  6. Fractionation (fraction of total dose given per unit of time)

ATOMIC AND MOLECULAR RESPONSE

- Excitation or ionization in the atoms of living tissue are a response to exposure of tissue to ionizing radiation.
- Excitation or ionization events may lead to subtle responses in tissues such as a small increase in temperature at the site or more overtly, in the breaking of chemical bonds.
- The energy of radiation used for imaging and radiation therapy likely leads to ionizing events.
- It is difficult to say whether the ionizing events are the consequence of direct or indirect effects; most likely they are a consequence of indirect effects.
- The atoms in living tissue come together to form molecules.
- A major molecule in the body is water (H_2O).
- Since the body is about 80% water, it is rational to believe that the encounters between water molecules and radiation are what lead to manifested responses in living tissue to radiation.
- The irradiation of water causes the breaking of the chemical bond between the hydrogen and oxygen atoms, leading to the production of *free radicals.*

- A free radical is an uncharged molecule that contains a single unpaired electron in its outer shell, making it unstable and carrying excess energy.
- The result is the development of an ion pair H^+ and OH^- and two free radicals H^+ and OH (Figure 4-1).
- Free radicals have a short life span but can interact with neighboring cells.
- OH, the hydroxyl free radical, and hydrogen peroxide (H_2O_2) cause the majority of all radiation damage.
- The effects of radiation exposure may also be demonstrated in encounters with other molecules such as proteins, lipids, carbohydrates, and nucleic acids.
- The largest organic molecules are nucleic acids: DNA and RNA.
- DNA and RNA are responsible for cellular structure and function; they provide the map for developing cells.
- One guaranteed means for cell death is to interrupt transcription and prevent the synthesis of DNA in the parent cell.
- DNA is the primary target for the greatest damage to the cell; a direct encounter with this molecule would be known as a direct effect.
- DNA is a small molecule and is located in the small cell nucleus and difficult to target during radiation therapy.
- The effect on DNA following irradiation can lead to a variety of consequences involving the nitrogenous bases or chromosomes (Figure 4-2).
- Some consequences of DNA damage may be repaired, leaving the cells to recover and resume normal function; this type of damage is known as sublethal damage.

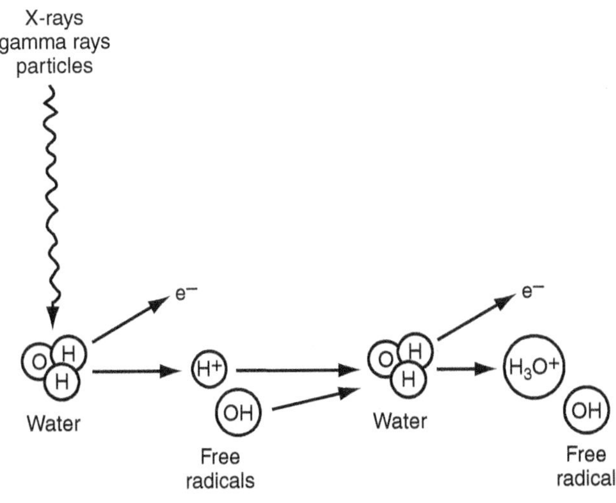

FIGURE 4-1 Breaking of water molecules to form free radicals.

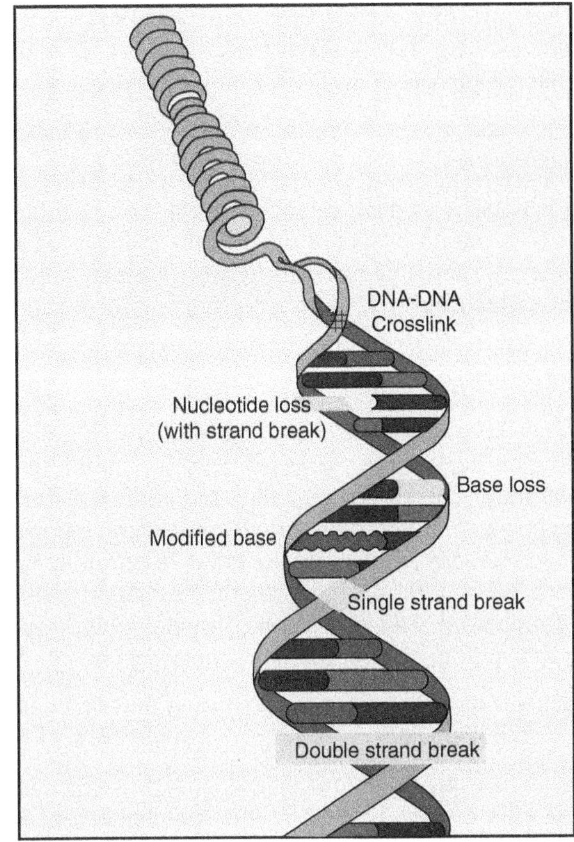

FIGURE 4-2 DNA strand showing nitrogenous bases following radiation damage.

- Other consequences of DNA damage may be permanent and may ultimately lead to cell death.
- Favorable effects of radiation therapy depend mostly on random encounters with other parts of the cell and not the nucleus, where DNA is located.
- Radiation interactions may lead to damage of the cell membrane and/or organelles in the cytoplasm.

CELLULAR RESPONSE

- The functional integrity of tissues depends on the organization and the parenchymal and stromal cells within it.
- Cells differ in their sensitivity to radiation.
- The *law of Bergonie and Tribondeau* states that cells that are rapidly dividing, have a long mitotic future, and are undifferentiated are the most responsive to radiation.
- The living cell periodically progresses through cell division so that new cells may take the place of old worn out or damaged cells.
- Cell division in germ cells is termed *meiosis,* whereas cell division in other types of cells is known as *mitosis*.

- There are four phases of division in nongerm cells: mitosis, Gap 1, DNA synthesis, and Gap 2; a fifth phase, known as Gap 0, indicates a period of rest.
- The phase most sensitive to radiation is the M phase; the most resistant is the S phase (Figure 4-3).
- It is possible to measure the percentage or fraction of cells in certain phases of the dividing cycle at a given time, and the time intervals between cellular mitosis, in research settings.
- The proportion of cells in mitosis is called the mitotic index.
- Being knowledgeable about the patterns of cellular division for certain types of cells is helpful when planning chemotherapy and radiation treatment regimens. This information influences whether chemotherapy is given in one bolus injection or with continuous infusion, and whether radiation will be administered using traditional fractionation, hyperfractionation, or hypofractionation schemes.
- Generation time, or interval between mitotic phases, for cell populations typically ranges from 8 to 30 hours.
- All cells do not have the same dividing frequency; some divide until maturation and others continue dividing for the entire life of the host.

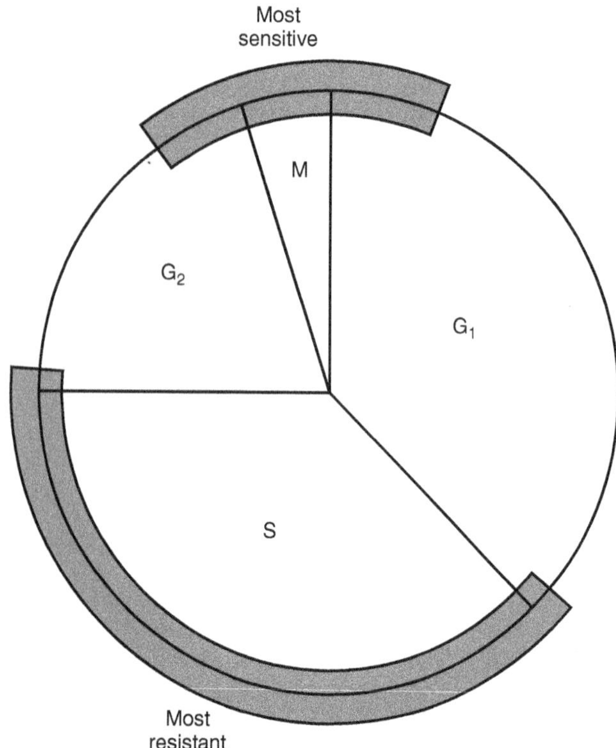

FIGURE 4-3 Phases of division showing the most sensitive and resistant phases in shaded areas.

- All cells are not in the same phase of division at the same time; therefore some cells in a population are more vulnerable to the potential damaging effects of radiation exposure than others during a single dose of radiation.
- Radiation may cause interphase death, delay in division, or reproductive failure, eventually causing the mitotic index to decline.
- The rate of decline becomes faster as radiation dose is increased and then reaches a saturation value.
- The decline eventually leads to cessation of increased cell number.
- A delay in reentering the mitotic phase increases as radiation doses accumulate; prolonged division delay will eventually lead to cell death.
- The *cell survival curve* describes the relationship between the radiation dose and the proportion of cells surviving.
- The relationship is logarithmic and therefore curves should be plotted on logarithmic graphs, with the dose along the *x*-axis and surviving fraction on the *y*-axis.
- The cell survival curve may introduce a third variable and show how the declining mitotic index and surviving fraction differs when:
  1. Radiation type varies
  2. Cell type varies
  3. Cell vasculature and oxygenation varies
  4. Phase of cellular division at time of exposure varies
- Two models have been widely used to plot cell survival and they are: single-hit, single-target theory and single-hit, multiple target theory.
- Primitive cells such as bacteria and viruses could be plotted on a single-target, single-hit model survival curve; there is likely no shoulder region and one hit would likely hit a critical part of the cell.
- Mammalian cells are plotted on a single-hit, multiple-target curve; these complex cells have many critical portions such as DNA, chromosomes, cytoplasm and its contents, water molecules, proteins, and gate-keeping membranes.
- Although radiation therapy is not usually administered using single doses (single-hit), we can extrapolate the consequence of exposed cells having multiple targets to a single dose forward to standard fractionation.
- When standard fractionated radiation is administered, target hits are random; if hits are uniform, a more rapid cell death could be observed.

- Important values to note when reviewing a cell survival curve (Figure 4-4) include:

  1. Dq = quasi-threshold dose; dose required to initiate a steady decline in the mitotic index; dose causing sublethal damage
  2. D_{37} = the dose required to leave 37% of cells surviving in the straight-line portion of the curve; single-hit, single-target theory
  3. Do = the dose range for death of 63% of cells in the straight line portion; most reliable value for determining cell sensitivity; multiple-target, single-hit theory
  4. N = extrapolation number; relative target number in the cells irradiated and a measure of the shoulder

- Using radiation with higher linear energy transfer (LET), and exposing cells that are rapidly dividing and well oxygenated during or near the M phase show a rapidly decreasing surviving fraction of cells as the dose accumulates.
- LET describes the average energy deposited per unit of path length to a medium by ionizing radiation as it passes through that medium.
- Particulate radiations have a high LET because of their charge and heavy mass; energy is deposited more densely and the biologic effect on both normal and cancerous tissue is greater.

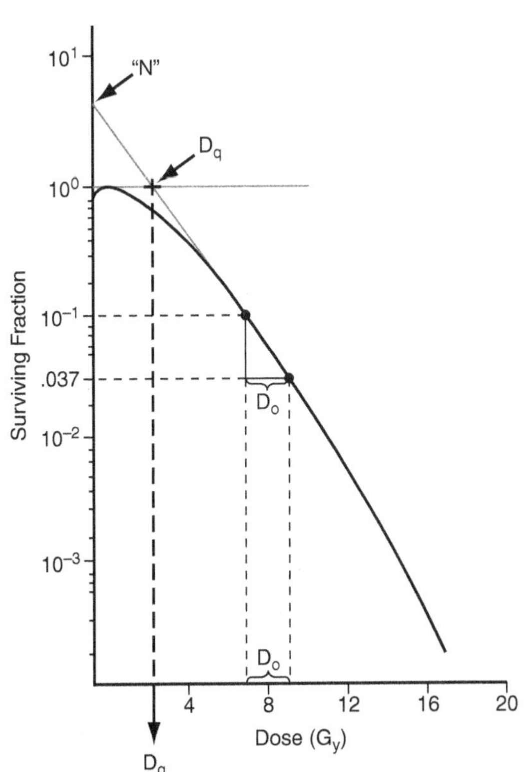

FIGURE 4-4 Cell survival curve with important values marked.

- Relative biologic effectiveness (RBE) provides a relative comparison of the effectiveness of a test radiation to the dose of 250 KV x-ray. It relates the ability of radiation with different LETs delivered under the same conditions to produce the same biologic effect.

$$\text{RBE} = \frac{\text{250 KV dose for a given effect}}{\text{Dose fo test radiation for same effect}}$$

- Equal doses of different LET radiations do not produce the same biologic effect.
- The oxygen enhancement ratio (OER) is a comparison of the doses required to reduce survival to a certain level in hypoxic and oxygenated conditions; hypoxic cells are radioresistant.

$$\text{OER} = \frac{\text{hypoxic dose needed to produce a biologic effect}}{\text{Oxygenated dose needed to produce a biologic effect}}$$

- As a tumor grows, a substantial portion of the tumor becomes hypoxic; this makes it critical to detect and begin treatment to tumors as soon as possible following a definitive diagnosis.
- Tumors that have good access to vasculature and are well oxygenated respond to radiation more readily than a poorly oxygenated cell population.
- The response of oxygenated cells to radiation exposure is most pronounced when sparsely ionizing radiation, such as x-ray, gamma, and electrons, are applied.

TISSUE RESPONSE

- There are several tissue types in the body.
- Epithelial, connective, muscle, nerve, and membranes are main tissue categories.
- As cells make up tissues, the sensitivity of certain cell types translate to the sensitivity of tissues the cells comprise.
- Changes in tissues following radiation are similar to changes we see following heat and cold exposure, infections, or traumatic injury.

Cardinal Signs of Injury
Redness
Swelling
Heat
Pain

- Changes may be seen immediately, within days or weeks (acute), or later as in months or years (latent).
- Changes seen within days or weeks may also be called deterministic or ***nonstochastic*** effects.
- Changes seen after months or years of exposure may be called ***stochastic*** effects.

- Immediate effects are rarely seen in therapeutic radiation but may be seen in nuclear accidents where total doses and exposure rates are extremely high.
- The response of tissues following significant doses of radiation may appear as vascular dilation, cellular inflammation, and at high doses, tissue necrosis.
- The four progressive stages of tissue response are easily observed in the skin of the irradiated patient where the absorbed dose to the skin exceeds 50 Gy.

Four Progressive Stages of Skin Response (standard fractionation)

1. Epilation
2. Erythema
3. Dry desquamation
4. Wet desquamation

- Beyond total doses fractionated doses of 50 Gy to the skin, tissue necrosis may occur; necrotic cells may shed and the area can repair and become repopulated
- Acute effects vary depending on the tissue irradiated and the fractionation and protraction (Table 4-1).
- Damage or radiation injury to tissues may be permanent and is greatly influenced by the total dose, fractionation, and protraction.
- During therapeutic radiation, doses high enough to cause tissue necrosis are avoided.
- When prescribing therapeutic doses of radiation necessary to kill malignant tumor cells, radiation injury to normal tissues in the area must be considered.
- Tolerance of normal mammalian tissues is expressed using *TD 5/5* or *TD 50/5* values.
- Tolerance doses (TD) are documented and referenced according to the sensitivity of tissue exposed, the volume of tissue exposed, and widely used fractionation schedules (i.e., 200 cGy per fraction, 5 fractions per week).
- TD 5/5 would be the dose that would likely cause 5% of an exposed population to realize an adverse late effect in 5 years following exposure (Table 4-2).
- TD 50/5 would be the dose that would likely cause 50% of an exposed population to realize an adverse late effect in 5 years following exposure.
- Any deviation from the standard fractionation scheme results in a different biologic response in both normal and cancerous tissue.
- Ellis developed an equation, known as the nominal standard dose (NSD) formula, in 1968. The formula was an attempt to design treatment schedules that resulted in optimal tumor response with acceptable normal tissue damage. This equation could also be used as a reference if the treatment schedule was interrupted.

  Ellis' formula: $D = NSD \times T^{0.11} \times N^{0.24}$
  D = total dose, T = elapsed time (protraction)
  N = number of fractions, NSD = 1800 rets

- Disadvantages to using Ellis' equation was that connective tissue was the reference tissue, so there was no accounting for more sensitive or more resistant tissues; neither was there a consideration for a variation in volume of tissue irradiated.
- Today, a similar equation may be used when standard fractionation is interrupted or varied. The modern formula is known as the biologic effective dose (BED) formula.

  BED = (nd) relative effectiveness
  nd = total dose
  Relative effectiveness $= 1 + d/\alpha$
  α = reference dose for early effects; accepted as 10 Gy
  **should substitute β for α for late effect; β = reference dose of 3 Gy

TABLE 4-1 Doses for Onset of Acute Effects (10 Gy/wk at 5 fractions/wk)

Tissue	Acute Effect	Onset Dose (Gy)
Skin	Erythema	20
	Dry desquamation	30
	Wet desquamation	40
Oral mucosa	Mild, patchy mucositis	30
	Confluent mucositis	40
Esophagus	Esophagitis	25
Salivary glands	Xerostomia	20
Rectum	Proctitis	30
Testis	Decreased sperm	0.25
Bone marrow	Lowered blood counts	4
	Extensive hypoplasia	50
Stomach	Gastritis	20

TABLE 4-2 Radiation Tolerance Doses—TD 5/5 (10 Gy/wk at 5 fractions/wk)

Tissue	Injury	TD 5/5 (Gy) Whole Organ
Skin	Ulceration/fibrosis	55
Intestine	Stricture	45
Salivary glands	Permanent xerostomia	40
Kidneys	Failure	23
Testis, ovary	Sterility	5-15
Bone	Arrested growth in child	20
	Necrosis in adult	60
Bone marrow	Reduced cellularity	20
Spinal cord	Necrosis	45
Lens	Cataract	5
Brain	Necrosis	50

From Emami B, Lyman J, Brown A. Tolerance of normal tissue to therapeutic irradiation. *Int J Radiat Oncol Biol Phys* 1991;21:109-122.

- Isoeffect lines show the relationship between total dose and overall treatment time for a specific tissue response, such as early skin reactions and other acute effects, or late tissue responses, such as necrosis or the development of secondary cancers.
- *Dose response curves* give another visual representation of tissue response to radiation exposure.
- Dose response curves may be linear or nonlinear, have a threshold, or no threshold.
- Dose response curves showing *deterministic,* or early effects typically have no threshold and are linear; the two variables on this type of curve would be dose and severity of the effect.
- Dose response curves showing *stochastic,* or late effects, typically have a threshold and may be linear or nonlinear depending on the endpoint; the two variables on this type of curve would be the dose and the probability of the late effect (Figure 4-5).
- Stochastic effects may be seen in the individual exposed or in the offspring.
- During radiation therapy, clinicians should monitor the acute or early effects of radiation.
- Monitoring of acute effects is easily performed by using an accepted toxicity scoring system (Table 4-3).

WHOLE BODY SYSTEM RESPONSE

- Whole body effects have only been able to be studied in small populations of people such as victims of nuclear accidents.
- Response to whole body radiation may progress through three phases: prodromal, manifest syndromes, and latent.
- A one-time dose of 300 to 500 cGy could lead to death within 30 to 60 days without medical intervention-LD 50/30 or LD 50/60.
- The likelihood of progressing through and the total time to progress through phases is influenced by total dose and dose rate.
- Prodromal symptoms include nausea, vomiting fatigue, fever, hypotension, and diarrhea.
- Prodromal symptoms exhibited and time frame is influenced by total dose and dose rate.
- Manifest syndromes are hematopoietic, gastrointestinal, and cerebrovascular (Table 4-4).
- Early effects to the unborn embryo or fetus may include spontaneous abortion or death in utero; doses as low as 0.05 Gy could be lethal to the embryo in the first trimester.

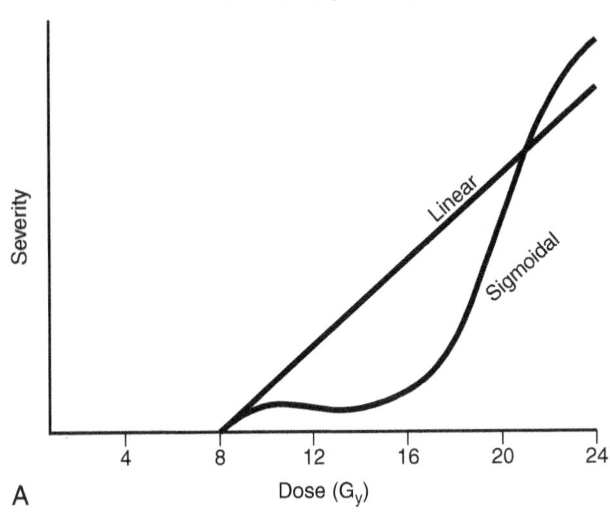

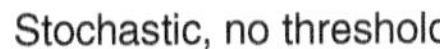

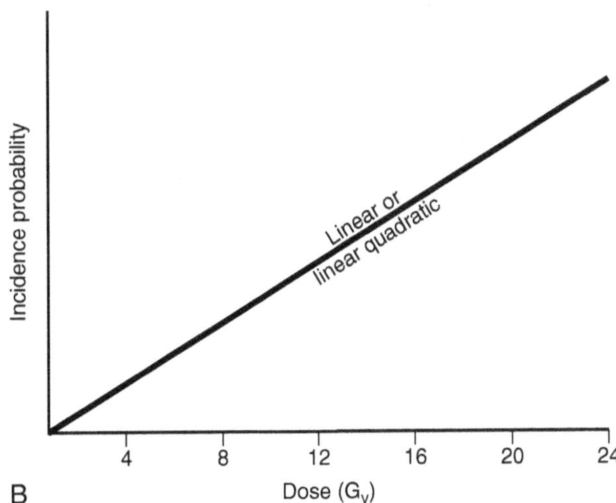

FIGURE 4-5 Dose response curves. **A,** Deterministic; **B,** stochastic.

- As cells mature during the second and third trimesters, lethal radiation doses to the unborn increase.
- Following birth, damage to the central nervous system and/or permanent damage to undeveloped germ cells may also be realized.
- Late *somatic,* or effects to the individual, may include radiation induced cancers, cataract formation, chronic bone marrow depression, shortened life span, and mutations in germ cells.
- Latent genetic effects may be seen in the offspring of whole body exposure victims.
- Both somatic and genetic, early and late effects of whole body radiation response must be considered when using whole body radiation therapeutically.
- Both somatic and genetic, early and late effects of whole body radiation response are considered when establishing annual dose limits for occupational radiation workers and the general public.

TABLE 4-3 Acute Radiation Morbidity Scoring Criteria

	0	1	2	3	4
Skin	No change over baseline	Follicular, faint, or dull erythema; epilation; dry desquamation; decreased sweating	Tender or bright erythema, patchy moist desquamation; moderate edema	Confluent, moist desquamation other than skin folds, pitting edema	Ulceration, hemorrhage, necrosis
Mucous Membrane	No change over baseline	Injection; may experience mild pain not requiring analgesic	Patchy mucositis that may produce an inflammatory serosanguinitis discharge; may experience moderate pain requiring analgesia	Confluent fibrinous mucositis; may include severe pain requiring narcotic	Ulceration, hemorrhage, or necrosis
Pharynx and Esophagus	No change over baseline	Mild dysphagia or odynophagia; may require topical anesthetic or nonnarcotic analgesics; may require soft diet	Moderate dysphagia or odynophagia; may require narcotic analgesics; may require puree or liquid diet	Severe dysphagia or odynophagia with dehydration or weight loss (>15% from pretreatment baseline) requiring N-G feeding tube, IV fluids, or hyperalimentation	Complete obstruction, ulceration, perforation, fistula
Upper G.I.	No change	Anorexia with $\leq$ 5% weight loss from pretreatment baseline; nausea not requiring antiemetics; abdominal discomfort not requiring parasympatholytic drugs or analgesics	Anorexia with $\leq$15% weight loss from pretreatment baseline; nausea and/or vomiting requiring antiemetics; abdominal pain requiring analgesics	Anorexia with >15% weight loss from pretreatment baseline or requiring N-G tube or parenteral support. Nausea and/or vomiting requiring tube or parenteral support; abdominal pain, severe despite medication; hematemesis or melena; abdominal distention (flat plate radiograph demonstrates distended bowel loops)	Ileus, subacute or acute obstruction, perforation, GI bleeding requiring transfusion/ abdominal pain requiring tube decompression or bowel diversion
Lower G.I. Including Pelvis	No change	Increased frequency or change in quality of bowel habits not requiring medication; rectal discomfort not requiring analgesics	Diarrhea requiring parasympatholytic drugs (e.g., Lomotil); mucous discharge not necessitating sanitary pads; rectal or abdominal pain requiring analgesics	Diarrhea requiring parenteral support; severe mucous or blood discharge necessitating sanitary pads; abdominal distention (flat plate radiograph demonstrates distended bowel loops)	Acute or subacute obstruction, fistula, or perforation; GI bleeding requiring transfusion; abdominal pain or tenesmus requiring tube decompression or bowel diversion
Lung	No change	Mild symptoms of dry cough or dyspnea on exertion	Persistent cough requiring narcotic, antitussive agents; dyspnea with minimal effort but not at rest	Severe cough unresponsive to narcotic antitussive agent or dyspnea at rest; clinical or radiologic evidence of acute pneumonitis/ intermittent oxygen or steroids may be required	Severe respiratory insufficiency; continuous oxygen or assisted ventilation

TABLE 4-3 Acute Radiation Morbidity Scoring Criteria—Cont'd

	0	1	2	3	4
CNS	No change	Fully functional status (i.e., able to work) with minor neurologic findings, no medication needed	Neurologic findings present sufficient to require home care; nursing assistance may be required; medications including steroids; antiseizure agents may be required	Neurologic findings requiring hospitalization for initial management	Serious neurologic impairment, which includes paralysis, coma, or seizures >3/wk despite medication; hospitalization required

From Radiation Therapy Oncology Group, at http://www.rtog.org/members/toxicity/acute.html. Accessed December 30, 2009.

TABLE 4-4 Whole Body Radiation Syndromes

Syndrome	Dose Range	Time Until Death Without Rescue
Hematopoietic	300-800 cGy	10-15 days
Gastrointestinal	1000-5000 cGy	3-10 days
Cerebrovascular	>5000 cGy	Hours-3 days

FOUR Rs OF RADIOBIOLOGY AND TIME/DOSE CONSIDERATIONS

- The rationale for planning radiation therapy regimens are explained by the 4 Rs of radiobiology.
- *Repair* is the first principle and refers to the repair mechanism built into all cells both normal and abnormal. Rest periods in standard fractionation schemes allow the normal cells to repair from sublethal radiation injury. Because tumor cells also have some capacity for repair, prolonged breaks in treatment are discouraged.
- *Reoxygenation* is the second principle and refers to the ability of both normal and tumor cell populations to revascularize as cells die in an attempt to continue thriving. This phenomenon is both a help and a hindrance. The presence of oxygen increases cellular sensitivity to radiation through greater potential of free radical formation. Revascularization improves the viability of the abnormal growth; increased vascular supply is good for the recovery of normal tissues in the area.
- *Repopulation* is the third principle and refers to the trigger of surviving cells in a tumor to divide faster in an attempt to live. This phenomenon is justification for repeated radiation injury events as provided by fractionated doses. Hyperfractionation and hypofractionation schemes are designed with this phenomenon in mind, with the specific growth and dividing pattern of the cells being irradiated.
- *Redistribution or reassortment,* the fourth principle, is the ability for the cell population to return to a more even distribution of younger, dividing cells following decreased surviving fraction. This phenomenon also justifies repeated dosing as in standard fractionation and establishes the importance of avoiding breaks in treatment.
- The use of chemical *radioprotectors* is founded on the principles of reoxygenation and repair. These chemicals may scavenge free radicals or facilitate direct chemical repair at sites of DNA damage in normal tissue.
- The use of chemical *radiosensitizers* is founded on the principle of reoxygenation as well. Instead of trying to force oxygen into the cell as in the use of hyperbaric chambers, chemicals developed as oxygen substitutes are used to make hypoxic tumor cells respond to radiation as though they were well-oxygenated; some drugs may selectively kill hypoxic cells.
- Radioprotectors and sensitizers have a finite period of effectiveness; it is important to administer radiation doses within an hour or two following these biologic modifiers.

BIBLIOGRAPHY

Bushong SC: *Radiologic science for technologists*, ed 9, St Louis, 2008, Mosby.

Clifford Chao KS, et al: *Radiation oncology: management decisions*, ed 2, Philadelphia, 2002, Lippincott Williams & Wilkins.

Forshier S: *Essentials of radiation biology and protection*, ed 2, Clifton Park, 2009, Cengage Delmar Learning.

Gunderson LL, Tepper JE: *Clinical radiation oncology*, ed 2, Philadelphia, 2007, Churchill Livingstone.
Hall EJ: *Radiobiology for the radiologist*, ed 6, Philadelphia, 2006, Lippincott Williams & Wilkins.
Lenhard R, Gansler T, Osteen R: *Clinical oncology*, ed 8, 2001, American Cancer Society.
Washington CM, Leaver D: *Principles and practice of radiation therapy*, ed 3, St Louis, 2010, Mosby.

REVIEW EXERCISES

1. TD 5/5 indicates the dose required to cause a 5% chance of injury to people irradiated within ________ following exposure.

a. 5 days
b. 5 hours
c. 5 years
d. 5 minutes

2. LD 50/30 indicates the dose likely to cause death in 50% of the population within ________ following exposure.

a. 30 days
b. 30 hours
c. 30 years
d. 30 minutes

3. The TD 5/5 for the whole kidney using standard fractionation is approximately:

a. 50 Gy
b. 30 Gy
c. 23 Gy
d. 0.5 Gy

4. The TD 5/5 for the whole brain using standard fractionation is approximately:

a. 60 Gy
b. 50 Gy
c. 45 Gy
d. 15 Gy

5. The period of organogenesis normally occurs during the ______week(s) of fetal development.

a. first two
b. second through eighth
c. twentieth
d. fortieth

6. The radiosensitivity in tissue may be enhanced by:

a. Increasing the oxygen in tissue
b. Increasing the dose given
c. Decreasing the fractionation size
d. Decreasing the volume of tissue irradiated

7. The phase of cellular division most resistant to radiation is the _______ phase

a. M
b. S
c. G0
d. G1

8. The immediate symptoms that appear after an acute radiation exposure are called:

a. Latent symptoms
b. Proportional symptoms
c. Chronic symptoms
d. Prodromal symptoms

9. The law of Bergonie and Tribondeau states that ionizing radiation is more effective against cells that are:

a. Actively mitotic
b. Undifferentiated
c. Have a long mitotic future
d. Well differentiated
e. a, b, and c
f. a, c, and d

Circle the correct word.

10. The development of a radiation-induced cancer is known as a (deterministic/stochastic) affect.

11. Nausea is associated with the (hematologic/prodomal) syndrome.

12. Radiation interacts with tissue (uniformly/randomly).

13. The (OER/RBE) describes the relative response to radiation in the presence or absence of oxygen.

14. Cells are most sensitive during the (M, G2, S) phase of division.

15. The fraction of cells actually progressing through cycles of division is known as the (growth, surviving) fraction.

16. The period over which radiation is delivered is referred to as the (protraction/fractionation).

17. Complete the table:

Type of Chromosomal Damage Caused by Irradiation	Consequences to Chromosomes	Consequences to the Cell
Single break, single chromosome		
Single break, two chromosomes		
Double break, one chromosome		
Double break, two chromosomes		

18. Complete the table to show cellular sensitivity to radiation:

Mitotic Rate	Differentiation	Sensitivity	Examples
High	Undifferentiated		
Moderate	Moderate differentiation		
Low	Moderate differentiation		
Low to none	Well differentiated		

19. Graph representative cell survival curves for high LET and low LET radiations. Label Figure 4-6 appropriately.

FIGURE 4-6 Cell survival curves.

20. Erythematous skin reactions during fractionated radiation therapy are seen as a result of:

a. Vascular dilation in the area
b. Loss of skin cells in the area
c. Regeneration of skin cells in the area
d. Extreme heat to the skin area

21. Epilation may initially be observed in patients receiving radiation under standard fractionation schemes at an approximate dose of:

a. 30 Gy
b. 50 Gy
c. 15 Gy
d. 5 Gy

22. The production of free radicals most often occurs from the irradiation of:

a. Water
b. RNA
c. Proteins
d. Salt

23. Protracted or fractionated dose are better tolerated by tissue than single doses because:

a. Tissue tolerance increases as dose increases
b. Tissue repair occurs between exposures
c. Fewer cells will be struck by radiation
d. Radiation damage cannot occur in previously killed cells

24. Which of the following is an effect of radiation on DNA?

a. Cross-linking
b. Increased viscosity
c. Free radical formation
d. Hydroxyl formation

25. As the dose of radiation increases:

a. The recovery rate in tissue remains unchanged
b. Tissue recovery time decreases
c. Tissue recovery time increases
d. Tissue recovery time increases until a certain dose threshold

26. In linear or nonlinear threshold dose-response curves, the following is true of the response:

a. Response will occur at all doses
b. Response may not occur at low doses
c. Response will never be realized
d. Response is proportional to dose

27. Radiation sickness symptoms associated with the reduced number of leukocytes is a major characteristic of:

a. Prodromal syndrome
b. Hematopoietic syndrome
c. Gastrointestinal syndrome
d. Cerebrovascular syndrome

28. The average energy deposited per unit of path length to a medium by ionizing radiation as it passes through that medium best describes:

a. Linear energy transfer
b. Radiation absorbed dose
c. Radiation equivalent
d. Tissue absorbed dose

29. The most radiosensitive tissue group among the following is the:

a. Central nervous system
b. Alimentary tract
c. Muscle
d. Cardiovascular system

30. The four Rs of radiation biology are:

a. Reoxygenation, repopulation, reimplantation, redistribution
b. Reoxygenation, repopulation, redistribution, repair
c. Reoxygenation, reimplantation, redistribution, repair
d. Reoxygenation, repair, repopulation, reduction

31. The whole body syndrome most likely to be observed following a single dose of 1-10 Gy is the:

a. Lethal dose syndrome
b. CNS syndrome
c. Hematopoietic syndrome
d. Gastrointestinal syndrome

32. Which of the following would be a stochastic or late radiation response?

a. Sterility
b. Bone marrow suppression
c. Skin erythema
d. Lung cancer

33. Which of the following is a more accurate representation of cell radiosensitivity?

a. Do
b. Dq
c. LD 50/30
d. D_{37}

34. The standard radiation used to determine RBE is:

a. 250 keV x-ray
b. 5 MeV alpha
c. 1 keV electrons
d. Cobalt-60 gamma

35. The central nervous system syndrome may be observed in those exposed to single whole body doses of:

a. 300 cGy
b. 5000 cGy
c. 500 Gy
d. 10 Gy

36. Without medical intervention, a person exposed to a single whole body dose of ___ may die within 10 days.

a. 10 Gy
b. 0.25 Gy
c. 1.0 Gy
d. 1.0 cGy

37. Normal tissue healing following radiation occurs by:

a. Regeneration
b. Repair
c. Revitalization
d. a and b

38. Irradiation of the salivary glands may lead to permanent xerostomia above doses of ___using the typical 2 Gy per treatment, 5 treatments per week fractionation scheme.

a. 10 Gy
b. 20 Gy
c. 30 Gy
d. 40 Gy

39. Exceeding the TD 50/5 for the spinal cord may lead to:

a. Perforation
b. Ulceration
c. Myelitis necrosis
d. Obstruction

40. Tissue injury ________ as the volume of tissue irradiated increases.

a. increases
b. decreases
c. is not influenced
d. manifests as erythema

Circle the correct word.

41. The TD 5/5 for the colon is (higher, lower) than the TD 50/5 for the colon.

42. The TD 5/5 is (higher, lower) for immature bone than for mature bone.

43. The TD 5/5 is (higher, lower) for bone marrow irradiation in a single dose than in fractionated doses.

44. An anticipated response to radiation dose above 55 Gy to the colon is (erythema, fistula).

45. The TD 5/5 for the ovary is (higher, lower) than the TD 5/5 for the lung.

46. Regarding nonstochastic effects:

1. The effects are never in the one exposed
2. The effects are never seen in future generations
3. The probability of occurring is related to dose
4. The severity of effects is related to dose

a. 1
b. 2
c. 3
d. 2, 4
e. 1, 2, 3, 4

47. The most radiosensitive tissue group is:

a. Central nervous
b. Alimentary tract
c. Lens
d. Urinary

48. The part of the cell between the membrane and the nucleus is known as the:

a. Plasma membrane
b. Cytoplasm
c. Cytoplasmic membrane
d. Golgi apparatus

49. The effect of radiation on tissue is influenced by:

1. Radiation type
2. Fractionation
3. Volume of tissue irradiated
4. Total dose

a. 1
b. 1, 2
c. 1, 2, 3
d. 1, 2, 3, 4

50. The primary function of the cell nucleus is:

a. Protein synthesis
b. Control the formation of the Golgi apparatus
c. Producing amino acids
d. Housing DNA and RNA

Find the following terms using the clues and definitions given. Use the numbered letters to unscramble a term for what may be known in radiobiology as the *liberated constituent of a molecule.*

51. The physical or mechanical restoration of damaged tissues.

___ ___ ___ ___ ___ ___
1 2

52. Redness of the skin caused by a change in permeability of the capillaries.

___ ___ ___ ___ ___ ___ ___ ___
3 4

53. Grade 1 toxicity for the skin caused by depopulation of clonogenic cells in the epidermis.

___ ___ ___ ___ ___ ___ ___ ___ ___ ___ ___ ___
5 6 7

54. Division of total dose into smaller doses given at intervals.

___ ___ ___ ___ ___ ___ ___ ___ ___ ___ ___ ___ ___
8 9 10

55. Acronym for average energy deposited per unit of path length.

___ ___ ___
11

56. Liberated constituent of a molecule

___ ___ ___ ___ ___ ___ ___ ___ ___ ___ ___

57. The occupational dose limit for deterministic effects to the lens of the eye is lower than the limit for the skin because:

a. The lens has a greater sensitivity to radiation than the skin
b. The skin has a greater sensitivity to radiation than the lens

c. The lens is easier to protect from radiation than the skin
d. The skin cells are more differentiated than the lens cells

58. The main objectives of radiation protection include:

a. Prevention of radiation-induced deterministic effects
b. Prevention of radiation-induced stochastic effects
c. Production of radiation-induced stochastic effects
d. a and b

59. A grade 1 morbidity score for the colon would indicate:

a. Diarrhea requiring parenteral support
b. Ulceration or perforation
c. Obstruction
d. Change in frequency or bowel habits

60. A grade 3 morbidity score for the skin would indicate:

a. Confluent moist desquamation
b. Swelling with dry desquamation
c. Mild redness and itching
d. Ulceration or necrosis

61. The onset dose for wet desquamation during standard fractionation is:

a. 15 Gy
b. 20 Gy
c. 30 Gy
d. 40 Gy

62. Somatic effects are:

a. The effects limited to the exposed individual
b. The effects manifested in subsequent generations
c. The effects seen after large doses only
d. The effects seen after small doses only

63. Ellis' NSD formula is:

a. $A = A_o e^{-\lambda t}$
b. $T^{0.11} \times NSD$
c. Total dose $= (NSD)\ T^{0.11}\ N^{0.24}$
d. NSD $=$ Total dose $\times N^{0.24}$

64. Ellis' formula did not accommodate:

a. Different tissue types with varying sensitivities
b. The variation in protraction
c. The number of fractions
d. A reference ideal dose

65. Conventional fractionation was based on experiments performed to:

a. Induce tumors in mice
b. Eradicate tumors in mice
c. Sterilize rams
d. Produce skin reactions in rams

Think About It

66. When irradiating the spleen for metastatic disease, hypofractionation may be employed, whereas certain primary head and neck cancers may employ hyperfractionation. Briefly explain the rationale for this difference.

67. An error has caused you to discover that your patient has received twice the prescribed dose during the first 2 weeks of treatment. Once you discover the error, what adjustments to this patient's treatment course are necessary?

68. Your patient has not yet received his radioprotector. It is time for his scheduled appointment and your two subsequent appointments have already arrived. In the essence of time, you could take him now and send him back to the waiting room to receive his injection later. Is this a feasible plan? Explain your answer.

69. You have a patient on a special hyperfractionation protocol. He is to receive two fractions per day. His first treatment was at 9:00 AM and his second

is scheduled for 3:00 PM. However, there has been a cancellation and you can squeeze him in at 1:30. Is this a feasible plan? Explain your answer.

70. There is a patient scheduled for 6 weeks of radiation using standard fractionation. After week 2 he informs you that he will be taking a 3 week cruise and plans to complete therapy when he returns. What would your counseling include?

71. The cardinal signs of tissue injury include:

1. Redness
2. Swelling
3. Heat
4. Pain

a. 1, 3
b. 2, 3, 4
c. 1, 3, 4
d. 1, 2, 3, 4

72. Regarding the tolerance of tissue, as the volume irradiated increases:

a. The tolerance dose increases
b. The tolerance dose decreases
c. The tolerance dose doubles
d. The tolerance dose decreases inversely by the square of the volume

73. The standard proposed unit for "rets" in Ellis' formula held the value of:

a. 1800
b. 4500
c. 1600
d. 1000

74. Lethal damage:

a. May be repaired by the body if circumstances are right
b. Is irreparable and leads to cell death
c. Is usually repaired by the body
d. Is shown in the shoulder of the survival curve

75. At doses above ______ Gy, you may see latent stricture in the esophagus during standard fractionation.

a. 5
b. 10
c. 40
d. 60

76. Ionizing radiation can disrupt chemical ______ in important biologic materials.

a. Balance
b. Distribution
c. Energy
d. Bonds

77. Which of the following is not a nitrogenous base found in DNA.

a. Phosphene
b. Adenine
c. Thymine
d. Guanine

78. The structure of DNA is referred to as a:

a. Single helix
b. Triple spiral
c. Double helix
d. Half spiral

79. Somatic cellular division takes place through the process of:

a. Symbiosis
b. Mitosis
c. Meiosis
d. Synthesis

80. Which phase of the cell cycle occurs between the two gap phases, G1 and G2?

a. Synthesis
b. Interphase
c. Telophase
d. Metaphase

81. The steps of cellular division in proper order are:

a. M, G1, G2, S
b. G1, M, G2, S
c. M, G2, S, G1
d. G1, S, G2, M

82. A cell survival curve:

a. Usually has a shoulder and straight portion
b. Cannot be drawn for human cells
c. Cannot show the effects of dose rate
d. Usually shows the fraction of surviving cells on a lincar scale

83. High LET radiation usually has:

a. An RBE of 1
b. An RBE of 0
c. High RBE
d. No relation to RBE

84. Which dose effect curve implies that if radiation dose is doubled, the biologic effect will be doubled?

a. Sigmoidal
b. Linear quadratic
c. Quadratic
d. Linear

85. When radiation exposure is fractionated:

a. The LET changes
b. There are more direct effects
c. The biologic effect is lessened
d. The time period is shortened

86. Cellular growth and development is called:

a. Differentiation
b. Proliferation
c. Mitosis
d. Meiosis

87. The key target in the human cell is the_______.

a. Cytoplasm
b. Mitochondria
c. Organelle
d. DNA

88. Cells are about ______water.

a. 50 %
b. 85%
c. 10%
d. 100%

89. On the cell survival curve, the "n" number denotes the:

a. Quasithreshold dose
b. Mean lethal dose
c. Extrapolation number
d. Median lethal dose

90. Radiation would have less effect on a cell if given

a. Over a short period of time
b. Over a long period of time
c. All at once
d. In the presence of oxygen

CHAPTER 5

Radiation Protection and Safety

Leia Levy

FOCUS QUESTIONS

- What organizations are responsible for setting the standards for radiation protection?
- What are the various sources of radiation exposure?
- What is the ALARA principle and how does it apply to occupational radiation workers?
- What are the dose limits for occupational workers, students, and general public?
- What are the advantages and disadvantages of the most common types of radiation monitors?
- What materials are most feasible to use as barriers?
- What factors are necessary for the calculation of primary and secondary barriers?
- How do brachytherapy safety procedures differ from safety procedures applicable to external beam?

GENERAL OBJECTIVES OF RADIATION PROTECTION

- Radiation protection involves physical, technical, and procedural factors used to protect patients, personnel, and the public from unnecessary radiation exposure.
- Before we protect ourselves, our patients, and others from the harmful effects of radiation exposure, we must identify potential sources of exposure (Table 5-1). These sources may be grouped into the following major categories:

Natural Background Radiation

a. Cosmic rays from nuclear reactions in space
b. Terrestrial radiation from natural, radioactive earth elements
c. Internal radiation from radioactive material always present in our bodies such as carbon-14, hydrogen-3, strontium-90, and potassium-40.

Man-Made Radiation

a. Medical x-ray equipment
b. Radioactive sources produced for nuclear medicine and brachytherapy
c. Television
d. Nuclear reactors and weapons

- Natural background radiation is the source of the majority of annual exposure. It is not possible to be totally protected from natural radiation; some amount of exposure is inevitable.
- We must make every attempt to limit exposure to man-made sources of radiation.
- The key to limited exposure is to follow the principle of ALARA.
- ALARA is an acronym for "as low as reasonably achievable"; refers to what must be done to keep exposure to potentially harmful radiation at a minimum.
- Remember three key terms for keeping exposures low: time, distance, and shielding.

  Time—limit your time in the area of exposure.
  Distance—keep the greatest distance possible between you and the source of exposure; inverse square law: $I_1 (D_1)^2 = I_2 (D_2)^2$.
  Shielding—use adequate, protective barriers between you and the origin of exposure.

RADIATION PROTECTION AND SAFETY ORGANIZATIONS

- The International Commission on Radiological Protection (ICRP) develops standards of protection for users of x-rays and other ionizing radiation. They are a group of experts interested in the safe use of all types of radiation; they publish recommendations for protection against exposure.
- The National Council on Radiation Protection and Measurements (NCRP) is a national group of experts who make recommendations for protection against exposure.

TABLE 5-1 Percentages of Annual Exposures from Various Sources

Source of Radiation Exposure	Yearly Exposure
Cosmic radiation	30 mrem
Terrestrial radiation	29 mrem
Internal sources	39 mrem
Radon to lungs	200 mrem
Nuclear medicine procedures	14 mrem
Nuclear power plants, consumer products	10 mrem
X-ray imaging	40 mrem

- The Nuclear Regulatory Commission (NRC) is the national group, which collaborates with individual states to establish regulations that are incorporated into federal and state laws.
- Other agencies involved in radiation safety include the Department of Transportation (DOT), the Food and Drug Administration (FDA), the Occupational Safety and Health Administration (OSHA), and the Environmental Protection Agency (EPA).
- Radiation dose limits were called skin erythema doses in the early days of radiation therapy.
- The term tolerance dose was used to describe exposure limits in the 1930s.
- From 1940 to 1991, following research and documentation of stochastic and deterministic effects due to high exposures, dose limits for occupational workers, students, and the general public were termed maximum permissible doses (MPD).
- Currently dose limits are simply referred to as recommended dose limits (DL).
- Dose limits are based on actual outcomes out of research that continues; this makes the recommendations fluid and apt to change over time.
- Dose limits for occupational workers are greater than those for the general public and are set at a risk level comparable to that for workers in other industries.
- Dose limits are established below the threshold value for deterministic effects and at a level to adequately limit the risk of stochastic effects.

UNITS OF EXPOSURE AND METHODS OF DETECTION

- Exposure is measured using units such as the Roentgen or coulomb/kilogram, the rad or gray, and the rem or sievert.
- The roentgen is one of the earlier units named after Wilhelm Roentgen and measures the amount of ionization produced by photons in the air per unit mass of air; the system international unit is the coulomb/kilogram.
- The traditional rad, system international unit gray, measures absorbed dose in a medium, such as tissue.
- The rem, system international unit sievert, measures equivalent dose and is appropriate for personnel exposure reporting. The conversion of this equivalent dose into absorbed dose requires the application of a quality factor assigned to the type of radiation and tissue weighting factor assigned to the specific organ exposed (Table 5-2).
- To detect exposure, several different tools may be used.
- Some tools are appropriate for personnel monitoring, while others are appropriate for surveying an area to detect the presence of radiation or for verifying adsorbed dose in the patient.

Common personnel exposure monitors (Table 5-3) include:

1. Film badge
2. Thermoluminescent dosimeters (TLD)
3. Optimal stimulated luminescence (OSL)
4. Pocket ionization chambers

- Personnel should be monitored if it is expected that the worker may receive $\frac{1}{10}$ of the recommended dose limit.
- Film badge monitor reports should be generated periodically and may specify "deep" or "shallow" dose equivalents. The sum of these doses would be the total effective dose equivalent (TEDE).
- Deep dose is measured at 1 cm depth and refers to external dose.
- Shallow dose is assigned to any internal dose received by ingestion or inhalation during the handling of radioactive materials.
- Exposure levels shown on film badge reports are given using units of equivalent dose: rem or Sievert.
- To calculate the effective equivalent dose as indicated by the equivalent dose value, the type of radiation and tissue exposed must be considered.

TABLE 5-2 Exposure Unit Conversions

Quantity	Traditional Unit	Conversion Factor to →	System International Unit
Exposure	Roentgen	2.58×10^{-4}	Coulomb/kilogram
Absorbed Dose	Rad	10^{-2}	Gray
Equivalent Dose	Rem	10^{-2}	Sievert

TABLE 5-3 Personnel Exposure Monitors

Film Badge	TLD Lithium Fluoride	Pocket Dosimeter	OSL Aluminum Oxide
+ Measures kV, MV photons, electrons, gamma; can detect approximate energy + Inexpensive + Provides permanent record of exposure − Excessive heat, humidity, or light exposure can damage − Has to be sent out for reading − Error margin ± 20%	+ Measures photons, electrons, other particles + Responds more like tissue; has similar atomic number so very accurate + Small enough to fit into ring badge + Humidity will not damage + Can be processed on site if equipment available − Cannot estimate the energy of radiation exposure	+ Reading is immediate + Initial cost is high but once obtained is inexpensive + Small enough to fit in pocket + Very accurate to within +2% − Humidity and mechanical shock will give erroneous readings	+ Wide range, accurate, and very sensitive + Can be reanalyzed for confirmation of dose + More sensitive than TLD − More expensive − New technology not well understood

+, advantages; −, disadvantages.

- The effective equivalent dose is calculated by the formula:

$$E = W_t(W_r) \times \text{absorbed dose}$$

E = effective equivalent dose
W_t = tissue weighting factor assigned to tissue type other than whole body
W_r = radiation weighting factor or quality factor

- Since the personnel monitors such as the film badge are intended to measure whole body exposure and the film badge is useful in detecting x-rays, gamma or electrons, the quality factor is assumed to be 1; therefore 1 rem = 1 rad and 1 Sv = 1 Gy
- If the effective equivalent dose is to be known for a specific organ, tissue weighting factors are given by their relative sensitivity to radiation.
- Tissues with the greatest sensitivity will have weights under the whole body weight of 1.

Example of Tissue Weighting Factors (W_t)
Gonads = 0.20
Bone marrow = 0.12
Bone surfaces = 0.01

- Special dose limits are expressed for the protection of the embryo/fetus of the radiation worker.
- Once pregnancy is known, the dose limit for the unborn takes precedence over the limit for the worker.
- Students under 18 would be subject to recommended dose limits to the general public.
- Students over 18 are subject to occupational limits.

WORK AREAS

- Work areas should be designated as restricted/controlled or unrestricted/uncontrolled.
- Restricted areas are ones in which exposure levels of personnel are monitored; barriers and other engineering controls should reduce exposure to less than 100 mrem/wk or 0.1 rem/wk or 1 mSv/wk.
- Unrestricted areas are ones that may be occupied by anyone; the maximum allowed exposure would be less than 1 mSv/yr or 2 mrem/wk or 0.002 rem/wk.
- Federal and state agencies require that signs be posted where there is radioactive material or radiation producing equipment.
- **Caution-Radioactive Material** is the required sign when the quantity of the radionuclide exceeds the activity specified by local law; appropriate locations would be the radioisotope inventory room or on source packaging.

Packaged and transported radioactive sources should also show:
Radioactive I white label—less than 0.5 mR/hr
Radioactive II yellow label—less than 1.0 mR/hr
Radioactive III yellow label—50 to 200 mR/hr and less than 10 mR/hr at 3 feet

- **Caution-Radiation Area** is the required sign necessary when an employee could receive more than 5 mrem/hr or 100 mrem in 5 days.
- **Caution-High Radiation Area** or **Caution-Airborne Radioactivity** is necessary when the dose rate is greater than 100 mrem/hr (not typical in the clinical setting).
- The radiation symbol required on radiation signs (Figure 5-1) is a three-bladed symbol in magenta on a yellow background.
- Protective barriers are designed to ensure that dose does not exceed the recommended dose limit to workers or the general public.
- Primary radiation, coming directly from the source, requires a primary barrier.
- Scatter or leakage radiation, coming from source housing or after interacting with the patient requires secondary barriers.

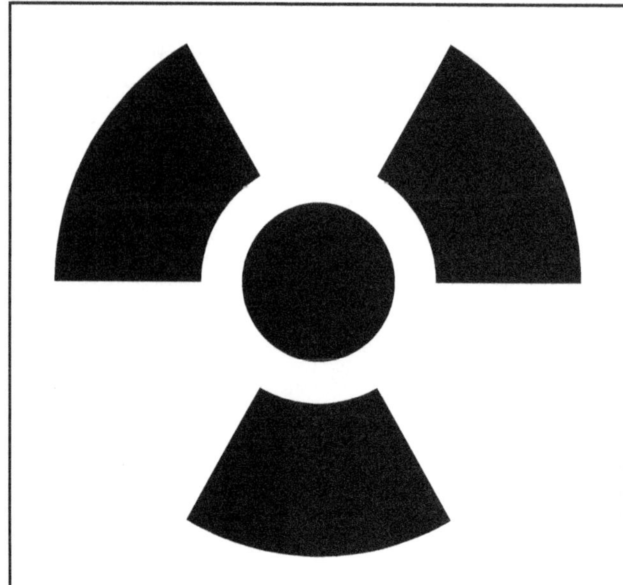

FIGURE 5-1 Radiation symbol.

- There are several factors to consider when designing protective barriers.

Factors to Consider for Protective Barriers

a. Workload—W: how much the primary beam is in use; number of patients × number of fields × average dose/field × dose rate × number of treatment days/week.
b. Use factor—U: the fraction of the workload in which a barrier is directly irradiated
c. Occupancy factor—T: the fraction of time during which an area is occupied
d. Maximum energy of the beam in use
e. Distance from the source—d

- The barrier material selected and thickness required is influenced by the maximum energy.
- Calculations for thickness of a barrier would include the linear attenuation coefficient and half value layer (HVL).

$$I = I_o e^{-M(X)}$$

I = intensity transmitted
I_o = original intensity on the absorbing material
M = linear attenuation coefficient
X = thickness of material

$$HVL = \frac{0.693}{M}$$

- For minimum exposure, the barrier material and thickness could not allow transmission of more than the recommended dose limit.
- Common materials used for barriers are concrete, iron, and lead; concrete is used widely as compared with lead because of minimal expense.
- Considering all other factors, primary barrier transmission factors could be calculated by applying the following formulas:

$$\text{Primary barrier factor} = \frac{0.1 \text{ rem } (d)^2}{W(U)(T)}$$

$$\text{Secondary barrier factor} = \frac{0.002 \text{ rem } (d)^2}{W(U)(T)}$$

- Work areas need to be monitored for the presence of radiation when equipment is in use and especially in areas of radioactive sources.
- There are a variety of changes that can be caused by ionizing radiation interacting with the air or other materials; the changes are what give indications of the presence of radiation.
- Combinations of change in material is potentially useful as a radiation detector.

Radiation Detection Mechanisms

1. Ionization-release of ion pairs by radiation
2. Biologic change in living systems
3. Chemical release of free radicals in solution
4. Heat/temperature rise from deposited energy
5. Scintillation-light flash in a special absorber
6. Thermoluminescence-light release on heating a phosphor
7. Super heated drop bubble formation in a gel matrix

- Ionization-based detectors are capable of high sensitivity as single ionizing events can be distinguished
- The ion chamber designed to measure the output of a therapy machine is not necessarily suitable for measuring low levels of radioactive contamination.
- Special surveyors are needed to measure low levels of radiation in leak testing.
- Biologic and chemical based detectors (Table 5-4) are relatively low in sensitivity; they require a lag time for results.
- It is appropriate to survey an area for radiation after brachytherapy procedures, after sources have been removed from a patient, when there are sources in storage, and after the installation of new equipment.
- Surveying equipment must be calibrated annually and following any repairs.

TABLE 5-4 Radiation Detectors and Applications

Ion Chamber Cutie Pie	Geiger Counter	Proportional Counters Scintillation Counters Neutron Counters (Rascal)	Silicone Diodes	Chemical-based Fricke Dosimeter	TLD
+ Measures dose rate in mR/hour + Cutie Pie good for measuring leakage from cobalt + Can detect x-rays, electrons on pulsed machines such as the linear accelerator (linac), and gamma + Special ion chambers filled with hydrogenous walls can detect photons and neutrons – Temperature and pressure corrections needed for free air chambers	+ More sensitive than ion chamber + Detects photons and particles + Has audible signal – Exposure rate with thin-window GM counters, otherwise can only detect presence and does not quantify – Not useful on pulsed linacs, has slow recovery time	+ Detects all particles, gamma and x-rays + Measures dose rate in mR/hour or mrem/hr + Good for measuring neutron contamination in and around accelerators + Good for measuring low levels of radiation	+ More sensitive than ion chambers + Measures absorbed dose + Get immediate results + Good for monitoring output constancy or dose monitoring in patients		+ Measures absorbed dose – Need special, expensive equipment for reading

+, advantages; –, disadvantages.

RADIOACTIVE SOURCES

- Sources must be stored in heavily shielded areas in an area secure from theft or loss.
- Proper ventilation is required, especially for encapsulated powdered sources.
- Inventory room should have a sink for cleaning applicators with a filter or trap to prevent loss.
- There should be a barrier behind which sources may be prepared; "L" block.
- Long forceps should be available in the room for handling of sources.
- Sources should be transported around the facility in lead containers or carts called "pigs."
- Trucks that transport must follow shielding regulations as dictated by the NCRP and DOT.
- Received packages should be visually inspected for damage or leaks.
- The appropriate radioactive content label should be present.
- Any packages containing more than 1 mCi and physical half-life greater than 30 days need to be wipe tested within 3 hours of receipt/18 hours outside of work hours.
- When disposing of radioactive waste NRC recommendations should be followed.

For Disposal of Radioactive Waste

1. Sewer system may include flushing; draining into a hold up tank for decay then flushing; emptying into an effluent pond or retention basin and holding for decay; placing in shielding container for delivery to a special chemical processing plant
2. Incineration requires a special license unless source is approaching background levels
3. Transfer to authorized recipient
4. Burial requires special license

- All waste receptacles should be close to the area they service, shielded, and out of the flow of traffic.
- A hot sink should be present and used only for discharge of radioactive wastes.
- Records of disposals should be maintained and readily available.
- Inventory of all sources must be performed for all sources quarterly, even if no sources have been used in that time frame; inventory records must be maintained for 3 years.
- In-patient rooms used for brachytherapy need to be private with dedicated restroom.
- Bed placement has to be such that neighboring patients would receive limited exposure.

- Nurses and other caregivers should wear monitoring devices and be instructed on how to care for the patient in a timely manner; bedside shields should be available.
- Other ancillary personnel needing to enter the patient room should be educated on exposure potential.
- Appropriate sign must be displayed on patient's room door.
- Visitors should be limited to adults; visits should be short; rule of thumb is 20 minutes or less.
- In case of an emergency, such as a radioactive spill or source loss: *evacuate, contain/isolate* area, *notify* and then appropriate personnel will *decontaminate*
- High dose rate (HDR) procedures should be performed in appropriately shielded rooms.
- Room surveys should be conducted following low dose rate (LDR) and HDR procedures to verify all sources have been returned to designated locations.
- Geiger-Müller counters may be used for room survey; keep in mind, Geiger counters can only detect the presence of radiation in the area but cannot quantify the amount of dose in the area.
- Afterloading procedures should be thoroughly preplanned to limit exposure of personnel and patients.

BIBLIOGRAPHY

Bushong SC: *Radiologic science for technologists*, ed 9, St Louis, 2008, Mosby.

Kahn FM: *The physics of radiation therapy*, ed 4, Philadelphia, 2010, Lippincott Williams & Wilkins.

Podgorsak EB: *Radiation physics for medical physicists*, ed 1, Berlin, 2006, Springer.

Stanton R, Stinson D: *Applied physics for radiation oncology*, ed 2, Madison, 2009, Medical Physics Publishing.

Washington CM, Leaver D: *Principles and practice of radiation therapy*, ed 3, St Louis, 2010, Mosby.

REVIEW EXERCISES

1. According to the current recommendations, which of the following will have the highest annual dose limit?
   a. The lens of the eye
   b. The hands of a member of the general public
   c. The embryo/fetus
   d. The hands of a pregnant therapist

2. According to the current recommendations, the guidance levels for cumulative exposures for a 30-year-old occupational worker with 3 years of experience is:
   a. 600 mSv
   b. 300 mSv
   c. 330 mSv
   d. 50 mSv

3. All of the following are advantages of the film badge personnel monitor except:
   a. Provides permanent record
   b. Exposure to interpretation delay
   c. Measure dose over large body area
   d. Radiation type can be determined

4. It is recommended that radiation exposure to the fetus should not exceed _____ for the entire gestation period.
   a. 0.1 rem
   b. 0.5 rem
   c. 1.5 rem
   d. 3.0 rem

5. Which of the following devices is not normally used to monitor occupational dose exposure?
   a. Film badge
   b. TLD
   c. Cutie pie
   d. Pocket dosimeter

6. The roentgen is a unit of measurement that specifies the ______ of air by x-rays or gamma radiation.
   a. excitation
   b. ionization
   c. absorption
   d. attenuation

7. When film badges are used for radiation monitoring, which of the following factors may affect the accurate reading of the badge?
   1. Exposure to excessive heat
   2. Submersion of the badge in fluids
   3. Damage to the film wrapper

   a. 1, 2
   b. 1, 3
   c. 2, 3
   d. 1, 2, 3

8. The term quality factor (Q):
   a. Varies with different types of radiation
   b. Varies with different types of tissue
   c. Varies as a function of age and gender
   d. Is measured in rem

9. Any container in which radionuclides are transported, stored, or used must have a label saying:

a. Caution - Breakable Container
b. Caution - High Radiation Area
c. Caution - Radioactive Material
d. Grave Danger - High Radiation Area

10. The organization in the United States that is principally responsible for recommending radiation dose limits is the__________.

11. The annual dose limit for the occupational worker's lens is__________.

12. The annual dose limit for the occupational worker's skin is__________.

13. The fraction of time that a radiation beam is directed at a specific barrier is termed the__________.

14. The annual radiation dose to the lung from radon gas is estimated to be__________.

Think About It

15a. If a survey meter shows an exposure rate of 300 mR/hour at 3 feet from the sources during the loading of a Fletcher intracavitary applicator, and the duration of the procedure is expected to be 6 minutes, what would be the exposure to the person standing 3 feet away from the sources?

15b. What would the exposure be to the same person if they stood just 2 feet away from the sources?

16. The dose rate is 0.5 rem/min at 40 feet away from a source. An office will be constructed 20 feet away from the source. An individual will occupy this office 8 hr/day, 5 days/wk and is allowed to receive 10 mrem/wk or less. How many tenth value layers of material are needed?

17a. A linear accelerator accommodates 35 patients/day, 5 days/wk. The average number of fields per patient is 4 and the average dose per field is 45 cGy. Calculate the workload.

17b. Calculate the primary barrier transmission factor at the console located at 1 m from the source for the restricted linear accelerator area in the previous question.

18. If the HVL for cobalt-60 is 1.1 cm of lead, what percent of transmission is expected using 4.4 cm of lead as a barrier?

19. Compare how dose is measured using the film badge and TLD.

20. Compare how exposure is measured using an ion chamber and Fricke dosimeter.

21. Dose equivalent is measured in units of:

a. roentgen
b. rad
c. sievert
d. curie

The following are TRUE/FALSE corrective statements. Put T on the line if the statement is true. If the statement is false, place an F on the line, then make the statement correct without changing the intent of the statement.

22. ___Maximum exposure rate at a specific distance from a patient following insertion of radioactive sources can be measured with TLDs.

23. ___Two half value layers of a material for a given radiation would decrease radiation intensity to 25%.

24. ____The requirement for barrier protection in walls/ceiling from primary radiation is reduced when there is a beam stopper on the treatment unit.

25. The agency that regulates the use of radiation producing machines is the:

a. AAPM
b. NRC
c. DOT
d. FDA

26. An example of a deterministic effect is:

a. Carcinogenesis
b. Genetic effects
c. Birth defects
d. Cataracts

27. The radiation detection device helpful in finding a lost radioactive source would be a/n:

a. Ion chamber
b. Geiger-Müller counter
c. TLD
d. Neutron counter

28. The largest dose from natural background radiation comes from:

a. Terrestrial
b. Radon
c. Cosmic
d. Internal

29. Which of the following was used first to measure radiation exposure and set limits:

a. Skin erythema dose
b. Tolerance dose
c. MPD
d. Dose limits

30. The amount of energy absorbed in a medium is expressed in units of:

a. Roentgen
b. Coulomb/kilogram
c. Sievert
d. Gray

Write the letter C for cosmic, T for terrestrial, or I for internal next to the statement that refers to the appropriate component of natural background radiation.

31. ______Product of interactions with the stars

32. ______Defined as "of the earth"

33. ______Increases with altitude

34. ______One major contributor is potassium-40

35. ______No shielding between the source and the person exposed.

36. ______Varies according to composition of the soil.

37. The two main types of background radiation are:

a. Natural and man-made
b. Cosmic and terrestrial
c. Confluent and regressive
d. Internal and external

38. The exposure from cosmic rays at sea level is lower than the exposure in Denver because:

a. The earth's magnetic field varies
b. The temperature is higher at sea level
c. The altitude is higher in Denver
d. There is more atmosphere to shield the individuals who live in Denver

39. Exposure from terrestrial radiation varies according to:

a. The thickness of the atmosphere
b. The magnetic field distribution of the earth
c. The number of diagnostic x-rays received
d. The composition of soil or rock in nearby areas

40. What quantity is measured directly by the TLD?

a. Exposure
b. Absorbed dose
c. Activity
d. Lag time

41. Following discharge of a patient who received low dose rate brachytherapy, a room survey should be conducted to:

a. Ensure patient care staff members have not been exposed
b. Make sure the former patient's roommate has not been exposed
c. Make sure that the survey meter has maintained a suitable charge between the procedure and patient discharge
d. Make sure that there are no remaining radioactive sources in the room

42. Appropriate disposal of radioactive sources include:

a. Transfer to an authorized recipient
b. Incineration
c. Burial
d. All of the above

43. Long forceps are required for direct handling of radioactive sources so that:

a. Exposure time to the handler's hands is decreased
b. Exposure time to the handler's hands is increased
c. Amount of exposure to handler's hands is decreased
d. Amount of exposure to handler's hands is increased

44. The radioactive source inventory room should have a sign that reads:

a. Caution Radioactive Material
b. Caution Radiation Area
c. Caution High Radiation Area
d. Grave Danger-High Radiation Area

45. The workload describes:

a. How much the primary beam is in use
b. The fraction of the workload in which a barrier is irradiated
c. The fraction of time during which an area is occupied
d. Energy of the beam in use

46. In the construction of a new radiation therapy center, the choices for primary barriers include concrete, lead, or iron. Measure for measure, I would need more________ for adequate absorption.

a. Concrete
b. Lead
c. Iron

47. The half value layer for a 6 MV beam is 22 mm of lead. Its linear attenuation coefficient is:

a. 31.7 mm^{-1}
b. 0.0315 mm^{-1}
c. 0.693 mm^{-1}
d. 15.24 mm^{-1}

48. When a radiation worker is away from work, it is best to store his personnel monitoring film badge:

a. In a safe place away from the source of radiation
b. In a locker inside the linear accelerator vault
c. In a drawer at the linear accelerator console
d. In the car for quick and easy access

49. High dose rate (HDR) brachytherapy procedures should be performed in:

a. A private surgical suite
b. In a private hospital room
c. In a patient examination room
d. In a shielded vault

50. Patients undergoing thyroid ablation with I^{131} should not be released to leave the facility until:

a. 2 hours have past since the swallow
b. 2 days have past since the swallow
c. Survey meter readings reach less than 5 mrem/hr at 1 m
d. Survey meter readings reach 0 mrem/hr at 1 m

51. Internal radiation exposure comes from radioactive materials always present in our bodies such as:

a. Xenon-131
b. Technetium-99
c. Hydrogen-3
d. Boron-12

52. Radioactive sources should be transported around the treatment facility in:

a. Sterile bags
b. Biohazard bags
c. Shielded containers
d. Sterile boxes

53. Nursing and other patient care staff caring for an admitted patient undergoing low dose radiation (LDR) brachytherapy should:

a. Wear gown and gloves to prevent radioactive spills
b. Wear a face mask to prevent inhalation of radioactive material
c. Wear goggles to prevent splashes of radioactive fluids to the eyes
d. Use standard precautions and perform duties as quickly as possible

54. A monthly radiation exposure report says an employee received 0.5 Sv. If the source of exposure were determined to be gamma radiation, the translation to absorbed dose would be:

a. 0.5 Sv = 0.5 Gy
b. 0.5 Sv = 0.5 cGy
c. 0.5 Sv = 10 Gy
d. 0.5 Sv = 100 Gy

55. The half value layer for a 6 MV beam is 32 mm of lead. The linear attenuation coefficient would be:

a. 46 mm^{-1}
b. 0.002 mm^{-1}
c. 22 mm^{-1}
d. 0.0216 mm^{-1}

56. How many half value layers reduce transmission to 2%?

a. 2 HVLs
b. 5 HVLs
c. 6.5 HVLs
d. 5.6 HVLs

57. Three tenth value layers (TVLs) reduce transmission to:

a. 10 %
b. 30%
c. 0.1 %
d. 0.3 %

58. The shielding around stored radioisotopes must be adequate to reduce radiation levels to:

a. less than 2 mrem/hr at 1 m
b. less than 5 mrem/hr at 1 m
c. less than 5 mSv/hr at 1 m
d. less than 5 rem/hr at 1 m

Think About It

59a. The half value layer for cobalt is 11 mm lead. What is its linear attenuation coefficient?

59b. How much lead would reduce this cobalt beam to 3 % transmission?

60a. The linear attenuation coefficient for a certain megavoltage beam using concrete as an absorber is 0.089 cm^{-1}. What is the half value layer?

60b. How much concrete is required to reduce transmission to 2% of the primary beam?

CHAPTER

6

Radiation Therapy Equipment and Quality Assurance

Leia Levy

FOCUS QUESTIONS

- How has radiation therapy treatment equipment evolved over time?
- What are the major components of the linear accelerator?
- Describe systems for treatment portal verification
- What benefits were there to introducing the computed tomography (CT) simulator to radiation therapy planning procedures?
- What benefits were there to introducing record and verify systems to radiation therapy treatment accelerators?
- How do the features of the conventional simulator differ from the CT simulator?
- Compare and contrast the conventional fan-beam CT and cone beam CT.
- What are some of the applicator devices used in brachytherapy procedures?
- Compare and contrast the linear accelerator, cyclotron, microtron, and betatron.
- Compare and contrast the characteristics of the x-ray beam to the heavy particle beam.
- List and compare some treatment portal verification systems.
- What quality assurance procedures are appropriate for treatment equipment?

THERAPY EQUIPMENT EVOLUTION

- Therapy machines operated in very low energy range in the early years of radiation therapy; x-ray tubes ranging from 5 to 800 kV were used.
- Grenz ray x-ray tubes operated in the range 5 to 15 kV.
- Low energy Crookes tubes operated in the range 50 to 100 kV and were also referred to as superficial therapy machines; treatment distance was at 15- to 20-cm source to skin distance (SSD).
- Medium energy tubes, developed by William Coolidge, also known as "hot cathode" tubes could generate higher energies in the range of 100 to 200 kV. They were also known as orthovoltage/deep therapy machines; treatment distance was at 50-cm SSD.
- Superficial and orthovoltage machines simply required an x-ray tube and mobile collimator system. Filters such as aluminum, tin, or copper would be required to be placed between the source and the patient to harden the beam.
- Coolidge paved the way for supervoltage units, also known as cascading tubes, in the 1930s. They operated in the range of 500 kV or greater; treatment distance was at 80- to 100-cm SSD.
- The first supervoltage machine operating as high as 1 MV was used in London. GE made a supervoltage unit installed at Mercy Hospital in Chicago in 1933.
- Other particle accelerators such as the betatron and cyclotron were used clinically in the 1930s.
- Megavoltage units (1 MV and greater), including the cobalt machine, and linear accelerator came on the scene in the United States in the 1940s.
- In the mid-1940s, William Hansen invented the linear accelerator. His research was based on work by Russ and Sigurd Varian, brothers who founded Varian Associates; 1954 marked the first medical use of the linear accelerator.
- In the meantime, radium (which had been discovered in 1898 by Marie and Pierre Curie) was being used to treat deep tumors
- 1949 L.G. Grummet, MD, designed a container for the use of cobalt-60 as a substitute for radium.

THE LINEAR ACCELERATOR (LINAC)

- The accelerator structure resembles a long pipe. The pipe is the path where charged particles (electrons) travel and gain energy from an alternating electromagnetic field.
- The typical accelerator consists of five main components: drive stand, gantry, patient support assembly (PSA), electronic cabinet, and console.
- The drive stand connects to the gantry; the gantry rotates on a horizontal axis on bearings within the drive stand, which is firmly secured to the floor; the stand contains the apparatus that drives the accelerator.
- The gantry is responsible for directing the beam out toward the patient. The major components in the gantry are the waveguides, electron gun, accelerator structure, and collimator head.
- The treatment gantry head (Figure 6-1) contains many intricate parts, including the bending magnet, target, primary collimators, monitor ion chamber, mirror and bulb assembly, secondary collimators, scattering foils, and flattening filter.
- The source of electrons is the electron gun; electrons start from rest in the gun and gain enough energy to approach the velocity of light after being assisted to intense acceleration by microwaves.
- Electrons enter the accelerator structure with relatively low velocity and experience progressive acceleration due to the introduced microwaves.
- The final electron energy is directly proportional to the length of the waveguide. Due to the limitations in the physical size of clinical linear accelerators (linacs), another technology has been developed that permits a shorter accelerating tube known as a standing wave accelerator guide.
- The design of the standing wave guide makes use of the concept of interference/Coolidge's cascading theory: when two electromagnetic waves are present at the same place, their energy potential increases across the tube.

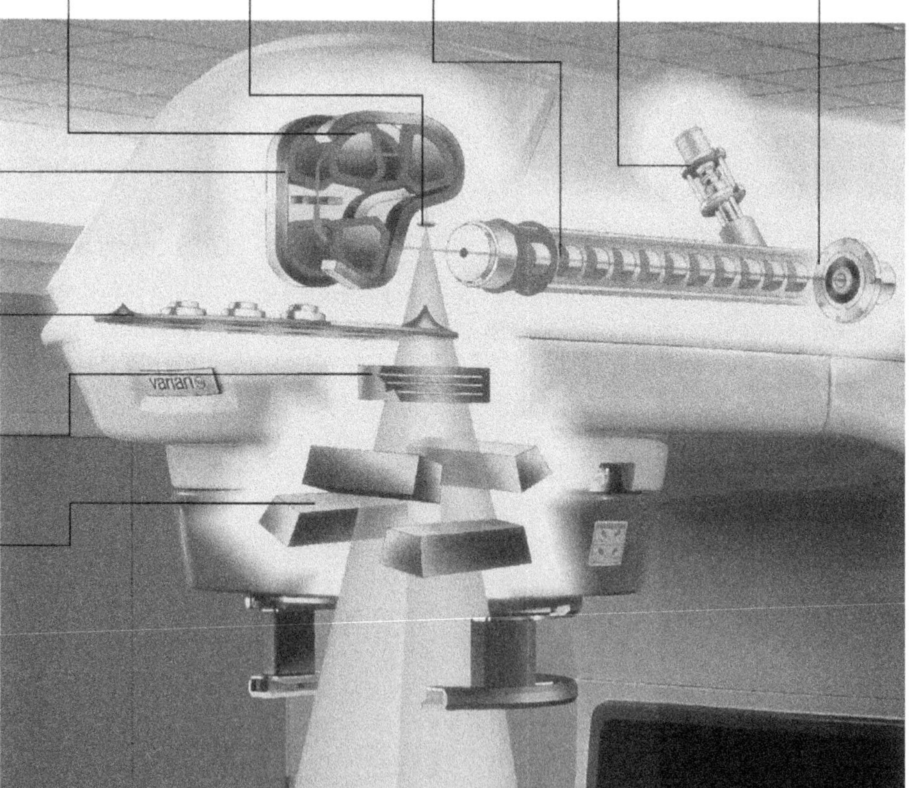

FIGURE 6-1 Linac gantry head cross section.

- The microwave power necessary to provide energy in the waveguide is provided by a magnetron or klystron.
- The magnetron is usually used in low energy linacs and generates high frequency microwave power.
- The klystron is required for higher energy units and is a generator of high frequency microwaves and also amplifies the microwaves.
- High energy machines have long accelerator tubes and need to be positioned horizontally. A bending magnet is therefore needed to direct the horizontal stream of electrons down and out toward the target and collimator opening.
- Two types of bending magnets are used: 90- or 270-degree bending magnets.
- The 90- and 270-degree bending magnets both serve the same purpose; however, the 270-degree magnet minimizes spatial dispersion of the beam.
- The electron beam is narrow in cross section—3-mm diameter. Its intensity is high in the center and drops quickly to nil as you move away from the center.
- The raw electron beam is referred to as a pencil beam.
- A scattering foil is used to spread the electron beam and achieve uniform electron fluence across the collimated area. This foil consists of thin metallic material, usually lead.
- The electron field size is typically defined by attachable cones; cones help control the free scattering of electrons in the air.
- For the production of x-rays/photons in the linac, the high energy electron beam is manipulated in a manner similar to electrons in diagnostic x-ray machines: the electrons are accelerated toward and collide with a heavy metal target, causing deceleration and conversion of energy to produce x-rays.
- The resulting photon beam has intense energy in the center and falls off as you move away from the central axis.
- The flattening filter is introduced into the path of photons to evenly distribute the energy of the photon beam; it is usually made of lead, tungsten, uranium, steel, aluminum, or a combination of heavy metals.
- The exiting beam is first collimated by a fixed primary collimator and then is incident on a monitoring ion chamber.
- Monitoring ion chambers keep track of dose rate and field symmetry.
- After passing through the ion chamber, the beam is further collimated by a mobile pair of collimators and/or multileaf collimators. The collimator area opening is typically limited to 40 cm × 40 cm.
- Field size setting is the actual measured field size at the isocenter of the linac and not at the location of the mobile collimators.
- The patient support assembly (PSA) is the apparatus that holds the patient and should have functions to move horizontally, vertically, and laterally and rotate on a stable axis around the isocenter.
- The operator's console is on the outside of the treatment vault and is where the patient may be monitored and the accelerator can be programmed to deliver a prescribed dose. Record and verify systems retain, recall, and display patient treatment data and record doses delivered.
- The electronic cabinet may be in the treatment vault or outside on an opposite wall and contains the auxiliary power distribution system and primary power distribution system, cooling system, and circuit breakers.

Quality Assurance for Linear Accelerators

- As the mechanics of the linear accelerator are very intricate and critical to the production of a quality beam and reliable output for dosing, regular quality assurance procedures are necessary.
- Values taken regarding output and performance are initially taken during acceptance testing.
- Acceptance testing requires comparison of output and performance values as measured against what the manufacturer has promised.
- After acceptance testing, commissioning takes place so that output and performance values are documented and used for treatment planning and dose delivery and for consistency in machine performance.
- Quality assurance procedures must include review of machine mechanics and reliability of indicators for beam direction and quality. What is most important is target accuracy and dose concentration with minimal effects on normal tissues.
- In addition, any built in interlocks in the R and V system instituted to keep patients, personnel, and the general pubic from unnecessary radiation exposure, must be reliable on a daily basis.
- Quality assurance procedures are grouped by priority: those of critical importance for accurate treatment delivery and patient/personnel safety should be verified daily. Other factors are recommended for review monthly and yearly during an equipment overhaul.
- Review the recommended quality assurance procedures published by the AAPM (Table 6-1).

TABLE 6-1 Daily Quality Assurance Procedures for Medical Accelerator*

Procedure	Machine Type and Tolerance		
	Non-IMRT	IMRT	SRS/SBRT
1. X-ray output constancy (all energies)	3%		
2. Electron output constancy (if special e-monitoring available for daily measurement, otherwise, weekly)			
3. Laser localization	2 mm	1.5 mm	1.0 mm
4. Distance indicator (ODI at isocenter)	2 mm	2 mm	2 mm
5. Collimator size indicator	2 mm	2 mm	1 mm
6. Door interlock		Functional	
7. Door closing safety		Functional	
8. Audiovisual monitors		Functional	
9. Stereotactic interlocks (lockout)	—	—	Functional
10. Radiation area monitor		Functional	
11. Beam on indicator		Functional	

*Refer to AAPM task group 142 report for monthly and annual QA. September 2009.

THE COBALT-60 MACHINE

- Before the use of linacs, the cobalt machine was the first high energy photon machine available in large numbers to the radiation therapy community
- The cobalt is a lot simpler in design but has some of the same basic components as the linac such as a drive stand, gantry, PSA, and operator's console.
- Since this machine uses a naturally decaying source of radiation, no AC/DC wiring is required. All that is needed is a source of electricity and motors to power the housing compartment containing the source.
- The cobalt-60 source is produced in a nuclear reactor by bombarding stable cobalt with neutrons. As the artificially created radioactive source decays, beta particles and two gamma photons are emitted with energies of 1.17 MV and 1.33 MV; the average of these two energies is 1.25 MV.
- The gantry head contains the source, source drawer or carrying wheel, stationary primary collimator, mobile secondary collimators, and field light source (bulb).
- Mobile collimators typically have an area opening limit of 35 cm × 35 cm.
- As natural decay is occurring, correction in the output for decay of about 1.09% per month has to be accounted for in treatment time calculations.
- The typical cobalt source is a cylinder ranging from 1 to 2 cm in diameter containing cobalt disks.
- The source is positioned in the gantry surrounded by protective housing made of lead filled steel or depleted uranium when the unit is off; housing should only allow 0.1% transmission.
- When the unit is on, the source is carried forward so that the circular end of the cylinder faces down and out toward the collimator opening. Timer error should be added to calculated treatment times to account for source traveling time on the drawer or wheel mechanism (Figure 6-2).
- The weight of the protective housing needs a counterbalance in the form of a beam stopper; the beam stopper also serves to absorb exiting beam and decreases the required amount of shielding opposite the primary beam.

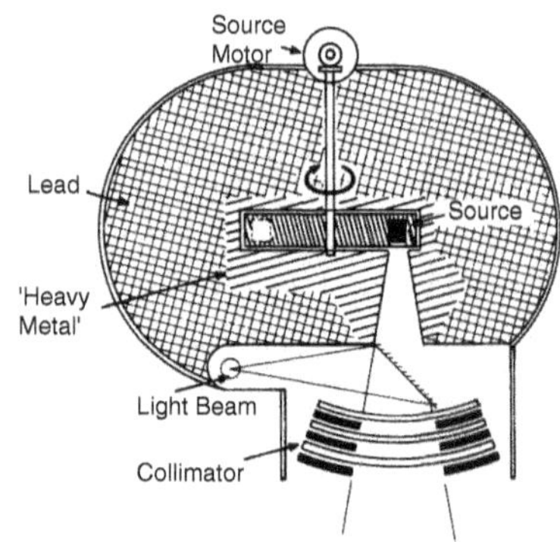

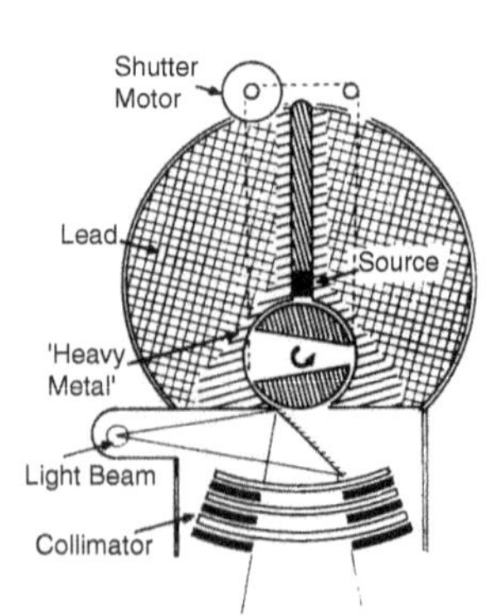

FIGURE 6-2 Cobalt gantry head cross section.

- Since the source is not a point source, the beam geometry is complicated by geometric penumbra.

$$\text{Penumbra} = \frac{s\,(SSD + d - SDD)}{SDD}$$

S = source size
D = depth
SSD = source to skin distance
SDD = source to diaphragm distance (collimator)

- Trimmer bars are tertiary collimators and are attachable to the collimator and help to minimize penumbra reaching the patient.
- Since the source is always in decay, the treatment room is never at background radiation levels. Therapists should minimize time in the treatment room and keep a reasonable distance from the gantry head containing the source.

Quality Assurance for Cobalt Teletherapy Unit

- As the cobalt units contain an active radioactive source, the quality assurance procedures must address safety of personnel and constancy of exposure to patients.
- Any safety interlocks would need to be checked daily; other mechanical details could be verified monthly or during yearly machine overhaul.
- Daily quality checks (Table 6-2) should be focused on limiting exposure to patients and personnel and beam direction.
- As you review quality assurance recommendations for teletherapy cobalt units, think about the most critical indicators for safety as those needed for daily verification.
- Think of the nature of nuclear transformation and how this phenomenon is associated with dose delivery. An acceptable time frame for fluctuations in dose would be at monthly intervals for a decaying source with a half-life of 5.26 years.
- Then, dose fluctuations and dose agreement with beam indicators such as the light field, collimators, and cross hairs should be verified monthly.

TABLE 6-2 Daily Quality Assurance Procedures for Cobalt Units*

Procedure	Tolerance
1. Door interlock	Functional
2. Radiation room monitor	Functional
3. Audiovisual monitors	Functional
4. Lasers	2 mm
5. Distance indicator (ODI)	2 mm

*Refer to AAPM task group 40 report for monthly and annual QA. April 1994.

OTHER PARTICLE ACCELERATORS

- To date, other particle accelerators have been used mostly in research.
- The betatron accelerates electrons and consists of a magnet fed by an alternating current of high frequency waves.
- Electrons are injected into an evacuated circular chamber and accelerated in a circular orbit in the presence of an electric field. Magnetic flux changes and keeps the electrons in the orbiting pattern, and the electron beam may be deflected out toward the collimator opening.
- A target may be introduced after the deflector to produce an x-ray beam.
- The betatron (Figure 6-3) was used in megavoltage radiation therapy in the 1950s, but it has very limited field sizes and low dose rates compared with the linac, making it unpopular for use in therapy today.
- The cyclotron has been and is still used in nuclear power plants to produce radioisotopes. Flourine-18 used in PET imaging is produced in proton cyclotrons.
- The cyclotron can produce deuteron, neutron, and proton beams and has been modified for more wide spread use in therapy.
- Particles are accelerated in a spiral pathway inside two evacuated D-shaped cavities, called dees (Figure 6-4), by a uniform magnetic field. The dees have a small space between them and have opposite polarity.
- An oscillating radiofrequency voltage with a constant frequency is introduced between the two dees and the charged particles accelerate while crossing the space between the two; more energy is gained as the particles continue to cross the space and the spiral diameter increases.

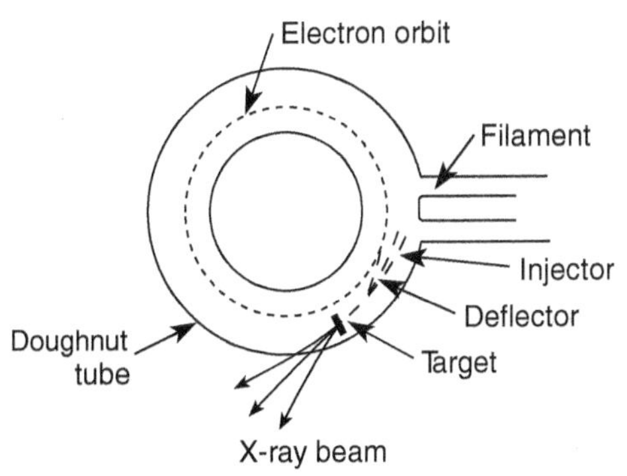

FIGURE 6-3 Betatron.

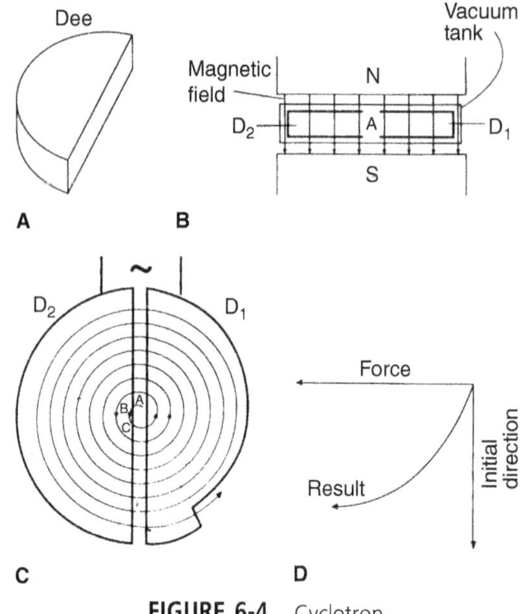

FIGURE 6-4 Cyclotron.

- Heavy particles can gain enough mass in the cyclotron that they go out of synch with the oscillating field; a special machine reduces the frequency of the voltage as the particle energy increases to keep this from happening. This is known as a synchrocyclotron.
- The microtron is an electron accelerator. The first microtron, used in 1972, generated a 10 MeV electron beam.
- A higher power microtron was later introduced and could produce a 22 MeV electron beam. It also had the ability to generate high power photons and multiple electron energies.
- In the circular microtron, electrons are accelerated by an oscillating electrical field of one or more microwave cavities. A magnetic field forces the electrons to move in a circular path and return to the "resonant cavity."
- As the electrons return, they receive higher energy and the orbits of increasing radius occur in the magnetic field similar to the betatron.
- A deflection tube of steel extracts the beam from the accelerating path. An electron or photon beam can be produced.
- The advantages of the microtron over the linac is that it has a simpler design and is physically smaller than the typical linac.

TOMOTHERAPY

- The tomotherapy machine, designed in the 1990s, has a ring gantry design such as the CT scanner and delivers radiation doses of 6 MV energy in a helical fashion.
- There is a binary multileaf collimator for beam shaping and intensity modulation.
- As the gantry rotates simultaneous with the advancing couch, helical fan-beam intensity modulated radiation therapy (IMRT) is delivered from all angles around the patient.
- The width of the fan beam is 40 cm and the maximum length the moving couch can accommodate is 160 cm.
- Delivery of modulated dose, 360 degrees around the patient, allows for more conformal delivery to small target volumes than accomplished with multiple angles and segments as in traditional IMRT regimens on a linear accelerator.
- During the treatment regimen, diagnostic quality sectional and/or three-dimensional images may be acquired using the tomotherapy unit (Figure 6-5) to verify accurate focus on the target volume.

BRACHYTHERAPY EQUIPMENT

- Radioactive sources used in brachytherapy are available sealed or unsealed.
- Sealed sources come in pellets, seeds, capsules, needles, buttons, or metal rods; pellets can be contained in small catheters with spacer material.
- Unsealed sources can be suspended in liquid for injection or ingestion; radioactive isotopes (Table 6-3) may also be electronically infused into dense materials known as plaques for surface applications.
- Traditional manual loading of sources require the use of special applicators/holders such as the tandem, ovoids, trocars, and in-dwelling catheters.
- Manually placed applicators historically would assure relatively stable placement of sources, after which placement could be verified with imaging.

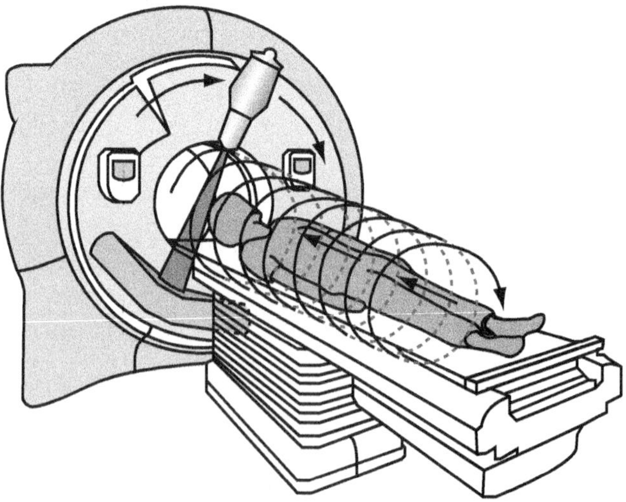

FIGURE 6-5 Tomotherapy unit with patient on PSA.

TABLE 6-3 Commonly Used Radioisotopes, Forms, and Applications

Isotope	Half-life	Source Form	Applications
Cesium-137	30 years	Tubes, needles	LDR intracavitary, interstitial
Iridium-192	73.8 days	Seeds	LDR interstitial, HDR interstitial, and intracavitary
Cobalt-60	5.26 years	Encapsulated spheres	HDR intracavitary
Iodine-125	60 days	Seeds	Interstitial
Palladium-103	17 days	Seeds	Interstitial
Gold-198	2.7 days	Seeds	Interstitial
Strontium-90	28.9 years	Plaque	Superficial ocular lesions
Strontium-89	51 days	IV solution	Diffuse bone metastases
Iodine-131	8.06 days	Capsule	Thyroid cancer

Modified from Clifford Chao KS, et al: *Radiation oncology: management decisions*, ed 2, Philadelphia, 2002, Lippincott, Williams, and Wilkins.

- Manually placed applicators and containers also facilitate ease of source removal in temporary brachytherapy procedures.
- Today, there are remote, afterloading applicators, such as accelerated breast irradiation devices (MammoSite, and electronic HDR units).

Quality Assurance for Brachytherapy

- When radioactive sources are used, dose rates are critical for reference at any point in time.
- Dose rates of radioactive isotopes are given by the use of radiation detectors.
- Radiation detectors need regular calibrating so that readings are reliable.
- Detectors should be calibrated monthly or after each repair.
- Sources themselves should be inspected for physical integrity by visual inspection, leak testing, and activity measurement.
- Physical integrity should be checked before each use.
- Source strength or activity should be checked upon receipt and then verified at an agreed upon interval depending on the half-life; activity should be checked against the stated manufacturer's value.
- Source strength calibrations have to be traceable to a national standards laboratory.
- Source uniformity and symmetry can be checked using radiographic procedures.
- All sources maintained in inventory are required to be wipe tested for leakage radiation semiannually at a minimum.
- Wipe testing should be performed upon receipt and then at 6-month intervals for sources with long half-lives.
- Afterloading devices can be checked using radiographic imaging for source position.
- Remote afterloaders should be checked for functional performance and source activity.
- Following implantation, radiation surveys must be performed immediately in and around the patients room.
- If the patient is to remain in the hospital, adjoining rooms must be lower than 0.2 mSv per hour.
- If the patient is to be released, with permanent implants, radiation levels need to be less than 0.5 mSv/hour at 1 m.
- If the patient is released following temporary implants, surveys must be performed of the room to assure that all active sources have been removed and returned to a safe location.
- Main objectives for the quality assurance program regarding brachytherapy should include appropriate documentation of written prescription, date, identification of the patient, treatment area and related calculations, and any deviations from standard practices or complications.

CONVENTIONAL SIMULATORS

- Conventional simulators are diagnostic-range x-ray tubes mounted in a rotational gantry that mimic the commonly used linear accelerator; there is a PSA that should also mimic all motor functions of the PSA used for treatment.
- Conventional simulators are used to localize the target volume using fluoroscopy and/or static two-dimensional radiographic imaging.
- Fluoroscopic and diagnostic imaging settings must be able to accommodate various patient thicknesses and tissue densities for accurate localization.
- An image intensifier positioned opposite the tube converts exiting photon energy to visible light to be viewed on a monitor.

- Treatment fields may easily be delineated by use of shutters and field defining wires, gradicule, and optical distance indicators.
- The conventional simulator room should also have a laser system that mimics the positioning laser system in the treatment room.
- Initial fields may be planned, postplanning fields may be verified, and manual beam shaping devices, such as lead or Cerrobend blocks, may also be verified on the conventional simulator.
- One limitation of the conventional simulator is that target localization can only be performed with visual representation of tissues at the ends of the density spectrum—bone versus air—unless contrast materials are used.

CT SIMULATORS

- CT simulators were invented to enhance target localization; conventional simulators only provided anatomic target data in two dimensions showing bone and air or contrast filled cavities, whereas the CT simulator brought the capacity to view anatomic data in three dimensions with all tissue densities easily visualized.
- CT simulators are modeled after the diagnostic CT scanner for the production of cross-sectional images; the cross-sectional image allows the planning therapist, dosimetrist, and physician to visualize the target volume and all other tissues around it.
- The CT simulator must have a large bore to allow for a variety of patient positions and positioning devices; room lasers and flat table top are also required.
- Acquisition of anatomic data can occur using axial or helical scanning.
- Helical scanning is thought to provide more data for the computer to use for image reconstruction; however, data for reconstruction can be controlled by setting appropriate slice thicknesses and scan intervals in either mode.
- Images from the CT simulator should be easily transferable to the treatment planning system.

Quality Assurance for Conventional Simulators

- Since conventional simulators were designed to replicate the movements of the linear accelerator, similar quality assurance activities are necessary.
- The conventional simulator needs image quality, field defining, and beam directional device-related quality assurance activities (Table 6-4).

TABLE 6-4 Daily Quality Assurance Procedures for Conventional Simulators*

Procedure	Tolerance
1. Lasers	2 mm
2. Distance indicator (ODI)	2 mm

*Refer to AAPM task group 40 report for monthly and annual QA. April 1994.

Quality Assurance for CT Simulators

- The more widely used CT simulators give more detailed information on tissue density and geometry; therefore, the quality assurance procedures for the CT simulator will focus on the interpretation and transfer of data and geometry.
- Patient and personnel safety cannot be ignored in quality assurance for CT simulators.
- As you review quality assurance for the CT simulator, note that safety switches, alignment of a gantry laser with the center of the image, image performance (to include CT number accuracy for water, image noise, and in plane spatial integrity per x and y directions) are daily recommended checks (Table 6-5).
- Orientation of gantry lasers, spacing of lateral wall lasers with respect to lateral gantry lasers, orientation of wall and ceiling lasers with respect to the imaging plane, mechanical table functions, image reconstruction, and exposure quality are recommended to be checked monthly.

DIGITAL IMAGERS FOR FIELD VERIFICATION

- In the early days of therapy, treatment field verification was achieved during therapy by placing film in special cassettes opposite the beam as it exited the patient (film-screen method).
- Special emulsion film in heavily screened cassettes or in oncology cassettes could be exposed with just a few monitor units to a couple hundred monitor units.

TABLE 6-5 Daily Quality Assurance Procedures for CT Simulators*

Procedure	Tolerance
1. CT number accuracy for water	0 ± 5 HU
2. Image noise	Manufacturer specifications
3. In plane spatial integrity for x or y direction	± 1 mm
4. Alignment of gantry lasers with the center of imaging plane	± 2 mm

*Refer to AAPM task group 66 report for monthly and annual QA. October 2003.

- Dark room or daylight processing of film was required before portal verification would be possible.
- Images using the film-screen method on megavoltage therapy machines had low contrast due to the high beam energy and low absorption in the patient.
- Today systems such as cone beam CT (CBCT) have improved treatment portal verification greatly.
- CBCT provides three-dimensional imaging for field verification; its cone-shaped kilovoltage beam captures a broader volume of data at each revolution around the patient (Figure 6-6).
- The cone-shaped beam makes it easier for the associated image translator to reconstruct anatomic data, producing a clearer and more accurate image.
- CBCT can be integrated into a linear accelerator system and mounted on the gantry so that three-dimensional or two-dimensional sectional target localization verification may be performed before treatment delivery.
- Onboard imaging (OBI) systems (Table 6-6) such as CBCT help therapists make adjustments to treatment fields more readily as reproducibility of setup fluctuates or patient external and internal anatomy changes throughout the treatment course.
- Another OBI device comes in the form of a kV x-ray tube, also available to be integrated into the linear accelerator; it is mounted on the gantry.
- The kV x-ray tube allows for the capturing of two-dimensional diagnostic quality images to verify field placement before treatment.
- Another OBI device consists of a simple image detection unit, digital image processor, and color monitor.

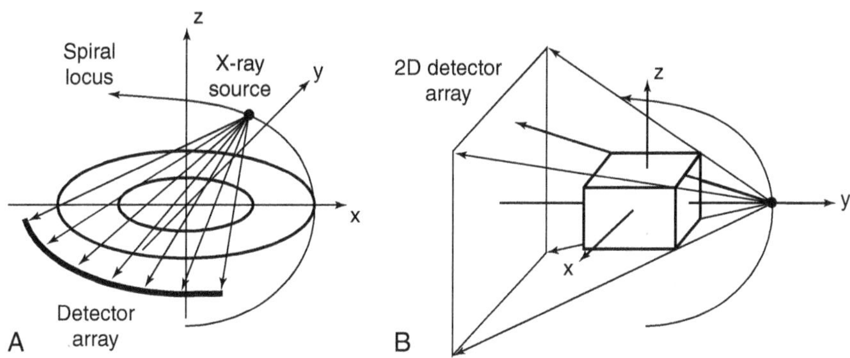

FIGURE 6-6 Fan beam versus cone beam CT geometry.

TABLE 6-6 Comparison of Various Online Electronic Portal Imaging Devices (EPID); Also Referred to as Onboard Imaging (OBI) systems

EPID/OBI System Types	Characteristics
Cone beam CT (CBCT)	- Three-dimensional, cross-sectional imaging - Visualization of the target volume location - Cone beam may be kV or MV rotating 360 degrees around the patient (kV requires a retractable arm positioned at 90 degrees to the MV treatment head) - A back projection algorithm reconstructs the images
Fluoroscopic portal imaging detector	- Detector has a metal plate and fluorescent phosphor screen, a 45-degree mirror and television camera - Plate converts the x-rays to electrons and fluorescent screen converts electrons to light photons - Mirror deflects light to the TV camera and camera produces an image
Ionization chamber detector	- Grid of ionization chamber type electrodes - Two metal plates spaced about 1 mm apart, with the space filled with isobutene - Electrodes on one plate are oriented 90 degrees to electrodes on the other plate - Voltage is applied between electrodes and ionization at the intersection is measured - Selection of each electrode on each plate produces a two- dimensional ionization map and is then converted into a gray scale image
Amorphous silicon flat panel detector	- Solid state array of amorphous silicone photodiodes and field effect transistors - Metal plate fluorescent screen combination - Light photons produce electron hole pairs in the photodiodes; quantity is proportional to intensity, allowing an image to be produced

- The detection unit and image processor are mounted to the linac gantry; images are captured, filed, and stored on disk for archiving and retrieval.
- The digital processor substitutes the poor contrast MV images with a high x-ray energy digital fluoroscopy imaging system, resulting in instant images of better quality.
- Small exposures of three monitor units or less are all required; an image is produced in 1 second, limiting motion while filming.
- The image is formed on the fluoroscopic screen and transferred to the camera via a high reflectance mirror positioned at 45 degrees under the fluoroscopic screen.
- The camera must be calibrated every few days and the detector should be calibrated monthly or whenever the detector may have been bumped or moved.
- The detector has a fluoroscopic screen and a high resolution video camera located near the gantry.
- Respiratory gating systems may also be used as a means toward portal verification but most appropriately as a means toward using the location of the target to focus the radiation from day to day.
- Image-guided radiation therapy (IGRT) is a concept introduced after it became apparent that some targets are mobile.
- To maintain small margins around target margins that are mobile, a method for daily localization is necessary.
- Respiratory gating was developed in Japan for use in heavy ion therapy; now it can be used with the linac and can be applied during treatment of any area where breathing may affect the location of the target.
- A reflective marker is placed on the patient, a video camera follows the marker and will track its position as the patient breathes.
- Marker movement sends a signal that is processed by a computer that initiates a beam hold when the target is out of preset parameters; parameters have to be set during simulation with markers in place.
- Another system uses breath hold for administration of dose; breathing patterns are monitored and measured by a mouthpiece and shown on a monitor.
- When optimal breath hold volume is achieved, a balloon blocks airflow to the patient for a brief period of time and dose can be delivered only during the breath hold periods.
- A mobile ultrasound unit was introduced to use sound wave imaging as a means toward IGRT.
- An ultrasound unit—B-mode acquisition and targeting (BAT) —positioned near the linac treatment table can be used to visualize the location of targets before treatment.
- The location of the target during each imaging session is compared with the location of the target during simulation and table and patient may be adjusted to bring the visualized target in line with the predetermined isocenter.
- Widest application for BAT has been for the localization of the prostate gland as it has been noted that the gland may move from day to day; ultrasound is performed transabdominally.
- Similar to BAT is the BrainLab system; it uses a reflective marker array attached to an ultrasound probe.
- The array is calibrated by an infrared tracking system relative to reflective markers on the patients body.

Quality Assurance for Portal Verification Devices

- Portal verification systems must be calibrated regularly to assure that quality images are produced, limiting the need for repeat imaging.
- OBI systems need regular calibration so that digital image processing is at an optimum.
- Systems such as the Theraview system sends a weekly message indicating that the fluoroscopic screen needs to be exposed so that adjustments may be made to the detector.

STEREOTACTIC RADIATION THERAPY DEVICES

- Stereotactic radiation therapy (SRT) or stereotactic radiosurgery (SRS) are techniques that use very small and highly conformal, non-coplanar beams to treat small target volumes while sparing neighboring tissues.
- The main characteristics that distinguishes SRT/SRS is the use of circular beams, arc angles, and often multiple isocenters through multiple planes to achieve high dose concentration.
- SRT can be performed in a single fraction or multiple fractions.
- When single fractions are used, the term appropriate is SRS; when multiple fractions are used, the appropriate term is SRT.

- Single-dose SRS procedures are performed on functional disorders, some benign tumors and metastatic lesions, and sometimes for dose boosting where doses range from 12 to 25 Gy.
- Multiple fraction SRT typical dose sizes are 7 Gy/fraction for a total of 42 Gy or 4 Gy/fraction for a total of 40 Gy.
- Techniques may make use of photons, electrons, or gamma radiation beams.
- During SRT/SRS margins are very small, requiring elaborate immobilization and targeting systems along with strict treatment planning.
- Stereotactic head rings/frames are surgically attached to the skull and have to be fitted to an indexed positioning device attached by brackets to the patient support apparatus (multiple fraction SRT would require this to be in place for a prolonged period).
- A gamma knife unit allows the positioning of up to 201 sources in a hemispherical helmetlike shield; the helmet only accommodates the skull for SRS to brain tumors. Stereotactic frame then fits tightly into the hemispherical helmet where the cobalt sources are collimated with beam channels; channels may be 4 to 18 mm in diameter.
- Linac based SRT uses strict localization of the target, stereotactic frame, PSA brackets, and focused circular fields (achieved dynamically or with attachable cones); beams may be arced or static.
- Attachable cones are typically made of Cerrobend encased in stainless steel; cones range in diameter from 5 to 30 mm.
- A miniature 6 MV linac on a robotic arm, known as Cyberknife, is another approach to SRS.
- No stereotactic frame is used for Cyberknife; rather, an image-guided target localization system is used so that treatment may be delivered to extracranial targets.
- Monitoring and tracking of a target position is continuous so that the beam is aimed accurately.

TREATMENT ACCESSORIES

- Treatment accessories are used to indicate beam direction and location of the isocenter, modify the absorption and scattering characteristics of the beam, or to aid in positioning and immobilization of the patient.
- Beam directional devices would include: front and back pointers, breast bridges, lasers, cross hairs, gradicule, BB trays, the field light and mirror assembly, digital readouts for gantry and collimator angles, and electron cones and collimators.
- Beam modifiers would include: standard wedges, dynamic wedges, custom tissue compensators, bolus materials, Cerrobend blocks, and multileaf collimators.
- Positioning aids help establish the desired patient position and would include: pillows and sponges, headrests, chin-straps, breast boards, and wing boards.
- Immobilization devices are intended to limit patient motion and would include: Aquaplast, vac lock systems, alpha cradle, bite blocks, casts, molds, and tape (simple immobilization).

Quality Assurance for Accessories

- Treatment accessories need to be checked for physical integrity and reliability.
- Latching mechanisms for interlocking accessories such as cones, trays, and standard wedges should be checked monthly.
- Fabricated Cerrobend blocks may be checked for voids using radiographic imaging; when pouring, care must be taken to prevent air bubble formation.
- Bolus materials should be checked regularly for cleanliness and voids, and for appropriate thickness.
- Positioning and immobilization devices should be regularly inspected for tears, leaks, and broken parts.

TREATMENT PLANNING AND RECORD AND VERIFY (R AND V) SYSTEMS

- There are several computerized treatment planning systems.
- Before computerized treatment planning, hand drawn isodose renderings had to be generated for customized planning.
- Single and multiple field atlas' were available to superimpose over hand drawn anatomic drawings to find the optimal plan for the patient.
- Early computerized planning systems only allowed two-dimensional representation of anatomy and isodose distribution.
- Systems needed to be programmed with special algorithms for the calculation of cumulative dose points and could only generate open field plans.
- Today's systems have programmed algorithms that allow for therapy planning with cumulative dose points throughout the treated volume, tissue density

heterogeneity recognition, visualization of dose points in 3 dimensions and ability to shape fields and reflect dosimetric influences on referenced output.

- Computers also brought the ability to store individual patient data for daily verification of field details.
- Record and verify systems (R and V) were developed to minimize treatment errors.
- Errors in treatment may be related to mechanical malfunction, patient variations, or technical variations.
- Before computerized R and V, therapists had to rely on hand-written documentation of treatment parameters and manual settings.
- R and V systems in its early stages would only show patient parameters as reference data without any interlocks or warnings if parameters did not agree.
- Today's systems not only show patient parameters but have safety interlocks that require an override when parameters do not match; moreover, daily doses are recorded on disk, making manual charting unnecessary.
- As R and V systems serve as both a quality control system and documentation tool, quality assurance processes must include a review of accurate translation of inputted data and accurate retention of daily treatment activity.

Quality Assurance for Treatment Planning Systems and R and V Systems

- Treatment planning systems are an integral part of accurate treatment delivery.
- Its fundamental performance must constantly be under scrutiny; this includes the interpretation of data and algorithmic calculations.
- As these computerized systems are relied upon for daily and cumulative dose information, it is imperative that a small tolerance of error is acceptable (2% tolerance for isodose distributions and monitor unit calculations).
- Some departments may employ a secondary calculation program to double check the primary treatment planning software for dose calculation; the double check may be computerized or manual.
- Input and output devices should be checked daily, prediction algorithms and transfer of data (i.e., from CT) should be checked monthly for reliability; it is acceptable to verify monitor unit calculation accuracy yearly.
- It should be noted that some treatment centers may also employ external dose measuring mechanisms to verify the accuracy of planning systems, such as TLD, and diode measuring for surface dose verification.
- IMRT systems should be checked for accurate dose delivery. Independent and individual plan verification is strongly recommended.
- A quality tool such as the "mapcheck" system, which produces portal intensity maps for each field using a phantom, is a good indicator for planned intensity across the treatment field.
- Record and verify systems are only as good as the data inputted.
- Quality assurance for the R and V systems may include a manual, labor intensive review of data.
- A thorough weekly review of the patient charts (Table 6-7) is recommended whether in written form or electronic.
- A relatively easy way to check the R and V system is for the therapist to review the treatment plan before the initiation of treatment.

TABLE 6-7 Sample Weekly Chart Review Checklist

Review Items	Date 5/10	Date 5/17	Date 5/24	Date 6/2
History and physical	√			
Pathology	√			
Operative reports	√			
Surgical reports	√			
Complete therapy prescription	√			
Stage of disease indicated	√			
Simulation note(s)		√		
Pain assessment		√	√	√
Physics/dosimetry check		√	√	√
Billing	√		√	√
Identification photos		√		
Intent of therapy indicated	√			
Discharge summary				√
Final physics check				√
Final billing review				√

- Review the computerized treatment plan to verify that field sizes, portal arrangement, beam shaping, and use of modifiers documented in the plan agree with the information shown in the R and V system; this quick review gives adequate opportunity to identify and intercept potential errors.

BIBLIOGRAPHY

Clifford Chao KS, et al: *Radiation oncology: management decisions*, ed 2, Philadelphia, 2002, Lippincott Williams & Wilkins.

Kahn FM: *The physics of radiation therapy*, ed 4, Philadelphia, 2010, Lippincott, Williams, and Wilkins.

Podgorsak EB: *Radiation oncology physics: a handbook for teachers and students*, ed 1, Vienna, 2005, International Atomic Energy Agency.

Report of AAPM Radiation Therapy Committee Task Group 40. April 1994.

Report of AAPM Radiation Therapy Committee Task Group 66. October 2003.

Report of AAPM Radiation Therapy Committee Task Group 142. September 2009.

Seeram E: *Computed tomography: physical principles, clinical applications and quality control*, ed 3, St Louis, 2009, Saunders.

Stanton R, Stinson D: *Applied physics for radiation oncology*, ed 2, Madison, 2009, Medical Physics Publishing.

Washington CM, Leaver D: *Principles and practice of radiation therapy*, ed 3, St Louis, 2010, Mosby.

REVIEW EXERCISES

1. In 1 month, the output of a cobalt machine would reduce by about:

a. 0.1%
b. 1%
c. 2%
d. 5%

2. The protective housing around the cobalt source in the cobalt machine should only allow transmission of ______ of the output.

a. 0.1%
b. 1%
c. 2%
d. 5%

3. The target of the linac must have:

a. A low melting point
b. A high melting point
c. The ability to bend
d. Low thermal conductivity

4. The source of electrons in a linear accelerator is the:

a. Klystron
b. Magnetron
c. Electron gun
d. Waveguide

5. What type of target is used in high energy linear accelerators?

a. Transmission type
b. Reflection type
c. Refraction type
d. None of the above

6. Trimmer bars are attached to the collimator of the cobalt machine to reduce the effect of:

a. Penumbra
b. Symmetry
c. Flatness
d. Dose

7. Calculate the width of penumbra at depth for a patient treated on the 80-cm SAD cobalt unit. The source diameter is 2.0 cm, the SDD is 40 cm, and the treatment SSD is 75 cm.

8. Change the source diameter to 3.0 cm in the above case and see what happens to the penumbra.

9. Change the SDD to 30 cm in the previous case and see what happens to the penumbra.

10. Increase the SSD to 77 cm and see what happens to the measured penumbra.

11. Which of the following machines does not accelerate electrons?

a. Microtron
b. Betatron

c. Cyclotron
d. X-ray tube

12. The purpose of the flattening filter in the linac is to:
    a. Direct the stream of electrons out toward the collimator opening
    b. Prevent deflection of microwaves
    c. Evenly distribute and spread out the raw electron beam across a specified area
    d. Evenly distribute the energy of the photon beam across a specified area

13. What is the purpose of the ion monitor chamber in the linear accelerator?

14. What is the purpose of the magnetron and klystron in the linear accelerator?

15. Why does the cobalt machine not have an electron gun?

16. Trimmer bars attached to the cobalt collimator system should not be allowed closer than 15 cm from the patient's skin. Briefly explain.

Circle the correct word.

17. As distance from the source increases, penumbra (increases, decreases).

18. As the SDD increases, penumbra (increases, decreases).

19. As the source size decreases, penumbra (increases, decreases).

20. The target in the linear accelerator is typically made of (tungsten, aluminum).

Think About It

21. Briefly explain why teletherapy cobalt units did not need a circulating cooling system.

22. Irregular surface contours may be compensated for by using standard wedges, using customized tissue compensators, or by appropriately placing bolus material on/in the irregular surface. What is the advantage of using standard wedges and customized tissue compensators over bolus materials for irregular surface contours?

23. Radium has an extremely long half-life and a relatively high average gamma energy-making the source easy to use repeatedly for a long period of time and suitable for delivering substantial, penetrating dose to tissue. Why is radium no longer used in brachytherapy procedures?

24. Which of the following radioisotopes is used for diffuse bone metastasis?
    a. Cesium-137
    b. Cobalt-60
    c. Strontium-90
    d. Strontium-89

25. Which of the following radioisotopes is a pure beta emitter?
    a. Cesium-137
    b. Cobalt-60

c. Phosphorus-32
d. Iodine-131

26. The field light on the linear accelerator is intended to represent:

a. The area of radiation exposure
b. The size of the target
c. The width, length, and depth of the treatment field
d. The distance from the source of radiation to the patient's skin

27. The teletherapy cobalt machine has a beam stopper. The purpose of the beam stopper is to:

a. Prohibit the primary beam from penetrating adjacent wall and ceiling
b. Prohibit scatter radiation in the treatment room
c. Act as a counter-balance to the heavy gantry head
d. a and c are correct

28. The scattering foil is placed in the path of the stream of electrons in the linear accelerator when programmed to operate in the ______ beam mode.

a. Proton
b. Electron
c. X-ray
d. Fluoroscopic

29. The klystron or magnetron is the source of ______ in the linear accelerator:

a. Microwaves
b. Alternating current
c. Accelerated electrons
d. Magnetic fields

30. The cyclotron may produce ______ beams.

a. Electron
b. X-ray
c. Proton
d. Gamma ray

31. The purpose of a positioning device is to:

a. Make the patient comfortable
b. Accommodate the most appropriate position for accurate treatment delivery
c. Prevent or limit patient motion during treatment
d. Limit the setup time

32. The energy range for the early generation superficial therapy machines is:

a. 50 to 150 kV
b. 150 to 500 kV
c. 600 to 1000 MV
d. 20 to 25 MeV

33. A long cylinder loaded with radioisotopes and placed in the vaginal space could be used to treat the:

a. Vaginal vault
b. Endometrium
c. Pelvic side wall
d. Vulva

34. The linear accelerator generates a high-energy photon or electron beam by:

a. Accelerating charged particles in a circular pattern
b. Accelerating charged particles in a linear path
c. Producing electromagnetic pulses used to accelerate protons and neutrons
d. Keeping photons in synch with a magnetic field

35. Output corrections must be made monthly when using cobalt sources. The correction is about:

a. 0.1 % per month
b. 1 % per month
c. 5 % per month
d. 10 % per month

36. Geometric penumbra, characteristic of the cobalt beam, increases with:

1. Increasing beam energy
2. Increasing source size
3. Increasing distance from the source
4. Decreasing beam energy

a. 2, 4
b. 1, 2
c. 3, 4
d. 2, 3

Matching

37. ____ Radium-226
38. ____ Iodine-125
39. ____ Cesium-137
40. ____ Gold-198

A. 74.2 days
B. 60 days
C. 30 days
D. 2.7 days
E. 30 years
F. 1622 years
G. 1622 days

41. Heyman capsules may be used to treat the:

a. Vaginal vault
b. Endometrium
c. Vulva
d. Prostate

42. The Fletcher's suite application is an example of:

a. Interstitial low dose rate brachytherapy
b. Intracavitary low dose rate brachytherapy
c. Permanent implant brachytherapy
d. Injected, unsealed source brachytherapy

43. The BAT system uses ______ energy to localize the treatment target.

a. x-ray
b. microwave
c. radiofrequency
d. ultrasound

44. The important QA test(s) associated with the light field are (circle all correct):

a. Field size accuracy
b. Beam output
c. Light and radiation field coincidence
d. None of the above

45. Functional performance of radiation therapy equipment can (circle all correct):

a. Not vary with time
b. Change due to malfunction of system electronics or component fault
c. Change due to wear and tear of the equipment
d. Change due to environmental conditions

46. The target to patient skin distance is measured using (circle all correct):

a. A meter scale
b. An SSD rod
c. An ODI indicator
d. None of the above

47. The collimator, gantry, and couch of a conventional simulator rotate about their respective axes. The recommended tolerance for locating the isocenter in these rotations is a sphere of dimension:

a. 2 mm radius
b. 2 mm diameter
c. 5 mm radius
d. None of the above

48. The tolerance for the localizing laser and the ODI indicator is:

a. 1 mm
b. 2 mm
c. 5 mm
d. None of the above

49. The constancy of linac output for photon and electron beams must be checked:

a. Daily
b. Weekly
c. Monthly
d. Only during commissioning

50. The constancy of linac output, when compared with the benchmark values established during commissioning, must be within:

a. 1%
b. 3 %
c. 5 %
d. None of the above

51. The symmetry and flatness of the clinical photon beam can be checked using (circle all correct):

a. Film
b. A beam profiler
c. A calorimeter
d. None of the above

52. The x-ray beam in the linac must exhibit flatness within about:

a. 1%
b. 2%
c. 5%
d. None of the above

53. Scan and couch vertical positional accuracy for CT planning must be:

a. <1 mm
b. About 2 mm
c. About 5 mm
d. About 1 cm

54. Which of the following checks must be carried out daily on the cobalt machine? (circle all correct):

a. Function of radiation room monitor
b. Function of door interlocks
c. Beam output
d. Timer error

55. Cobalt beam output must be checked:

a. Daily
b. Weekly
c. Monthly
d. Annually

56. Full calibration and overhaul of treatment equipment must be carried out:

a. Daily
b. Weekly
c. Monthly
d. Annually

57. In the case of brachytherapy sources:

a. All sources must be leak tested
b. Short half-life sources need never be tested for leakage
c. Sources not in use need not be tested for leakage
d. Long half-life sources only need leak testing annually

58. The exact position of the source in the applicator can be checked by (circle all correct):

a. Visual inspection
b. Measuring the AKS strength of the source
c. Taking a radiograph
d. None of the above

59. Brachytherapy sources must be calibrated (circle all correct):

a. By the manufacturer only
b. By the accredited dosimetry calibration laboratory only
c. Before being used for clinical dosimetry
d. By a user using a chamber with calibration traceable to an accredited dosimetry calibration laboratory

60. In a brachytherapy procedure room, the following items must be available all the time (circle all correct):

a. A radiation survey meter
b. A temporary storage container
c. A cutter and long-handled tongs
d. All of the above

61. The tolerance for the coincidence of light and radiation field, in the case of the medical linac is:

a. 2 mm or 1% of field length being measured, whichever is greater
b. 3 mm
c. 5 mm
d. None of the above

62. Localizing lasers on simulators must be within ______ of isocenter.

a. 1 mm
b. 2 mm
c. 3 mm
d. 2 cm

Below are 13 components of the linear accelerator. In the statements that follow, indicate which components are used. Some may be used more than once.

A. Electron gun B. Accelerating guide C. Waveguide D. Bending magnet
E. Target F. Scattering foil G. Flattening filter H. Ion chamber
I. Field light J. Collimator jaws K. Klystron L. Modulator
M. Radiofrequency driver

63. Microwave power is produced to accelerate electrons. ______

64. Microwave power is directed toward the accelerator guide. ______

65. Reference signal is provided for generation of microwave power. ______

66. Electrons are produced. ______

67. Electrons are accelerated to high energy. ______

68. At the end of acceleration, high energy electrons are focused toward the collimator opening. ______

69. X-rays are produced by bremsstrahlung and characteristic radiation process. ______

70. The electron beam is spread out uniformly over the field area. ______

71. X-ray beam intensity is made uniform over the field size at the isocenter. ______

72. Monitors radiation output. ______

73. Monitors radiation beam uniformity by monitoring and controlling symmetry and flatness.________

74. Produces high voltage and high power electrical pulses to generate microwave power.________

75. These components, through which electrons travel, are under very high vacuum. ________

76. Microwaves travel through these components and are prevented from reflecting backward. ________

77. During a split field test for longitudinal displacement of the collimator for jaw symmetry, the collimator is rotated through an angle of:

- **a.** 360 degrees
- **b.** 270 degrees
- **c.** 180 degrees
- **d.** 90 degrees

78. To check the accuracy of gantry digital readouts, one could use:

- **a.** Closed collimators
- **b.** A spirit level at 45-degree angle increments
- **c.** A breast bridge at 90-degree angle increments
- **d.** A spirit level at 180-degree angle increments

79. A short exposure is taken on a radiographic film aligned with metallic marks on the borders of a collimated light field. This describes testing for:

- **a.** Light field/radiation coincidence
- **b.** Field flatness
- **c.** Collimator symmetry
- **d.** Field intensity

80. The linear scales on the treatment table are useful as an aid for:

1. Daily treatment setup
2. Translation of patient positions from simulation to treatment
3. Providing information regarding filament voltage

- **a.** 1
- **b.** 3
- **c.** 1, 2
- **d.** 1, 2, 3

81. Safety door interlocks should be checked:

- **a.** Annually
- **b.** Monthly
- **c.** Weekly
- **d.** Daily

82. Which of the following verifies the accuracy of radiation dose delivery?

- **a.** Back up timer, radiation off switch, door interlock, and emergency off switch
- **b.** Back up timer, door interlock, and override switch
- **c.** Radiation off switch and override switch
- **d.** Door interlock, radiation off switch, and collision ring

83. To ensure the patient's safety during treatment on a megavoltage linear accelerator, the patient must be monitored by:

- **a.** Directions given before treatment
- **b.** Intercommunication systems
- **c.** Watching the patient through a window
- **d.** Instructing the patient to yell out for help as needed

84. The process for testing a new accelerator against manufacturer's specifications before putting it into service is termed:

- **a.** Insurance calibration testing
- **b.** Acceptance testing
- **c.** Error correction testing
- **d.** Quality assurance testing

85. A high energy photon unit will require daily quality checks for the determination of:

- **a.** Light and radiation field coincidence
- **b.** Dose rate constancy
- **c.** Field symmetry and flatness
- **d.** Crosshair centering

86. Gantry and collimator indicators should be accurate to within ________ degree (s).

87. The common acceptable value for field flatness is about ________ % over the central 80% of the largest field size at isocenter.

88. All of the following might account for a beam's flatness deviating outside specifications, except:

- **a.** Flattening filter shift
- **b.** Target position shift
- **c.** Incorrect mirror angulation
- **d.** Fluctuation of current

89. While treating a patient using a rotational arc technique, the gantry rotates beyond the endpoint. This is likely a malfunction of the:

a. Operator's console
b. Limit switch
c. Collision ring
d. Override switch

90. A mechanical distance indicator is used to verify:

a. Gantry rotation
b. Collimator rotation
c. Field size congruence
d. Accuracy of optical distance indicator

91. If the mirror and bulb assembly has to be replaced, it is critical to perform the following quality check(s) before using the machine:

a. Dose rate
b. Light field and radiation coincidence
c. Collimator angle readout
d. Gantry angle readout

92. Which of the following has the shortest half-life?

a. Cesium-137
b. Gold-198
c. Iridium-192
d. Radon-222

93. The average gamma energy for cobalt-60 is:

a. 1.33 MV
b. 1.25 MV
c. 1.17 MV
d. 0.66 MV

94. Superficial therapy machines used short treatment distances because:

a. More precise positioning of the beam is provided than at longer distances
b. Less shielding against leakage radiation is required than at longer distances
c. Shorter distances are more biologically effective than longer distances
d. Percent depth dose falls off rapidly
e. Secondary radiation augments the skin dose

95. In early generation kV therapy machines, the quality of the photon beam could be increased by:

a. Increasing the mA
b. Decreasing the half value layer of material
c. Increasing the filtration
d. Decreasing the kVp

Write T for true and F for false for the following:

The effective energy of a photon beam can be increased by:

96. Increasing the beam on time. ______

97. Increasing the tube current. ______

98. Increasing the tube potential. ______

99. OBI is an acronym for:

a. Onboard imaging
b. Off beam indicator
c. Optical beam indicator
d. Off baseline measurement indicator

100. The machine that consists of a short metallic cylinder divided into two D-shaped cavities is known as the:

a. Cyclotron
b. Betatron
c. Microtron
d. Van De Graaf

101. The gantry head of the linear accelerator contains all of the following except:

a. Flattening filter
b. Ion chamber
c. X-ray target
d. Klystron

CHAPTER

7

Treatment Planning

Michael Hosto

FOCUS QUESTIONS

- What means are there for target localization during radiation therapy planning?
- What are the steps in the planning process using conventional simulation equipment and CT simulation equipment?
- How are appropriate patient positioning and immobilization techniques determined?
- What is the importance of acquiring both internal and external anatomy information for planning?
- What considerations are there for selection of treatment parameters, such as geometric field size and shape, modality, energy, and portal arrangement?
- What basic dosimetric calculations are necessary for everyday practice?
- How are diagnostic imaging modalities used in therapy planning?
- How are beam modifiers such as bolus, custom compensators, wedges, and modulation technologies used to customize treatment plans?
- What are key directional terms used in the interpretation of treatment plan data?
- What information is gleaned from the DVH, plan data sheet, and fluence map?
- What are some common beam arrangements?
- What types of clinical situations make certain beam arrangements appropriate?

CONVENTIONAL SIMULATORS

- A conventional radiation therapy simulator is a diagnostic x-ray unit in which the control features and functionality duplicate that of a therapeutic linear accelerator.
- Radiographs are taken documenting the gantry angles, field sizes, collimator angles, and table angles that will be used for treatment.
- Some simulators are equipped with fluoroscopy tubes to reduce the amount of film usage, decrease overall x-ray exposure to the patient, and hasten the planning process.
- A graduated scale or grid is located in the head of the gantry (Figure 7-1) and broadcasts an image of two perpendicularly crossed axes onto the skin of the patient.
- The grid is displayed onto the patient's skin with a light and mirror assembly in the gantry head representing the path of the x-ray beam.
- The intersection of the crossed axis is the central axis (CAX) when viewed on the patient's skin or on a radiograph; it denotes isocenter.
- The grid is graduated with hash marks or dots 1.0 to 2.0 cm apart.
- Linear accelerators require the use of a grid that is placed into the gantry head for use with port films so that the grid pattern visualized may be easily used as reliable reference to preceding simulation images.
- These removable grids are referred to as BB trays, fiduciary trays, or graticules.
- The grids/graticules on the conventional simulator and linear accelerators aid in target localization, determination of field size, and provide reference for treatment accuracy.
- There are mobile field-defining wires that are also reflected onto the patient's skin.
- Following determination of all treatment parameters, the patient's skin may be marked so that the isocenter and geometric field area is easily visualized.

CT SIMULATORS

- A computerized tomography machine (CT) is the most commonly used simulation modality today.
- They are used in conjunction with a three-dimensional treatment planning computer (3-D TPC) to virtually simulate the patient before treatment.

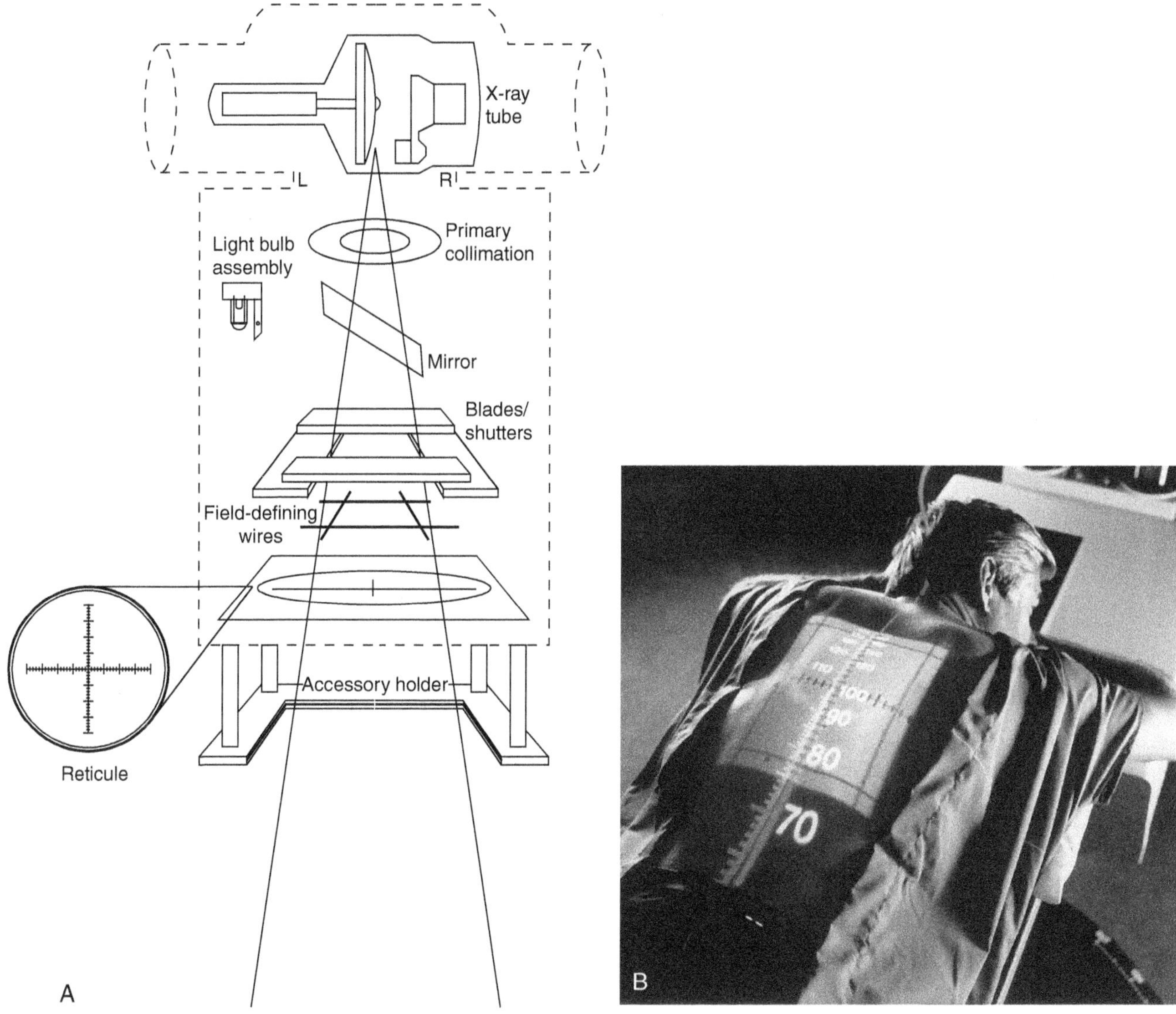

FIGURE 7-1 **A**, Cross axes demonstrated by reticule and **B**, projected on the patient's skin.

- A standard diagnostic CT or a dedicated CT simulator can be used.
- When using a diagnostic CT, the standard concave patient table top must be replaced with or adapted to a flat table top as found on a linear accelerator.
- The transverse or axial images created by the CT are fed into a 3-D treatment planning computer (TPC), which creates digitally reconstructed radiographs (DRRs) that are used as radiographic simulation reference images.
- DRRs can be printed to paper, x-ray film, or maintained digitally on a record and verify system.
- A grid is electronically placed on the DRR image by the 3-D TPC just as the grid seen on conventional simulation radiographs.
- Before scanning, slice thickness and pitch is selected based on established protocol.
- Helical or axial scanning should also be selected based on established protocol.
- Helical scanning lessens the possibility of skipped anatomic data collection.
- When simulating a patient for intensity modulated radiation therapy (IMRT), the CT slice thickness should be 2 to 3 mm to provide enhanced detail and optimal density differentiation for heterogenic dose calculation.
- A 5-mm slice thickness may be used for non-IMRT treatment planning to reduce the amount of computer contouring of anatomy.
- Keep in mind that as slice thickness is increased:
  1. DRR resolution declines
  2. Small structures may not be articulated well on the reconstructed images
- Images may be visualized in any anatomic plane; axial, coronal, or sagittal.

XYZ COORDINATE SYSTEM

- During simulation, isocenter localization is accomplished by using a three-dimensional XYZ coordinate system (Figure 7-2).
- Delineation of the treatment target and the placement of the isocenter relative to the target is referred to as localization.
- x is the transverse axis that extends right to left in the patient.
- y is the longitudinal axis extending head to foot.
- z is axis extending upward from the table top.
- When referencing an isocenter movement during simulation or reproducing the isocenter location for treatment, the XYZ localization method is most effective.
- The XYZ coordinates are fixed relative to the simulator, CT, TPC, or linear accelerator table top.
  1. If the patient is laying supine and head first on the table, the positive x axis is on the patient's left while the positive y axis is cephalic and the positive z axis is anterior.
  2. If the patient is laying prone and head first on the table, the positive x is at the patient's right, the y axis is unchanged, and the positive z axis is posterior.

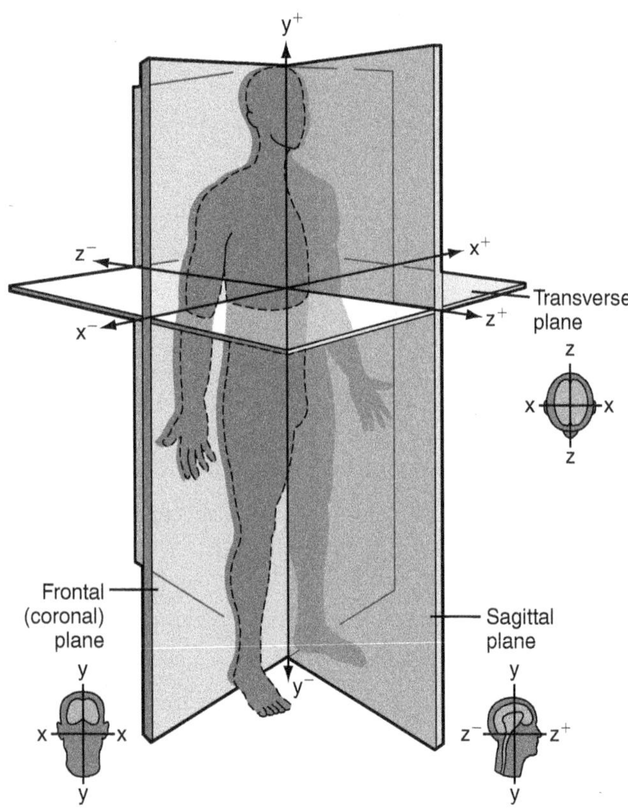

FIGURE 7-2 Diagram of XYZ coordinates.

  3. If the patient is laying supine and feet first, the positive x is on the patient's right, the positive y is caudal, and the z axis is unchanged.

LASERS USED FOR LOCALIZATION

- Lasers mounted on the walls and ceilings of simulation rooms and treatment rooms assist in localization.
- Laterally mounted wall lasers in conjunction with sagittal ceiling or wall mounted toe lasers are designed to converge at the point of SAD or isocenter.
- Lasers broadcast a very narrow beam of light onto the patient.
- Patient marks are placed on the laser light to indicate where the isocenter is located.
- For conventional simulators, isocenter localization is done with table movement.
- For CT simulators, isocenter localization is done either with laser movement or in the treatment planning computer after simulation.

GENERAL SIMULATION PRACTICES

- During the simulation process, the location of the isocenter is determined.
- Patient should be positioned in a manner that is suitable for the area of treatment and in a manner that can be accurately reproduced on the treatment table.
- Properly placed marks, photographs, and detailed descriptions aid in reproducibility.
- Patient marks can be applied with felt pens, paint pens, carfusion, or tattoos.
- To assure the patient maintains a level position, place marks using all laser lines.
- Sagittal alignment can be maintained by placing two marks 10 cm to 20 cm apart along the sagittal laser lines.
- If a conventional simulator is used or a treatment machine is used for initial simulation, the crosshairs provided by the gradicule can serve the same purpose as the sagittal lasers.
- When administering IMRT or conformal 3-D therapy, margins are tight leaving little room for setup error; patient marks alone are often too unstable to be solely relied upon.
- Verify patient setup radiographically as often as is feasibly possible.
- Soft and pliable head holders, pillows, sponges, and table mats should be avoided whenever possible; these devices foster setup inconsistency.

- Firm, commercial positioning aids provide more consistent setup.
- A firm knee support reduces the lordotic curvature of the spine and makes the patient more comfortable on the hard treatment couch.
- Knee supports should be avoided for treatment areas below the level of the diaphragm because leg elevation is seldom consistent. Leg elevation can cause variation in the location of the internal anatomy in the abdomen and pelvis.
- Immobilization devices help maintain patient position.

POSITIONING, POSITIONING AIDS, AND IMMOBILIZATION DEVICES

- Positioning aids should help facilitate a certain position consistently; these aids do not immobilize the patient.
- Whatever position is determined for your patient should be comfortable and easily accommodate the treatment strategy.
- A few examples of positioning aids include commercial head holders, custom head holders, knee sponges, wing boards, prone pillows, Duncan masks, chin straps, and shoulder pulls.
- Immobilization devices help limit movement of the patient during treatment.
- The proper use of immobilization devices can decrease setup and targeting errors significantly.

Head and Neck

- The position for treatment in the head and neck area is usually supine. Supine is comfortable for most patients and portal arrangements typically include the use of lateral beams. Supine position also makes it easy to clinically verify that the sensitive lens is excluded from treatment fields.
- Head and neck positioning and immobilization should include a rigid plastic head holder that cradles the head while supporting the neck at the required chin extension or flexion.
- Thermoplastic molding products such as Aquaplast, which when warmed in water becomes pliable, can be fitted and contoured over the patient's head and secured to the table top.
  1. A size that covers only the head works well for treatment areas above the clavicles.
  2. A longer style (S-frame) that covers the head and shoulders works well for treatment areas in the head, neck, and supraclavicular regions.
  3. Aquaplast dries quickly and becomes rigid.
  4. Positioning marks can be applied to the mask avoiding skin marks.
  5. While the mask is cooling, use your fingers to mold at the glabella, chin, and entry of the auditory meatus.
- The use of shoulder pulls/adjustable straps tends to be controversial. Their use lends to setup variability.
- More precise shoulder retractor apparatuses come with some head and neck immobilization systems; the position of retractors should be carefully documented and referred to for daily setup.
- When planning for intensity modulated radiation therapy (IMRT) in the area of the head and neck, two methods may be used to compensate for no shoulder straps. They include:
  1. Computer contouring of the shoulders from the distal clavicle to the lateral aspect of the shoulder then set dose constraints on the shoulders.
  2. Set gantry angles above or below the shoulders.
- Bite block systems can be both a positioning aid and immobilizer. Bite block systems that are mountable to the table top or to a head holder can lock into place and assure consistent chin extension. Free bite blocks can be used to position and immobilize the tongue, and upper and lower jaw.

Breast

- Typical position for treatment of the breast is supine. The prone position using a special prone breast board is useful for patients with large breasts.
- Make sure legs and ankles are not crossed because this causes rotation of the torso.
- Wing boards are suitable for treatment of the breast. They allow the patient to raise both arms above the head with comfortable resting platforms for the elbows.
- For the breast especially, a wing board can be used along with a breast board at a slight incline to reduce the slope of the chest.
- Use of the wing board for treatment of the breast allows the patient to raise both arms above the head, making the torso more symmetric, thus reducing many of the setup variables associated with a "one arm up" setup technique.
- Breast boards with attachments to help reproduce elbow, wrist, and hand positions are also suitable.
- With 3-D treatment planning computers, breast board elevation can be kept at a minimum 5 to 10 degrees. The TPC can be used to optimize dose distribution and reduce hotspots on a sloped surface.

- The chin should be raised and the head turned away from the treated breast.
- A myriad of devices have been created to secure the breast in a fixed position, but their effectiveness is questionable. Allowing the breast to find its natural position tends to be more reproducible than any breast tissue immobilizer regardless of breast size.
- Skin folds that occur around the breast area are areas prone to erythema and desquamation, but the severity can be reduced by adjusting the position of the arm(s) or chest slope; various computerized treatment planning techniques can help reduce high dose accumulation in areas of buildup.
- A Vac-Loc system used with or without a wing board is a viable alternative to a breast board for breast setups.
- A Vac-Loc bag is filled with Styrofoam beads. When air is removed from the bag, it retains the shape and contour of the patient.
- Vac-Loc bags are reusable.
- An alternative to the Vac-Loc system is the alpha cradle system that uses two liquids, which when mixed together create a thermal reaction.
- When placed in a plastic bag and sealed, the chemicals expand and conform to the patient's body and then solidify.

Chest, Abdomen, Pelvis, and Extremities

- The Vac-Loc or alpha cradle systems work well for supine treatments of the chest, abdomen, pelvis, and extremities.
- The wing board is also appropriate for treatment of the chest and abdomen, especially when the use of lateral or posterior oblique fields are anticipated.
- Chin extension is determined based on the upper limits of the treatment fields.
- For treatments in the pelvic region, the Vac-Loc bag should extend from the buttocks to the feet. Supplementing the Vac-Loc bag with a large rubber band around the feet helps to keep the legs from rotating laterally. The exact position of the feet should be easily replicated.
- Although supine position is comfortable, prone position helps decrease the volume of small bowel in the pelvis and decreases gluteal folds where dose easily builds.
- For prone treatments of the pelvic region, belly boards are desirable.
- A 30 × 30 cm whole cut into the belly board with the bottom edge at the level of the iliac crest allows the small bowel to move anteriorly out of the treatment area.
- Planning for lower extremities is typically simple with the patient positioned supine, with reproducible positioning and immobilization of the legs.
- Positioning and immobilization can become more complex and will need to be tailored to individual cases to avoid opposite limbs and neighboring tissues when using high dose therapies for such cancers as soft tissue sarcoma and primary osteosarcoma.
- Alpha cradle and Vac-Loc systems have appropriately sized units for extremity radiation therapy.
- Planning techniques including bladder/rectal filling or voiding assist in tissue sparing and minimizing side effects; status of these organs should remain consistent throughout simulation and then throughout treatment.

TREATMENT PLANNING WITH CONVENTIONAL SIMULATION

- Conventional simulators have taken a back seat to the CT simulators but are still viably used.
- Target localization can be achieved through the use of boney and surface landmarks.
- Boney anatomy and low density cavities are easily visualized using the x-ray tube on the conventional simulator.
- Visualization of soft tissue targets is optimized by using contrast agents such as barium sulfate, iodine-based solutions, and air in or around the area of interest (Figure 7-3).
- Barium is inert and should only be used in the gastrointestinal tract; if perforation is suspected, barium-based contrast should be avoided.
- It is important to obtain orthogonal films before and after contrast is administered when using conventional simulation so as not to obscure important anatomy on planning films.
- Iodine-based contrast is very versatile and is easily absorbed and excreted by the liver and kidneys.
- Liver and kidney function should be tested before administering iodine-based contrast (remember to check BUN and creatinine before iodine contrast).
- Anaphylactic shock is a strong possibility for iodine-based contrast; ask patients for known allergies, especially to shellfish.
- Field size, gantry angle, collimator angle, table angle, treatment depths, and blocking can be determined during the conventional simulation session.

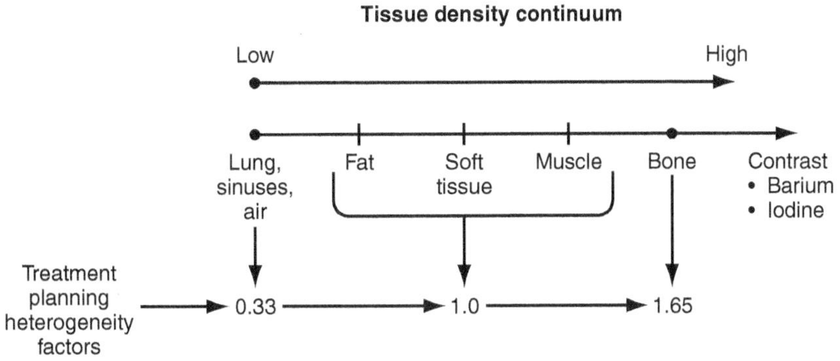

Tissue density continuum

Low
High

Lung, sinuses, air
Fat
Soft tissue
Muscle
Bone
Contrast
• Barium
• Iodine

Treatment planning heterogeneity factors
0.33
1.0
1.65

FIGURE 7-3 Tissue density continuum and treatment planning heterogeneity factors.

- Contouring of external anatomy can be accomplished by using manual methods using plaster of Paris or solder wire; mechanical contouring is performed with a pantograph or similar system.
- Manual contouring can be done through the plane of converging fields (Figure 7-4); for example, if lateral and vertex fields are anticipated, then the contour has to be done through the coronal plane or if an anterior and lateral are anticipated, then the contour should be taken through the axial plane.
- Contouring of internal anatomy can be accomplished by translation of anatomy from a diagnostic image or contrast filled cavities visualized on simulation film.
- This process can be carried through to treatment without the benefit of treatment planning computers for simple planning; if computer planning is necessary, manual contour data can be digitized into a planning computer for isodose distribution.

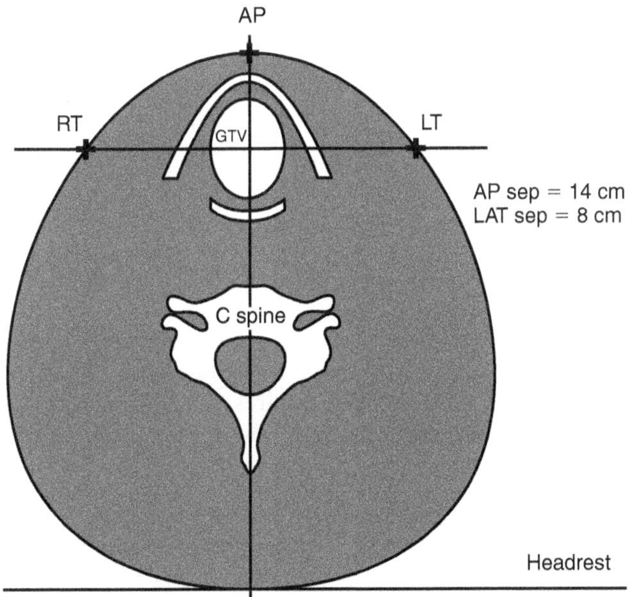

FIGURE 7-4 Manual contour sample.

- For simple planning without the TPC, where dose calculations and monitor units would be provided, each field will require calculations to be done by hand.
- When simulations and their subsequent treatments are done without the use of a treatment planning computer, optimized dose distributions and heterogenic density considerations (as shown in Figure 7-3) cannot be made.
- The physics staff at each oncology center provides calculation tables pertinent to each machine for manual calculation.
- Factors needed for manual calculations:
    1. Field size factor (FSOF = field size factor × reference dose rate)
    2. Reference dose rate/output/conversion factor (cGy/minute or cGy/MU)
    3. Tissue air ratio (TAR)/tissue maximum ration (TMR)
    4. Percent depth dose/%DD/Depth dose fraction
    5. Inverse square factor (ISF)
    6. Attenuating factors for block trays (TF), wedges (WF), other compensators
    7. Back scatter or peak scatter factor (BSF/PSF)
    8. Mayneord factor
    9. Prescribed dose/target dose

For Isocentric (SAD) Setup Techniques

- Target dose ÷ FSOF × TMR or TAR × WF × TF = Monitor units (MU).
    1. Target dose is the amount of dose each field is to receive from the daily total dose.
    2. FSOF is the field size output factor derived from the field size at treatment depth.
        a. Use the Sterling formula to calculate equivalent square.
        2 (field width × field length) ÷ field width + field length = equivalent square.
        b. Using the FSOF tables, find the correct output factor for the given equivalent square.

3. TMR is tissue maximum ratio derived from the effective square crossed referenced to treatment depth.
   a. Effective square is the equivalent square of the unblocked portion of the treatment field.
   b. Using the TMR tables, find the correct TMR by cross referencing the effective square to treatment depth.
4. TAR is tissue air ratio derived from the effective square cross reference to treatment depth (your center will tell you whether to use TMR or TAR in manual calculations).
5. WF is wedge factor also found in the calculation tables.
   a. WF is dependent on wedge angle, field size, and beam energy.
6. TF is tray factor, which refers to the acrylic tray that supports any blocking that may be required in the field.
   a. TF is dependent on the type of tray, beam energy, and the number of holes it has.
   b. If MLC is used, no tray is required. TF = 1.0.

For Nonisocentric (SSD) Setup Technique

- SSD treatment techniques were at the genesis of radiation therapy treatment delivery.

1. Began with source-based teletherapy and bridged into electronic teletherapy.
2. Unlike isocentric (SAD) treatment techniques, SSD techniques use a setup point on the patient's skin set to that specific unit's designed SSD.
   a. SSD is usually 80 or 100 cm.
3. The setup point is not isocentric.
4. For source-based teletherapy units, an output factor is used as a measure of the source activity.
   a. When using the output factor for dose calculation, the final answer will be in minutes and seconds as opposed to MUs.
   b. For electronic teletherapy units, the output factor is (1) and the resulting dose calculation is in MUs.

- There are disadvantages to using SSD treatment techniques:

1. The patient has to be moved and repositioned for each gantry angle.
2. Rotational therapy is not possible.
3. A slight setup error can result in a potentially more drastic target miss than with SAD techniques.

- There are advantages to using SSD treatment techniques:

1. More clearance exists between the patient and the gantry head.
2. A larger field size is achievable.

- Instead of using "tissue maximum ratio" in the denominator of the dose calculation, percentage depth dose is used.
- An inverse square factor referencing Dmax is used in the dose calculation.
- Target dose ÷ %DD × FSOF × BSF × Inv. Sq. factor × source output factor × TF × WF = Time/MU

1. Percentage depth dose is commonly written as PDD or %DD.
   a. %DD = (dose at depth ÷ dose at a static reference depth) × 100
   b. As with TMR, to find %DD, cross reference treatment depth with effective square
2. The BSF (backscatter factor) or patient scatter is typically found on the same reference table as %DD.
   a. BSF is referenced by effective square.
3. FSOF (field size output factor) considers scatter from the collimation system.
   a. Equivalent square is used to reference FSOF.
4. An inverse square factor is often incorporated into the formula to compensate for depth of Dmax. $(\text{SSD} \div \text{SSD} + \text{Dmax})^2$
5. If using a source-based treatment unit, use the appropriate source output factor.

- For an extended distance, a few factors must be considered.

1. The %DD is based on the field size at the new distance.
2. Inverse square $[(\text{old SSD} + \text{Dmax}) \div (\text{new SSD} + \text{Dmax})]^2$
3. Mayneord factor must be used in the denominator of the calculation.

$$[(\text{new SSD} + \text{Dmax}) \div (\text{old SSD} + \text{Dmax})]^2 \times [(\text{old SSD} + \text{depth}) \div (\text{new SSD} + \text{depth})]^2$$

Keep In Mind—Manual calculations may be required for emergency radiation therapy or clinical treatment setups where there is limited time for computer planning.

TREATMENT PLANNING WITH CT SIMULATION

- A computerized tomography simulation, unlike a conventional simulation, requires a three-dimensional treatment planning computer to virtually simulate the patient once the scan is done.
- Small radiopaque wires of a density that does not cause any undesirable artifact on the axial images are placed on the patient corresponding to the XYZ coordinates. These may be referred to as surface fiducials.

1. Wires allow the location of the preliminary isocenter to be viewed on the CT images.
2. Placement of fiducials allows target localization using the XYZ coordinate system with the marks placed on the patient during simulation as the origin.
3. Radiopaque markers are commercially available or can be made from expired arterial catheter wire.

- The scan should begin and end at reasonable margins above and below the area of interest and anticipated treatment volume.
- Consideration of likely treatment strategies and target volume, optimal patient position, position aids, and immobilization must come before scanning and computer planning.
- Final isocenter markings may be placed on the patient before the end of the CT simulation or the position of the radiopaque wires can be marked on the patient's skin indicating a starting point for any required shifts after a suitable plan is approved.

COMPUTERIZED TREATMENT PLANNING

- Treating a target with a multifield approach is preferable.

1. Provides a more homogenous dose distribution around the target.
2. Reduces a potentially high dose in any one area.
3. Minimizes side effects.

Choosing the Proper X-ray Energy/Modality

1. A higher energy for deeper targets and lower energies for more shallow ones.
   a. Higher energy photons have a deeper Dmax and are more penetrating. They are better suited for pelvic and abdominal treatment areas.
   b. Lower energy photons have a shallower Dmax and dispense their energy more rapidly with depth. Tumors of the head and neck region, breasts, and superficial targets are better served with a lower energy.
   c. Dmax is the depth of electronic equilibrium or the maximum build up depth.
   d. Skin sparing is a result of Dmax.

Consider this: 6 MV photon beam has a Dmax of 1.5 cm while an 18 MV photon beam has a Dmax of 3.5 cm.

2. Electron beams are used to treat superficial targets.
   a. Rapid fall off in tissue with some skin sparing; bolus may be used with electrons to reduce skin sparing.
   b. Appropriate electron energy is determined by the depth of the area of interest and which dose line is selected by the physician.
   c. Rules of thumb E/2 = the range of the electron beam in cm

E/3 = the depth of the 80% isodose line
E/4 = the depth of the 90% isodose line
E= electron energy

Choosing the Proper Gantry Angles

1. Avoid dose limiting organs or at least reduce exposure to them.
2. Beams arranged in a symmetrical manner tend to provide a more symmetrical target coverage.
3. Avoid using beam angles that are not executable due to lack of clearance with either the table or the patient.
4. Too many beams may have a diminishing return; increased integral dose.
5. When using electron fields, the horizontal axis should be parallel to the treated surface; en face.

- Using wedges (Figure 7-5) and bolus to manipulate dose distribution

1. The thicker the wedge angle, the more dose distribution is effected.
2. The angle of the wedge is described as the angle of the 50% isodose line at the central axis for low energy beams or the angle of the dose line located at 10 cm beneath the surface at the central axis for high energy beams.
3. Rule of thumb when using a pair of wedged fields Hinge angle = 180 − 2 (wedge angle)
4. Wedges have a beam hardening effect with polyenergetic beams such as those from a linear accelerator.
5. Avoid placing wedges any closer than 15 cm to the patient to prevent undue electron scatter skin contamination.

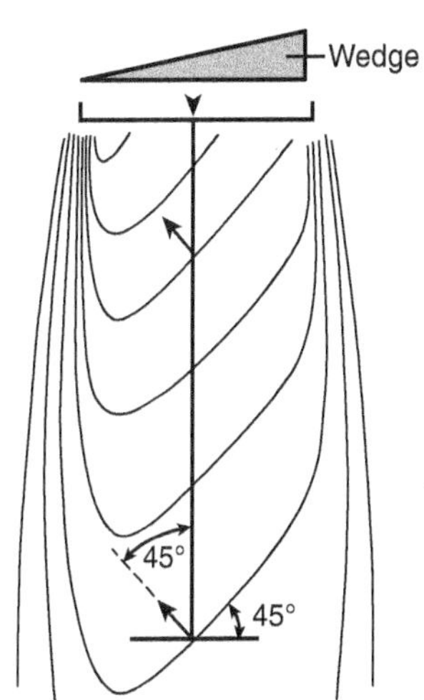

FIGURE 7-5 A 45-degree wedge isodose chart.

6. An alternative to standard, universal wedges is virtual wedging achieved by dynamic collimators. Gradual progression across the treatment field achieves the same dose line tilting as seen when using standard wedges.
7. Bolus can be any tissue density equivalent material.
   a. Fills in deficits to have a more homogenous dose distribution
   b. Shifts dose lines and brings Dmax closer to the skin surface when skin sparing not desirable.

Determining Field Shape and Size

1. Field shaping is dictated by the tumor size, local extensions, and regional metastasis.
2. When determining field size, do so dosimetrically and avoid guessing target margins.
3. Expand the field size as needed to cover the target with no less than 95% of the prescribed dose.

Target Volume Terminology

1. Gross tumor volume (GTV) is only the tumor visible by imaging such as CT, MRI, or PET; fusion of images (Figure 7-6) from PET, MRI, and CT are especially helpful in determining the GTV.
2. Clinical target volume (CTV) is the GTV plus a margin of up to 2.0 cm that encompasses an area where an unseen tumor or disease may be harbored. This margin is variable based on the radiation oncologist's perspective about a specific pathology and protocol requirements.
3. Internal target volume (ITV) compensates for physiologic movements and variations in size and shape or position of the CTV during therapy. Determination of this volume establishes feasibility of image-guided radiation therapy (IGRT) techniques, including surgical fiducial marker localization, BAT (ultrasound localization), and respiratory gating.
4. Planning target volume (PTV) is the CTV with additional margin of 0.5 cm to allow for patient movement and setup error.
5. Treated volume includes additional margins to allow for limitations in the treatment technique.
6. Irradiated volume is any tissue receiving greater than 50% of the specified target dose.

INTERPRETING THE TREATMENT PLAN

- The treatment plan data sheet should explain the treatment strategy, the number of fields, orientation of fields, field weights, and modifier factors along with monitor unit calculation factors.
- Plan summary sheets (Figure 7-7) can also provide information regarding regions of interest and their total doses.
- Shifts from the preliminary setup markings placed at simulation time should be indicated on the plan data sheet in XYZ coordinate language, on the summary sheet, and/or on a representative cross-sectional image

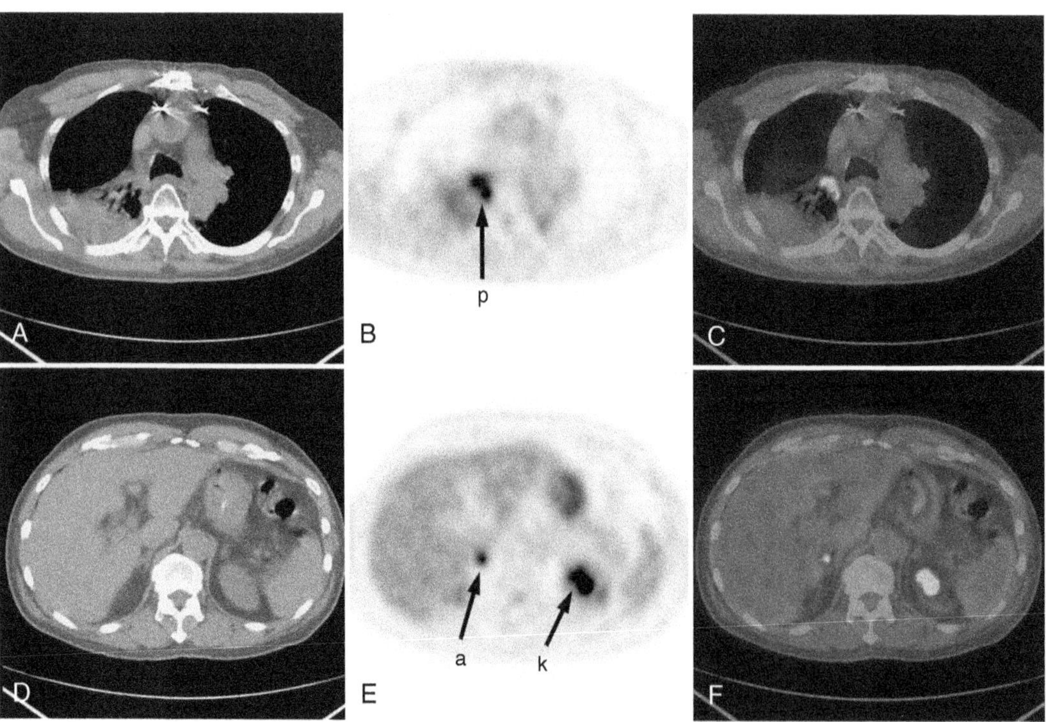

FIGURE 7-6 CT/PET scan fusion in patient with lung cancer **A**, Transaxial CT scan. **B**, Transaxial PET scan at same level as A. **C**, A and B images fused. **D**, Transaxial CT scan at a level inferior to set A, B, and C. **E**, Transaxial PET scan at same level as D. **F**, D and E images fused. a = adrenal gland; p = primary lung tumor; k = kidney.

04 Ap - IMRT **44 MU**

Machine:	MEVMLC		Isocenter X	−1.0 cm
Model:	Siemens_PRIMUS		Isocenter Y	1.0 cm
Energy:	6X		Isocenter Z	−2.0 cm
Technique:	STATIC		Field SAD:	100.0 cm
Gantry:	0.0 deg		Field SSD:	89.4 cm
Collimator:	0.0 deg		Point SSD:	88.8 cm
Couch Rtn:	0.0 deg		Depth (equiv):	12.1 cm (12.0 cm)
Parent	X1: +4.2 cm	Y1: +3.0 cm		
Fld Size:	X2: +5.0 cm	Y2: +4.8 cm	Relative Weight	1.027
Scale:	Siemens IEC		Dose Contribution:	26.7 cGy
MLC:	Siemens 58 MLC		MLC Type:	Dose Dynamic
Action Points:	12			

05 Lao 50 - IMRT **48 MU**

Machine:	MEVMLC		Isocenter X	−1.0 cm
Model:	Siemens_PRIMUS		Isocenter Y	1.0 cm
Energy:	6X		Isocenter Z	−2.0 cm
Technique:	STATIC		Field SAD:	100.0 cm
Gantry:	50.0 deg		Field SSD:	87.6 cm
Collimator:	0.0 deg		Point SSD:	86.9 cm
Couch Rtn:	0.0 deg		Depth (equiv):	14.7 cm (14.3 cm)
Parent:	X1: +3.4 cm	Y1: +3.0 cm		
Fld Size:	X2: +5.4 cm	Y2: +4.8 cm	Relative Weight	1.018
Scale:	Siemens IEC		Dose Contribution:	26.7 cGy
MLC:	Siemens 58 MLC		MLC Type:	Dose Dynamic
Action Points:	14			

06 Lao 100 - IMRT **43 MU**

Machine:	MEVMLC		Isocenter X	−1.0 cm
Model:	Siemens_PRIMUS		Isocenter Y	1.0 cm
Energy:	6X		Isocenter Z	−2.0 cm
Technique:	STATIC		Field SAD:	100.0 cm
Gantry:	100.0 deg		Field SSD:	84.0 cm
Collimator:	0.0 deg		Point SSD:	84.1cm
Couch Rtn:	0.0 deg		Depth (equiv):	17.1 cm (17.4 cm)
Parent:	X1: +3.4 cm	Y1: +3.0 cm		
Fld Size:	X2: +4.4 cm	Y2: +5.0cm	Relative Weight	0.977
Scale:	Siemens IEC		Dose Contribution:	20.9 cGy
MLC:	Siemens 58 MLC		MLC Type:	Dose Dynamic
Action Points:	12			

07 Lpo 150 - IMRT **43 MU**

FIGURE 7-7 Plan data sheet.

- Composite plans are two or more plans combined to show summative doses for all phases of the treatment regimen.
- Treatment planning using composite plans can optimize the quality of the therapy regimen by accurately depicting dose limitations to vital organs and, if need be, gives early alert for adjustments to assure tolerance doses are not exceeded.
- Composite plans showing dose distributions on cross-sectional data sets can be quick reference for dose points.
- Dose volume histograms (DVH) are graphs showing the volume of a particular organ and the amount of radiation that organ will be exposed to by percentage of volume (Figure 7-8).
- Fluence maps (Figure 7-9) are quick reference tools for concentration of dose when IMRT is used

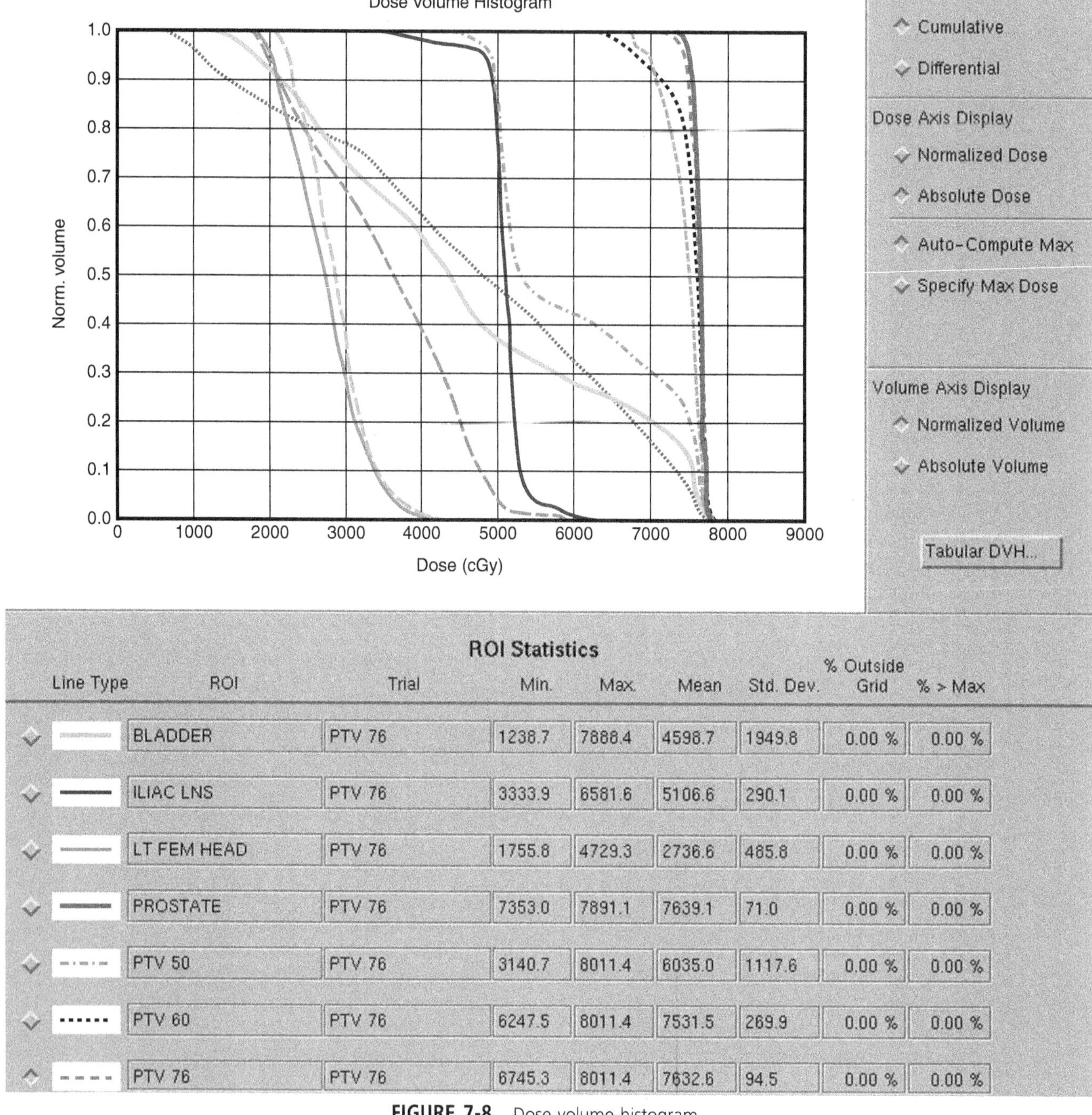

Line Type	ROI	Trial	Min.	Max.	Mean	Std. Dev.	% Outside Grid	% > Max
	BLADDER	PTV 76	1238.7	7888.4	4598.7	1949.8	0.00 %	0.00 %
	ILIAC LNS	PTV 76	3333.9	6581.6	5106.6	290.1	0.00 %	0.00 %
	LT FEM HEAD	PTV 76	1755.8	4729.3	2736.6	485.8	0.00 %	0.00 %
	PROSTATE	PTV 76	7353.0	7891.1	7639.1	71.0	0.00 %	0.00 %
	PTV 50	PTV 76	3140.7	8011.4	6035.0	1117.6	0.00 %	0.00 %
	PTV 60	PTV 76	6247.5	8011.4	7531.5	269.9	0.00 %	0.00 %
	PTV 76	PTV 76	6745.3	8011.4	7632.6	94.5	0.00 %	0.00 %

FIGURE 7-8 Dose volume histogram.

Common Fixed Fields Versus Dynamic Field Arrangements

- Fixed fields are still widely used. Certain fixed field arrangements are appropriate when the optimal dose needs to be delivered to the target and adjacent tissues kept under tolerance (TD 5/5) using simple techniques.
- Dynamic therapy, such as IMRT, rapid arc, and tomotherapy, are most appropriate when a very high dose needs to be delivered to areas in very close proximity to relatively low tolerance tissues. It attempts to lessen acute side effects and decrease the risk of late effects as compared with conventional, fixed field techniques.
- Tumor localization, localization of adjacent organs, and consideration of tolerance doses aid in determining whether conventional, fixed fields or dynamic fields are appropriate (Table 7-1).

Leaf Sequencing

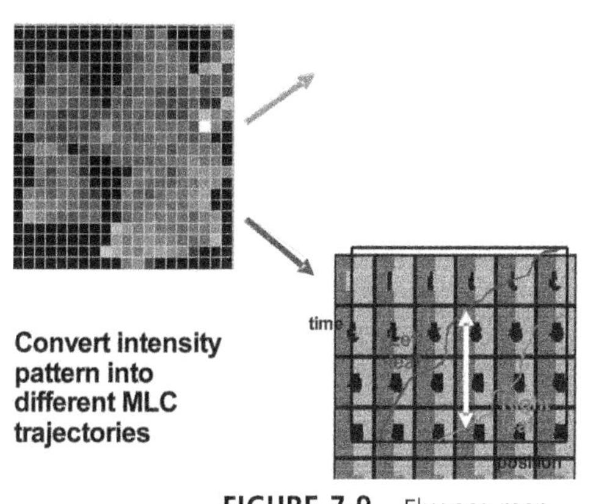

FIGURE 7-9 Fluence map.

Deviations from the Treatment Plan

- Therapists should be prepared for possible changes in the treatment plan during the course of therapy.
- Deviations without appropriate adjustments can adversely affect the clinical outcome.
- Deviations should be acknowledged and documented and adjustments made immediately (Table 7-2).

Adjacent Fields

- Special care is required when radiation needs to be administered in areas adjacent to each other.
- Computerized treatment planning can produce accurate representations of overlapping, high dose regions.
- Adjustments to the plan may be made to reduce or eliminate overlapping dose regions.
- Three methods to reduce or eliminate overlapping dose regions are: calculation of surface skin gaps, calculation of beam divergence with implementation of couch kicks or gantry angles, and the use of the half-field technique.

1. Skin gap formula: ½ A1 × (d/SSD) + ½ A2 × (d/SSD)
   A1 and A2 = dimension(s) of the treatment fields along the gap axis
   d = depth at which beams will overlap
2. Beam divergence formula: $\tan^{-1}$ (A/2SSD)
   A = dimension of the treatment field for which divergence is computed
3. The half-field technique uses asymmetric jaws or fabricated Cerrobend blocks to block fields up to the central axis. This allows us the opportunity to take advantage of no divergence at the central axis. When half-field techniques are used, adjacent fields may be directly abutted.

TABLE 7-1 Common Field Arrangements and Rationale

Field Arrangement	Features of Dose Distribution	Application
Parallel opposed pair 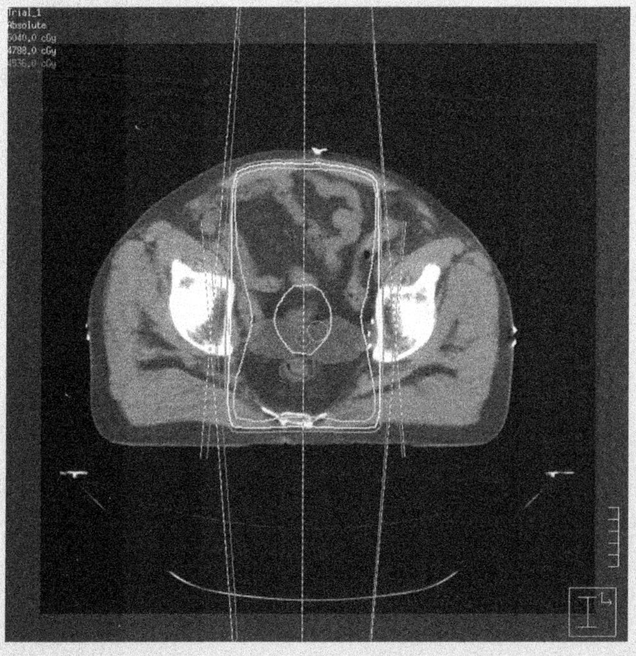	Assuming homogenous patient contour, even distribution throughout	Centrally located targets with no dose limiting structures in the path such as the whole brain, humerus, femur, breast

Continued

TABLE 7-1 Common Field Arrangements and Rationale—Cont'd

Field Arrangement	Features of Dose Distribution	Application
4 field box 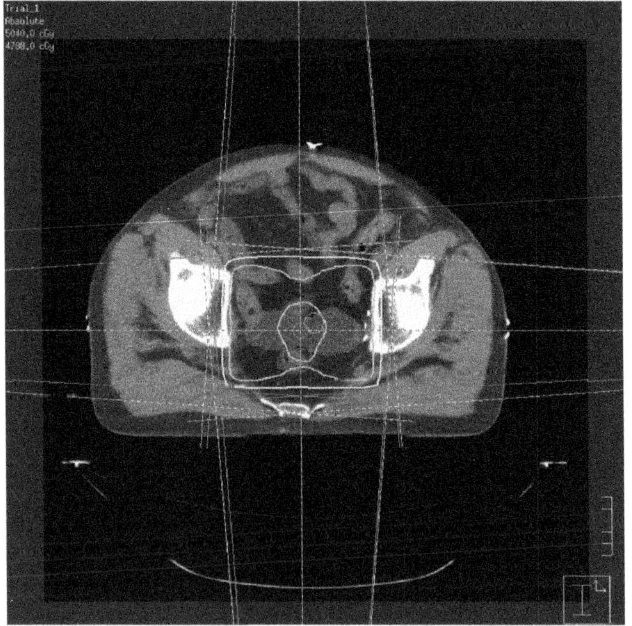	Concentration of dose near the intersection; sparing of tissues peripherally	Deep-seated targets with dose limlting tissues surrounding such as the prostate, bladder, endometrium
3 field with 90-degree hinge 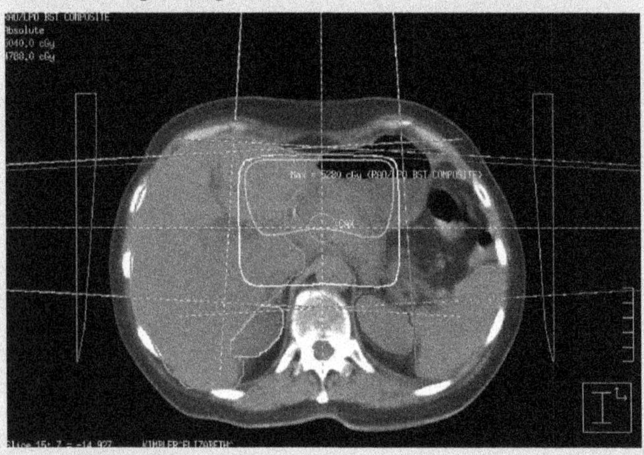	Concentration of dose near the intersection; sparing tissues peripherally and especially tissues on either side of the target	Deep targets with dose limiting tissues on one side, such as in treating the pancreas with sensitive kidneys posterior, rectum with sensitive small bowel and bladder anterior
2 field with 90-degree hinge 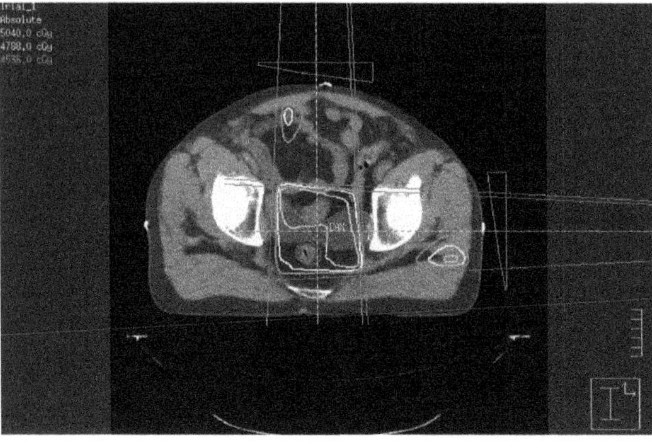	Concentration of dose in or near the hinge; manipulated with modifiers such as wedges	Unilateral targets such as laterally located primary brain tumors, maxillary sinus

Continued

TABLE 7-1 Common Field Arrangements and Rationale—Cont'd

Field Arrangement	Features of Dose Distribution	Application
Arcs or multiple field IMRT 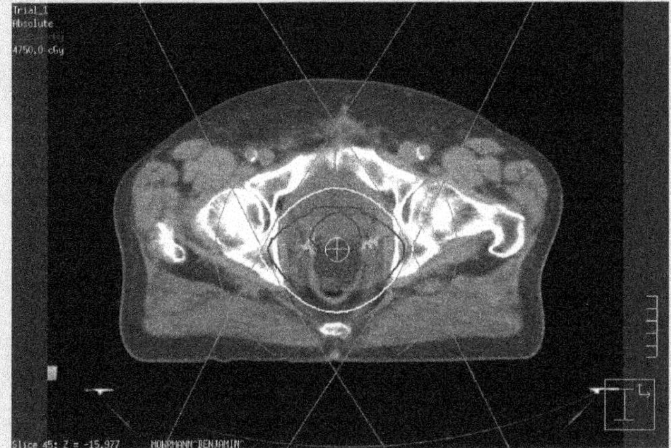	Concentrated dose toward the center sparing tissues in the periphery	Small, deep targets like the prostate, cervix, pituitary gland with sensitive tissues all around
Single field photon 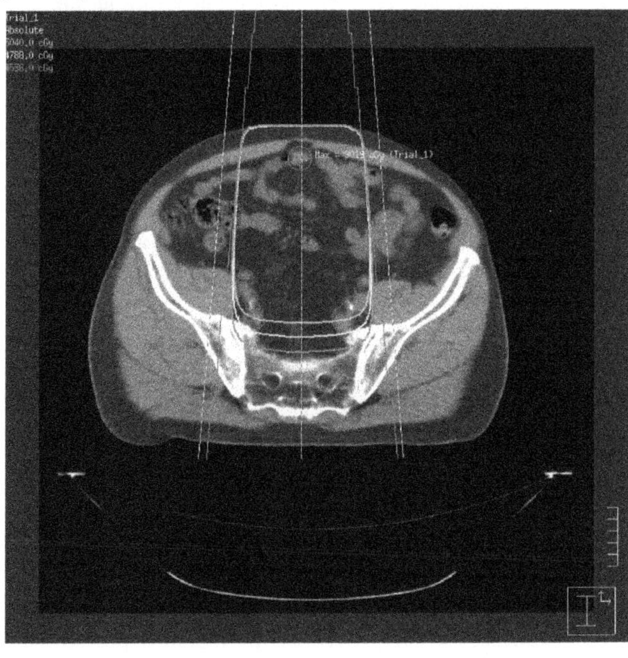	Dose fall off with increasing depth; sparing tissues beyond the interest point	Targets near the surface such as thoracic spine, upper lumbar spine, superficial supraclavicular lymph nodes
Single field electron 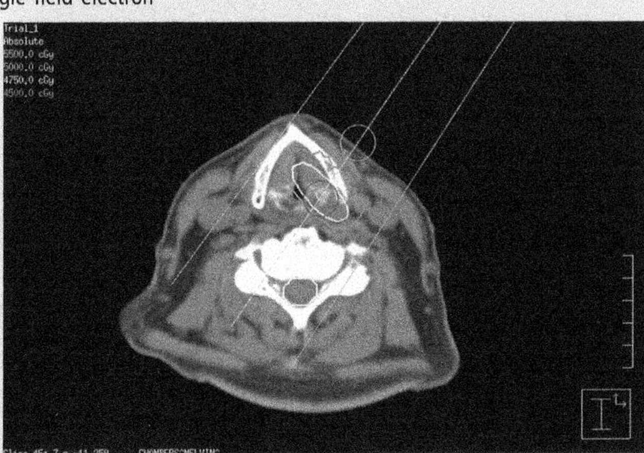	Rapid dose fall off; maximum dose near the surface	Treatment of superficial targets; bolus may be applied to eliminate skin-sparing at the surface

TABLE 7-2 Sample Treatment Plan Deviations, Impact, and Adjustments

Deviation	Possible Impact	Suggested Adjustment(s)
Physician ordered change in field size or MLC position	Target volume, output has changed, absorbed dose is changed	Recalculation of monitor units to comply with prescription
Physician ordered change in dose per fraction or total dose	Absorbed dose is changed	Recalculation of monitor units to comply with prescription
Machine malfunctions and patient treatment incomplete	Absorbed dose is changed	Document actual monitor units given; calculate absorbed dose and adjust for missing dose per physicist
Isocenter is moved, geometric size changed due to new clinical findings	Target volume, absorbed dose is changed	Recalculate monitor units, recontour to include new areas included in field
Patient loses or gains weight or is misaligned	Absorbed dose is changed, position of isocenter is changed	Recontour, remeasure, adjust isocenter placement; monitor unit recalculation may be necessary
Incorrect field treated	Target volume changed, absorbed dose changed	Replan to document dose to area treated; compensate for missing dose to intended target
Too many fractions treated	Absorbed dose changed; tolerance threshold compromised	Establish and document absorbed dose; find BED, and document
Too few fractions treated	Absorbed dose changed	Establish and document absorbed dose; add fractions if feasible
Missing accessory	Absorbed dose changed; isodose distribution changed	Calculate actual absorbed dose, replan with accessory missing and adjust accessories for the remainder of treatment
Incorrect accessory	Absorbed dose changed; isodose distribution changed	Calculate and replan with incorrect accessory; modify subsequent treatments
Treatment schedule interruption by noncompliance or patient illness	Biologic effect changed	Find BED; adjust fraction size or total dose to complete regimen

- Special care is required, especially when photon and electron fields are adjacent.
- The electron beam's bell-shaped isodose presents another challenge in attempting to avoid high dose areas beneath the surface for adjacent fields.
- Computer planning is best to visualize isodose distribution for adjacent electron fields or matched photon and electron fields.
- Physicians may order periodic match line changes/ feathering when adjacent fields are treated.

BRACHYTHERAPY TREATMENT PLANNING

- Brachytherapy is a radiation therapy delivery system in which radioactive sources are placed on or near the intended target.
- A higher dose can be delivered to the target area while significantly reducing exposure to the surrounding tissues.
- Radioactive sources used in brachytherapy may be applied for seconds, hours, days, or permanently—depending on the type of cancer, its location, and the half-life of the radioactive isotope.
- Areas of common usage are the mouth, tongue, prostate, brain, uterus, bronchus, and vagina.
- There are three general categories of brachytherapy: HDR, LDR, and MDR.
- HDR (high dose rate) uses an isotope that delivers a dose rate equal to 20 cGy/min.
- LDR (low dose rate) uses an isotope that delivers a dose rate 0.5 to 2.0 cGy/min.
- MDR (medium dose rate) is anywhere between 2.0 cGy/minute and 20 cGy/min.
- Therapeutic isotopes can be naturally occurring or artificially made.
- Artificial isotopes tend to have higher gamma energies and shorter half-lives.
- The common types of radioactive decay are:
- *Alpha decay*—occurs in elements that have atomic numbers greater than 82 in which a pair of protons and a pair of neutrons are emitted. Consists of two neutrons: a helium nucleus.
- *Beta decay*—where a positive or a negative electron from the nucleus is given off. Can be called a positron of a negatron.
- *Electron capture*—where an orbital electron is taken in by the nucleus and changes a proton into a neutron and in turn, the nucleus emits a beta particle.
- *Internal conversion*—where the energy within the nucleus is great enough to be passed on to one of the orbital electrons, and is then ejected from the atom.
- Common radioactive isotopes used are cobalt, cesium, palladium, gold, iridium, iodine, phosphorus, ytterbium, and strontium.

- With few exceptions, most radioactive isotopes for therapeutic use are sealed in a double layer of steel or similar metal and referred to as sources.
- The double layering of metal on a radioactive source is to ensure containment of the isotope and to filter out low energy alpha and beta particles.
- The source sizes vary depending on the treatment location and the type of applicator that is available.
- Gynecologic brachytherapy procedures can use many types of source applicators, but the most commonly used are tandems and ovoids; they are referred to as a Fletcher suite when used together.
- A tandem is a long tube placed into the uterus, containing a source such as cesium-137 for LDR therapy or a 10-Ci iridium source for HDR therapy.
- Ovoids are devices used in pairs and placed side by side in the distal vagina for treatment of the vagina and/or cervix. They typically require one cesium-137 source each for LDR or a 10-Ci iridium source for HDR.
- Afterloading is the practice of installing an applicator into the patient first and then loading the sources at a later time.
- Afterloading allows time to verify appliance placement and/or create a treatment plan. Excess dose to personnel is also avoided.
- Remote afterloaders further reduce exposure to personnel.
- Sources can be placed into tumors with long needles referred to as trocars.
- Sources can be imbedded into plastic ribbon to maintain a specific spacing and placed into tumors using trocars.
- Noninvasive prostate gland tumors are commonly treated with small sources placed by trocars via a template.
- Single plane implants are used for narrow target volumes.
- Double plane implants are used for larger target volumes.
- Volume implants are implants that require more than two planes.
- To determine the type of isotope to use, one must consider the following:

   a. Activity
   b. Energy
   c. Half-life
   d. Shielding
   e. Capsular attenuation
   f. Exposure rate

- To find exposure rate from a single source divide activity in mCi by the distance of the point of interest squared. Then multiply by the exposure rate constant for the particular isotope used.

$$\frac{\text{Activity (mCi)}}{D^2 \times \text{Exposure rate constant}}$$

- Most brachytherapy treatments are planned on treatment planning computers with three-dimensional capabilities.
- Before treatment planning computers, several systems used to calculate dose and dose distribution to the irradiated volume were devised, such as:

   1. Patterson-Parker or Manchester system
      a. Uses a nonuniform source distribution to give a uniform dose distribution.
      b. Gynecologic implants using tandems and ovoids (Figure 7-10) commonly use this system to calculate the dose to a point "A."
   2. Quimby system
      a. Uses a uniform source distribution that yields a nonuniform dose distribution, with the highest dose usually in the center of the implant.
   3. Memorial system
      a. A version of the Quimby system
      b. Is described in Kahn's as a complete dose distribution around a lattice of point sources of uniform strength spaced 1.0 cm apart.
   4. Paris system
      a. Used for line sources, such as plastic ribbon with imbedded Ir^{192} or I^{125}.

- Types of implants include:

   1. Intracavitary such as a uterus implant
   2. Interstitial such as a prostate implant
   3. Intraluminal such as a bronchial implant or accelerated partial breast brachytherapy using the MammoSite system, for example

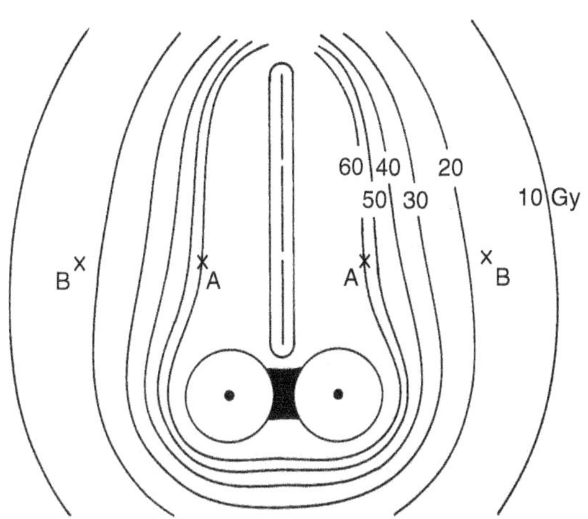

FIGURE 7-10 Points A and B for gynecologic brachytherapy.

- Before planning an implant, the patient usually has an orthogonal set of films taken that are used as a planning database.
- Prostate implants are preplanned using an ultrasound database.

BIBLIOGRAPHY

Bentel GC: *Patient positioning and immobilization in radiation oncology*, ed 1, New York, 1999, McGraw-Hill.

Bentel GC: *Radiation therapy planning*, ed 2, New York, 1996, McGraw-Hill.

Blackburn B, Shahabi S: *Blackburn's introduction to clinical radiation therapy physics*, ed 1, Madison, 1989, Medical Physics Publishing.

Bomford CK, Kunkler IH: *Walter and Miller's textbook of radiotherapy*, ed 6, London, 2003, Churchill Livingstone.

Hendee WR, Ibbott GS, Hendee EG: *Radiation therapy physics*, ed 3, Hoboken, 2005, Wiley-Blackwell.

Kahn FM: *The physics of radiation therapy*, ed 4, Philadelphia, 2010, Lippincott Williams & Wilkins.

Washington CM, Leaver, D: *Principles and practice of radiation therapy*, ed 3, St. Louis, 2010, Mosby.

REVIEW EXERCISES

1. The removable grids used in therapeutic linear accelerators to broadcast crosshairs onto a portal image are referred to as all of the following except:
   - a. BB tray
   - b. grating
   - c. fiduciary tray
   - d. graticule

2. Source axis distance (SAD) is measured from the _______ to a _______ around which the gantry rotates 360 degrees.
   Choose the correct answers from the following list:

Image intensifier	Thetatron	Point
Table top	Electron gun	Isodose line
Modulator	Focal spot	Gantry

3. The most commonly used axial image database for a 3-D treatment planning computer is:
   - a. MRI
   - b. PET
   - c. CT
   - d. US

4. Which of the aforementioned modalities can be used as a fusion study?
   - a. None
   - b. b, c, d
   - c. a, b, c
   - d. All of them

5. The XYZ coordinate system works well when localizing a target volume.
   True False
   If false, correct the statement to make it true.

6. Thinner CT slices ↑ or ↓ resolution of digitally reconstructed radiographs.
   Circle the correct answer.

7. List three things that help set up reproducibility.

8. The contour of a CT simulator tabletop should look like this.
   Choose the correct answer.
   - a. __
   - b. ⌴
   - c. ∩

9. Patient marks can be effectively applied by all of the following except:
   - a. Tattoo
   - b. Ballpoint pen
   - c. Felt pen
   - d. Paint pen
   - e. Carfusion

10. IMRT is a sophisticated method of radiation delivery to a target area and does not require port film verification.
    True False
    If false, correct the statement to make it true.

11. *Fill in the blank*. For treatments in the chest, head, and neck regions, _______ straightens the lordotic curvature of the spine, making the patient more comfortable during the treatment.

12. A good method for breast immobilization that often affords the best daily reproducibility is:
    - a. A plastic cup with straps
    - b. Nylon bra
    - c. Aquaplast cast
    - d. Nothing

13. For nonisocentric treatment techniques, ________ is the factor of choice to demonstrate central axis dose at a given depth.

a. TMR
b. TPR
c. TAR
d. %DD

14. When looking up the %DD or TMR for a given depth and field size, _______ should be used when there are blocks or MLC.

a. Equivalent square
b. Effective square

15. Mayneord factor is the formula used to find the equivalent square for a given field size. True False

If false, correct the statement to make it true.

16. List the pros and cons of SSD setup techniques.

17. List the advantages SAD setup techniques have over SSD setup techniques.

18. What invention allowed IMRT to become a reality?

a. Cerrobend
b. %DD
c. Tomotherapy
d. MLC
e. CT

19. The Sterling formula is a method to determine:

a. Extended distance
b. Equivalent square
c. Skin gap
d. Inverse square
e. Dmax
f. Penumbra

20. When an extended distance is required for a nonisocentric treatment technique, what changes and additions are needed in the calculation?
More than one answer is correct.

a. Include Mayneord factor in the denominator.
b. Change inverse square to reflect new SSD.
c. Find new %DD for field size at a new distance.
d. Change FSOF for different Sc.

21. Explain how the treatment planner can see the patient marks when viewing the axial images on the treatment planning computer.

22. Which of the following is not an advantage of using a multifield approach?

a. Minimizes side effects
b. Increases integral dose
c. Reduces a potentially high dose in any single area
d. Provides more homogeneous dose distribution around the target

23. Choosing the proper x-ray energy is critical for optimizing a treatment.
Associate the following treatment areas with the most probable beam energy used.
Write 6 MV or 18 MV behind each area.

Lung tumor ________
Nasopharynx ________
Prostate ________
Cervix ________
Pancreas ________
Breast ________
Upper arm sarcoma ________

24. *Circle the correct answer.*

Field size determinations should be done (dosimetrically/geometrically).

25. When choosing gantry angles, which of the following is not a valid consideration?

a. Avoidance of dose limiting organs
b. Angles that expedite treatment time
c. Unexecutable gantry positions
d. Too many beams
e. Symmetrical arrangements

26. Dmax is defined as: *(More than one answer is correct.)*

a. Skin to isocenter distance
b. Depth in which 20% of dose is absorbed
c. Point of peak dose in an irradiated medium
d. Depth where electronic equilibrium occurs
e. Area of maximum penumbra

27. Label the following descriptions as either GTV, CTV, or PTV.

A volume with typically a 0.5-cm margin to allow for patient movement and/or setup error. ______

Tumor volume encompassing visible tumor as seen on a diagnostic study or simulation images. ______

A volume with a variable margin of 1.5 to 2.5 cm that includes any suspected or unseen disease.______

28. Standard wedges can have a beam hardening effect when the radiation is monoenergetic.

True False
If false, what is the correct answer?

29. Name the two primary reasons for a bolus to be used.

30. TD 5/5 means:

a. 5% chance of complications at 50 cGy.
b. 5% chance of complications at 5 Gy.
c. 5 of every 5 patients will experience complications.
d. 5% chance of complications in 5 years.

Think About It

Using Figure 7-11 below, answer the following questions.

31. GTV is located at 10-cm depth. A dose of 100 cGy is delivered to the GTV using 4 MV single anterior photon beam. The bladder is at 7 cm deep. Assuming SSD technique, which of the following is true? *Circle all that are correct.*

a. Rectum will get more than 100 cGy
b. Bladder will get more than 100 cGy

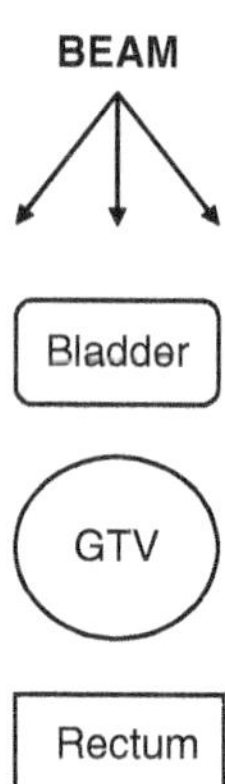

FIGURE 7-11 Primary beam incident on a GTV.

c. Rectum will get less than 100 cGy
d. Bladder will get less than 100 cGy
e. All of the above are correct

32. If 10 MV photons were used to treat the above tumor to 100 cGy, then compared to 4 MV beam treatment plan, which of the following would be true if all other factors remain the same? *Circle all that are correct.*

a. Rectum will get higher dose
b. Bladder will get higher dose
c. Rectum will get lower dose
d. Bladder will get lower dose
e. There would be no difference in rectum or bladder dose

33. A high energy x-ray beam is incident on the surface of water in a water tank. Indicate which one of the following statements is correct.

a. Maximum dose is at the water surface
b. Maximum dose is at a depth dependent on the x-ray energy
c. Maximum dose is always at a fixed depth, independent of x-ray energy
d. Dose increases with depth beyond the depth of maximum dose

34. Concerning 6 MV and 18 MV x-ray beams:

The depth of maximum dose for ______ MV is 1.5 cm; and depth of maximum dose for ______ MV is 3.5 cm. At 10 cm depth, the ______ MV beam will have a greater percent depth dose.

35. A deep seated tumor is treated posteriorly with a high energy photon beam. The tumor is at 13 cm depth and the percent depth dose is 65%. The

spinal cord is in the field and is at 5 cm depth. Percent depth dose at the spinal cord is 85%. If 200 cGy is delivered to the tumor, the calculated dose to the spinal cord would be:

36. A patient is delivered a dose of 150 cGy at a depth of 13 cm with 10 MV photons at 100 cm SSD. The percent depth dose is 60%. Calculate the dose delivered to the depth of maximum dose.

37. The energy loss of megavoltage electron beams in water is approximately ______ MeV per centimeter.

38. Electron arc therapy has what effect on the D_{max} position, as compared with a stationary electron field of the same energy?

a. Moves D_{max} towards the surface
b. Does not move D_{max} position
c. Moves D_{max} away from the surface

39. What two purposes do the metallic sheaths surrounding radioactive isotopes serve?

Label the following implant types as interstitial, intracavitary, or intraluminal

40. A prostate seed implant ______

41. An accelerated partial breast treatment such as MammoSite ______

42. Au 198 seeds imbedded into the tongue ______

43. When more than two planes of sources are used, it would be called a:

a. Stereo implant
b. Single-plane implant
c. Orthogonal
d. Volume implant

44. Demonstrate the generic formula for calculating an exposure at a specific distance for a particular isotope.

45. Match the following brachytherapy system with its distinguishing feature.

___	Patterson-Parker/ Manchester	A. Sources of uniform strength spaced 1.0 cm apart
___	Quimby	B. Uniform source distribution with nonuniform dose distribution
___	Memorial	C. Often used for calculating line sources
___	Paris	D. nonuniform source distribution with uniform dose distribution

46. When planning a GYN implant, which point is dose calculated to?

a. W
b. A
c. J
d. F

Fill in the blanks in questions 47-49.

47. Alpha particles are similar to the ______ (element) nucleus? It has a ______ charge.

48. When an element has an excessive number of neutrons, in order to achieve stability, it is likely to experience ______ emission.

49. The radioactive decay process that results in the ejection of a positive or negative electron would be referred to as ______ decay.

50. Considering the weight/size and charge of alpha, beta, and gamma particles, what simple device could be used to separate them?

51. List five of the most commonly used brachytherapy isotopes.

52. Prostate implants are preplanned on a treatment planning computer using a/an_______ database.

a. MRI
b. CT
c. Ultrasound
d. PET

53. HDR isotopes deliver at a dose rate = _______ cGy/minute.

54. LDR isotopes deliver at a dose rate between _______ and _______ cGy/min.

55. If the physician changes the field size after the treatment plan has been approved, the therapist should:

a. Record the new field size and follow the plan as approved
b. Record the new field size and submit the change to physics for new calculation
c. Reduce the monitor units by 1 if the field size has increased by 1 cm
d. Increase the monitor units by 1 if the field size has increased by 1 cm

56. Once it has been discovered that too many fractions have been delivered to the preliminary treatment fields, the therapist should:

a. Document the error and submit it to physics for necessary adjustments
b. Document the error and give less fractions to the boost fields
c. Document the error and continue the plan as approved to total dose
d. Document the error and skip the boost fields

57. Late Friday afternoon, the physician orders treatment to the whole brain for a recent consult. After field size, collimator, and gantry angles have been determined. The next step would be to:

a. Split the prescribed fraction dose in half and administer equivalent monitor units
b. Split the prescribed total dose in half and administer equivalent monitor units
c. Acquire patient separation data, refer to written prescription, and calculate monitor units
d. Acquire the patient separation data and administer monitor units from another whole brain patient chart

58. Your patient has been hospitalized for blood transfusion and infection and has missed three consecutive weeks of treatment. Upon the patient's return, the therapist should:

a. Relocalize the treatment area, remark the patient, and resume treatment
b. Remeasure, relocalize, remark, and resume treatment
c. Remeasure, relocalize, remark, and ask for BED adjustments in fraction size or total dose
d. Remeasure, relocalize, remark, and ask for OER for adjustments in fraction size or total dose

59. The wedge angle is determined by the tilt of the isodose lines at (select two):

a. The 50% isodose line in low energy beams
b. A depth of 10 cm for high energy beams
c. The depth of the 20% isodose line in high energy beams
d. The depth of 5 cm for low energy beams

60. A spinal cord compression at the level of T5-T6 is being treated emergently. The most likely field arrangement would be:

a. Two parallel opposed lateral fields
b. Two parallel opposed AP/PA fields
c. A single posterior electron field
d. A single posterior low energy photon field

61. The entire right breast will be treated in your patient diagnosed with T1 N1 M0 infiltrating ductal carcinoma. The most likely field arrangement would be:

a. Tangential fields with subsequent tumor bed boost
b. Tangential fields with internal mammary and supraclavicular fields
c. Parallel opposed AP/PA fields with spinal cord blocked
d. Single field electron field to the entire breast with bolus

62. A primary brain tumor located in the right temporal lobe will likely be treated with:

a. Two parallel opposed equally weighted photon beams
b. A wedged pair consisting of anterior and RPO fields
c. A wedged pair consisting of vertex and right lateral fields
d. Four field box technique with wedges on the lateral fields

63. Beam modifiers such as wedges would most likely be used in a treatment plan for:

a. Metastatic bone lesion in the femur
b. Primary cancerous lesion in the rectum
c. Metastatic bone lesion in the cervical spine
d. Primary cancerous lesion in the prostate

64. Manual contouring can be achieved by using all of the following tools except:

a. Solder wire
b. Calipers
c. Plaster of Paris
d. Bite block

65. Shoulder retractors are feasible for positioning and immobilization when treating the:

a. Lung
b. Whole brain
c. Thoracic spine
d. Neck

66. The optimal hinge angle for a 45-degree wedged pair is:

a. 30 degrees
b. 45 degrees
c. 60 degrees
d. 90 degrees

67. The angle between two beams is known as the:

a. Arc angle
b. Hinge angle
c. Wedge angle
d. Divergent angle

68. A suitable wedge angle for two fields separated by 90 degrees is:

a. 30 degrees
b. 45 degrees
c. 60 degrees
d. 90 degrees

69. What is the equivalent square for a 15 × 6 field?

a. 9.5 × 9.5
b. 8.6 × 8.6
c. 10 × 10
d. 2.1 × 2.1

70. An entire spine is treated by matching two fields both treated at 100 cm SSD. Field number 1 measures 8 × 20 and field number 2 measures 8 × 25. In order to match these fields at a depth of 5 cm, a ______ cm skin gap would be required.

a. 1.1 cm
b. 2.0 cm
c. 5.0 cm
d. 3.2 cm

Refer to the plan data sheet (Figure 7-7) to answer the following.

71. The reference field size for the AP field is:

a. 7.2 × 9.8 cm
b. 9.2 × 7.8 cm
c. 8.0 × 9.0 cm
d. 9.0 × 8.0 cm

72. The gantry angle for the LPO treatment field should be:

a. 100 degrees
b. 84 degrees
c. 50 degrees
d. 87.6 degrees

73. Assuming the patient is positioned supine with the head into the gantry, referencing an axial image view, the shift from the original planning isocenter should be:

a. 1.0 cm to the patient's right
b. 1.0 cm to the patient's left
c. 2.0 cm to the patient's right
d. 2.0 cm to the patient's left

74. Assuming the patient is positioned supine with the head into the gantry, referencing a sagittal image view, the shift from the original planning isocenter should be:

a. 2.0 cm cephalad
b. 2.0 cm caudal
c. 2.0 cm anterior
d. 2.0 cm posterior

75. Prescription for boost dose to a soft tissue sarcoma tumor bed at a depth of 5 cm reads: 200 cGy/fraction to the 90% dose line. The appropriate electron energy for this case would be:

a. 10 MeV
b. 15 MeV
c. 20 MeV
d. 25 MeV

CHAPTER

8

Oncology Patient Care

Leia Levy, Elva Marie Dawson and Jayme Leavy

FOCUS QUESTIONS

- What are the principles of body mechanics, patient transportation, and assistance methods needed to provide for the comfort and safety of the patient?
- What are the principles of patient rights and informed consent?
- How are the principles of medical ethics supported by the law?
- Define the principles of asepsis-surgical and medical.
- What procedures and methods constitute standard precautions?
- List the drugs commonly used in radiation oncology.
- Differentiate between disinfection and sterilization.
- List the rates of temperature, pulse, respiration, and blood pressure that are considered to be within normal limits for an adult.
- What are some potential hazards when administering oxygen?
- List the symptoms of anaphylactic shock.
- Define the five rights of drug administration.
- Explain effective patient education regarding radiation and chemotherapy related side effects.
- List the factors needed to communicate infectious disease.
- Define the category specific methods of isolation.
- Demonstrate the correct method of entering and leaving an isolation unit using strict isolation technique.
- What are the appropriate procedures for handling common medical emergencies such as cardiac arrest, respiratory distress and arrest, stroke, seizure, anaphylactic shock, and syncope?

ETHICAL AND LEGAL ASPECTS

- Law and ethics are inseparable.
- Ethics include character, customs or manners; ethics are what society defines as mannerable and depends on its mores or values.
- Mores are unwritten and accepted laws and values are those things regarded as good and desirable and can be learned from parents and others; both help us decide what's right or wrong.
- What we perceive as ethical is influenced by our personal mores and values.
- Medical ethics and health law have been born out of society's accepted customs, character and things it presently regards as good.
- There are seven ethical principles that shape how we behave and problem-solve in the medical community. The principles are:
- Beneficence—always act for the good of another/patient.
- Nonmaleficence—avoid harm to another
- Autonomy—ability to make independent decisions
- Justice—what's considered fair
- Veracity—tell the truth
- Role fidelity—operate in your scope; be true to your role
- Confidentiality—protection of privacy
- Each of the seven medical principles of ethics are supported by federal and state laws that have been passed and certain standards, rules, and procedures established by professional societies and other medical governing bodies.
- The American Registry for Radiologic Technologists (ARRT) is one professional, administrative organization that has established ethical policy as contained in the professional code of ethics.
- The code of ethics for radiation therapists contains language that supports beneficence and other ethical principles.
- Laws supporting beneficence may be found under tort law.
- A tort is any wrongful act against another; wrongs can be intentional or unintentional.
- Unintentional torts—negligence and malpractice

- Intentional torts—battery, assault, false imprisonment, infliction of emotional distress
- Quasi-intentional torts—defamation of character, invasion of privacy in some cases
- Elder Abuse and Neglect Act is an example of a federal law that supports beneficence.
- Nonmaleficence is also supported by tort law; this principle is most evident in the establishment of intentional and quasi-intentional tort liability.
- Our national and state rules about credentialing is a good example of administrative laws that support the principle of nonmaleficence.
- Competence as shown through certification, registration, licensure, and continuing education are included in credentialing.
- Autonomy is supported by the Patient's Bill of Rights Act of 1998.
- Autonomy is also supported by documents such as the DNR, living will, power of attorney, other advanced directives, and informed consent.

Autonomy Documentation

DNR

- Do not resuscitate is a request not to have cardiopulmonary resuscitation if your heart stops or if you stop breathing.

Living Wills

- Written legal documents stating the medical treatments or life-sustaining treatments the patient wants if they were seriously or terminally ill

Durable Power of Attorney

- States whom you have chosen to make health care decisions for you
- Becomes active any time you are unconscious or unable to make medical decisions
- Also called *health care proxy*

Advance Directives

- Tells your doctor what kind of care you would like to have if you become unable to make medical decisions

Informed Consent

- Physician provides the patient with information so that the patient can make an informed decision regarding whether to consent to treatment/procedure including:
  1. Nature of procedure, treatment, or disease
  2. Expected outcomes and likelihood of success
  3. Reasonable alternatives
  4. Known risks

- There are limits to the principle of autonomy such as:
  1. If an autonomous decision might cause harm to others such as the unborn
  2. In instances of "physician's privilege" where the physician does what he/she feels is best when the patient's personal choice has not been expressed
  3. If the autonomous decision may cause harm to society (legal moralism)
  4. If the patient is incompetent and does not have the capacity to make an independent decision
- The constitution and its amendments support the principle of justice
- Antidiscrimination laws, civil rights laws, labor laws, and due process also support the principle of justice.
- The Hippocratic Oath and codes of ethics contain language supporting justice
- A special relationship develops at the first encounter between the patient and clinician. Once responsibility for the care of another is accepted, then the relationship becomes fiduciary. Each one commits to being truthful, faithful, and to hold information confidential.
- The law of informed consent and HIPAA laws support the fiduciary relationship.

INTERPERSONAL COMMUNICATION

- Communication is critical to building helping relationships with patients and co-workers.
- Patients undergoing treatment for cancer likely have both psychological and social needs.
- Helping relationships in cancer care should address the physiologic, psychological, and social needs of the patient and their caregiver(s) (Table 8-1).

Challenges in Communication

Languages

- Translators should be provided by hospital before patient's appointment.

Hearing and Speech Impairments

- Interpreters should be provided by hospital before patient's appointment

Impaired Cognition

- Adjust communication strategies to match comprehension level of patient

Literacy

- Read information to patient
- Provide video with information

TABLE 8-1 Physiologic, Psychological, and Social Considerations of the Cancer Patient

	Considerations and Response
Physiologic Maslow's hierarchy a. Food, water, sleep b. Safety, security c. Love, belonging d. Self-esteem e. Self-actualization	The patient's disease may hinder the very basic need to consume and use food and water; the main objective of cancer care is to restore normal function. Once therapy begins, practitioners should make every attempt to accommodate patients when they need assistance obtaining transportation, being available to receive in-home health care/meals/medications, making dates with friends, visiting with family, continuing work, and enjoying hobbies. Therapists should introduce patients to key personnel who may offer assistance in these areas, invite them and family members to support groups and open houses, and/or engage in everyday conversations.
Pain relief	Pain may be caused by the tumor directly or by therapeutic interventions. 75% of patients with advanced disease report pain. 30%-50% of patients undergoing treatment report pain. Therapist should be active in regularly assessing pain and then communicating pain to the attending physician for appropriate management. The report of pain differs for each patient. It is advisable to use a reliable pain assessment tool that gives the patient the opportunity to be as descriptive as possible about pain. If patients are not able to report verbally, look for signs of pain such as facial expressions, temperament, and body posture.
Psychological Five stages of grief/coping a. Denial b. Anger c. Bargaining d. Depression e. Acceptance	Following diagnosis of a life-threatening disease such as cancer can induce responses similar to the stages of grief described by Dr. Elisabeth Kübler-Ross. Every patient does not go through all stages, nor do they go through each stage in progressive order. Therapist should be prepared to listen to patients without judging or discrediting patient responses. Be prepared to give appropriate referrals to experienced and credentialed counselors when you feel uncomfortable addressing psychological needs. Family members and caregivers may also go through similar stages of coping with the illness of their loved one.
Anxiety	Anxiety may come following diagnosis or during therapy. Patients who exhibit signs of increased anxiety should be referred to the physician.
Social a. Support from family/friends/people with similar illness b. Participation in normal life activities c. Intimacy	Invite and involve family in consultations, physician visits, and discussions with patient permission. Direct patients and family to local support groups and other health care facility activities such as fairs, screenings, and promotions. Encourage patients to continue daily activities as appropriate. Discuss intimacy and provide resources and referrals for patients who have specific questions or need suggestions on how to resume/continue in intimate relationships. Avoid labeling with terms such as "undersexed" or "impotent."

Modes of Communication

- Verbal
- Written
- Nonverbal
- Nodding
- Eyebrow movement
- Hands making a fist while laying down
- Eyes closed
- Tears
- Smiles
- Laughing

Tools Used for Effective Communication

- Handouts
- Videos
- Books
- Personal testimony
- Other patients
- Support groups
- Solid and honest communication
- Solidify trust between patient and RT
- Allow patient to ask questions
- Compassionate and straightforward

- Assess patient's comprehension level
- Repetition of information

ASSESSMENT OF ACUTE SIDE EFFECTS

- Onset doses for side effects caused by radiation may vary depending on fractionation schemes and volume of tissue irradiated
- Chemotherapy side effects also vary depending on the type of chemotherapy and/or dose
- Side effects may be acute or latent; the objective is to minimize acute effects, manage them when they occur, and prevent latent effects whenever possible

Acute Radiation-Related Side Effects

Skin Reaction. Skin reactions may persist 6 months to 5 years following completion of treatment. Certain areas are more sensitive than others such as:

- Sites where two skin surfaces are in contact
- Sites where epidermis is thin and smooth
- Areas where the integrity of the skin has been disrupted due to surgical incision/trauma
- Areas of inflammation

Progressive Stages of Skin Reactions

- Epilation—15 Gy (damage to hair follicles and subsequent hair loss)
- Erythema—20 Gy (damage to cells of the skin in minimal and treatment continues)
- Dry Desquamation—30 Gy (skin becomes dry and scaly due to destruction of sebaceous gland in the treatment area)
- Moist Desquamation—40 Gy (inflammation, edema, and blister formation and peeling of the epithelial layers of the skin)
- Necrosis—greater than 50 Gy (cell death)

Mucositis/Stomatitis

- Dose 3000 to 4000 cGy

Mucositis is an alteration in the mucous membranes of the oral cavity, which manifests as inflammation, desquamation, and ulceration.

Early Signs and Symptoms of Mucositis

- Dryness of mucous membranes
- Red, inflamed areas of the mucus membranes
- Presence of white or yellow membrane
- Mild burning sensation

Late Signs and Symptoms of Mucositis

- Ulceration
- Necrotic tissue
- Pain
- Bleeding

Esophagitis. Dose—2000 cGy

- Produces difficulty in swallowing and pain on swallowing
- Pain may mimic the type of pain associated with a myocardial infarction

Early Signs and Symptoms of Esophagitis

- Difficulty in swallowing
- Pain during swallowing
- Vomiting food or blood
- Chest pain
- Inflammation of esophageal lining

Nausea

- Dose—1000 cGy to 3000 cGy

Occurs when the epithelial cells lining the esophagus, stomach, and/or intestines are destroyed in response to radiation

- Never deny or overestimate the expectation that nausea may occur
- Maintain a positive approach

Signs and Symptoms of Nausea

- Usually begins 1 to 6 hours after radiation treatment
- Queasy stomach
- Belching
- Watery mouth
- Sour belch

Diarrhea

- Dose—40 Gy and above
- Epithelial cells in the large colon are destroyed in response to exposure

Signs and Symptoms of Diarrhea

- Watery stools
- Frequent bowel movements

Fatigue

- Fatigue is a feeling of discomfort, which results in a decrease in motor and mental skills.
- Usually begins after the first week of treatment and reaches its peak in 2 weeks, then gradually disappears 2 to 4 weeks after the treatment ends
- Results from destruction of cancer cells and normal cells with the release of waste products into the bloodstream

Myelosuppression

- Occurs when a high volume of bone marrow reserves are irradiated to doses above 20 Gy

- Of greatest concern when irradiating the chest, pelvis, and extremities

Signs and Symptoms of Myelosuppression

- Fatigue
- Easy bruising, nosebleeds
- Repeated infection
- Lowered blood counts

Xerostomia (dry mouth)

- Occurs when doses above 20 Gy are delivered to salivary glands
- Permanent damage to salivary glands may be seen above doses of 40 Gy

Signs and Symptoms of Xerostomia

- Patient complains of cotton mouth
- Difficulty swallowing food
- Sensation of dehydration/feeling thirsty
- Increased viscosity of saliva

Acute Chemotherapy-Related Side Effects

- Considering chemotherapy drugs differ in their mechanism of action, they impose a number of different side effects.
- Combination chemotherapies commonly increase the risk of patients experiencing overlapping side effects such as myelosuppression (low blood counts).
- A toxicity profile is reviewed and taken into consideration by the oncologist when the chemotherapy treatment approach is decided. Toxicity is graded using a scale of 1 to 4; the higher the grade, the higher the risk for anticipated side effects.
- Experienced side effects are particularly related to a person's pathophysiology. Coincidental factors include body surface area measurement (height and weight proportion), comorbidities of other medical disorders or diseases, gender (women are more prone to nausea and vomiting than men—likely related to hormone ratios).
- For acute side effects, the management goal is prevention. Premedications are given to prevent the occurrence.
- Subsequently, when the toxic effect occurs, the management goal becomes supportive.

Dermatologic Effects

- Some chemotherapy agents are classified as vesicants; that is, are toxic to soft tissue and may lead to long-term, local tissue damage (obvious at the injection site).

  Manifestations of local tissue damage:

  1. Blisters
  2. Desquamation
  3. Necrosis

  Examples of vesicant chemotherapy drugs:

  1. Vincristine
  2. Doxorubicin
  3. Etoposide
  4. Mitomycin

- Hand-foot syndrome is a painful skin irritation that would include pain, fissures, redness, and ultimately hyperpigmentation to the palms and soles of the feet; 5-FU and capecitabine may be culprits.
- Monoclonal therapy, also known as immunotherapy, may cause acne-appearing rashes to the face, shoulders, back, and chest.
- Late effects to the skin—referred to as "Radiation Recall"—may be seen in patients who are receiving alkylating agents after a radiation regimen or in the case of disease recurrence for which chemotherapy is given followed by a second course of radiation.

Mucositis, Stomatitis, Esophagitis

- During or after chemotherapy, a patient may have some sort of mouth problem, ranging from dryness to ulcerations.
- Usually 3 to 10 days following chemotherapy, patients experience mucosal burning sensation, followed by ulcers. When ulceration develops, treatment is mostly supportive until the cells regenerate themselves. This takes approximately 7 to 14 days.
- Basic hygiene is of primary importance and should be initiated before chemotherapy or radiation therapy start.
- Patients should brush their teeth three to four times a day; a suggested schedule is after meals and at bedtime. A soft toothbrush or sponge is recommended. Patients at higher risk for this occurrence should rinse their mouth frequently with salt water or baking soda.
- Chemotherapies that put patients at a higher risk for experiencing mouth sores are fluorouracil (5-FU) and methotrexate.

Nausea and Vomiting

- Nausea and vomiting result from stimulation of the chemoreceptor trigger zone of the medulla (brain). Some chemotherapy drugs are worse offenders than others.
- In most cases, patients are given antinausea and vomiting medication (antiemetics) to prevent and control this response.
- It is important to understand that some antiemetics may also have some side effects of their own that patients may experience. Common medications given

to prevent and treat nausea and vomiting are listed below.

- Patients who have been prescribed antiemetics for an extended period of time, beyond the period of chemotherapy, may continue to take this medication due to the continued sensation or as a preventative measure against the anticipated episodes of nausea and/or vomiting.

Antiemetic Drug Names

- Compazine (prochlorperazine)—Side effects of this medication consist of sleepiness, dystonia reactions (sluggish muscles), lockjaw
- Benadryl (diphenhydramine)—Side effects are drowsiness and dry mouth
- Lorazepam (Ativan)—Side effects consist of sleepiness and confusion
- Ondansetron (Zofran)—Side effects consist of headache and constipation
- Granisetron (Kytril)—Side effects consist of headache and constipation
- Dolasetron (Anzemet)—Side effects consist of headache and constipation
- Dronabinol (Marinol)—Side effects consist of sleepiness, appetite stimulation, and confusion
- Dexamethasone—Side effects consist of insomnia, stomach upset
- Metoclopramide (Reglan)—Side effects consist of diarrhea, anxiety, sleepiness
- Delayed nausea and vomiting can occur after cisplatin, carboplatin, and cyclophosphamide chemotherapy.
- The most effective antinausea for delayed nausea and vomiting are Reglan and dexamethasone.

Diarrhea

- Diarrhea occurs in 75% of cancer patients receiving chemotherapy due to the destruction of replicating epithelial cells of the gastrointestinal (GI) tract. This alteration causes inadequate digestion and absorption of nutrients.
- The degree and duration of diarrhea depends on the chemotherapy. Some chemotherapy drugs associated with diarrhea are fluorouracil (5-FU), methotrexate, cytarabine (Ara-C), capecitabine (Xeloda), and irinotecan (Camptosar).

Constipation

- Patients may experience constipation due to a number of cancer management medications such as narcotic analgesics for pain, calcium containing antacids such as Tums, and *vinca* chemotherapies.
- To maintain normal bowel functioning, a bowel regimen should be implemented for patients receiving any of the listed medications:
- Morphine (MS Contin)
- Oxycodone (OxyContin)
- Fentanyl (Duragesic)
- Hydrocodone (Vicodin)
- Hydromorphone (Dilaudid)
- Vinca alkaloid chemotherapies have the potential to cause neurotoxicity of the smooth muscles of the GI tract, leading to decreased peristalsis or paralytic ileus.
- The onset of constipation is usually within 7 days
- Vinca alkaloid chemotherapies include:
- Vincristine (Oncovin)
- Vinblastine (Velban)
- Vinorelbine (Navelbine)
- Elderly patients are particularly susceptible to constipation from both narcotic analgesic use and vinca chemotherapy.

Myelosuppression

- Myelosuppression is considered to be the most frequent and most serious chemo-related toxicity.
- Patients should be counseled that it is not uncommon to experience some degree of myelosuppression during their course of treatment.
- The majority of chemotherapy agents produce some degree of myelosuppression; however, the severity depends on the drug, the dose, administration frequency, and the route.
- Patients at greater risk for developing myelosuppression would be: (1) the elderly (less resilient bone marrow); (2) those who have been previously irradiated to the bone marrow target areas (sternum, pelvis, extremities, ribs); and (3) patients who received high doses of radiation and/or chemotherapy at an earlier date
- Cell-cycle nonspecific drugs, such as antimetabolites, cause a more acute myelosuppression.
- Cell-cycle specific drugs, such as nitrosoureas, cause a delayed myelosuppressive effect.
- More severe degrees of myelosuppression are seen in patients receiving alkylating agents
- Most myelosuppression occurs 7 to 14 days following chemotherapy administration
- Myelosuppression includes neutropenia, anemia, and thrombocytopenia

- Neutropenia is a decrease in the number of white blood cells (WBC); low WBC increases the potential for infection since they are the primary defenders for infection prevention

Important: Patients with decreased WBC should maintain adequate nutrition and fluid intake, avoid crowds and persons with known infections, and report any signs of infections such as fever, cough, sore throat, and stiff neck.

- Anemia is the decrease in the number of red blood cells (RBC), hemoglobin (HGB), and hematocrit (HCT). Fatigue is the most common symptom of anemia due to lack of circulating oxygen in the blood cell. Other signs of anemia include shortness of breath, headache, dizziness, irritability, pale nail beds and palms, and pale oral cavity.

Important: Patients with anemia should maintain adequate hydration.

- Thrombocytopenia is a decrease in the number of platelets (PLT). Bleeding tendencies are the most common sign of low platelet count since platelets are supportive of normal clotting mechanisms. Nosebleeds, bleeding of the gums, petechiae (small red, generalized spots), bruising, and urinary or intestinal bleeding are manifestations of low platelets.

Important: Patients with thrombocytopenia should limit falling risks, use soft bristle toothbrushes or sponge for teeth cleaning; avoid aggressive nose blowing; avoid aspirin, ibuprofen, and rectal suppositories.

Dry Mouth (xerostomia)

- Dry mouth can occur as a result of chemotherapy.
- Often dry mouth precludes oral mucosa ulcers.

MANAGEMENT OF ACUTE SIDE EFFECTS

Interventions for Radiation-Related Skin Reactions

- Gently cleanse skin in the treatment area
- Expose the area to the air as often as possible
- Avoid tight fitting clothing over the skin
- Avoid wearing harsh fabrics such as wool or corduroy
- Use gentle detergent to wash clothes
- Avoid exposure to cold temperatures
- Avoid swimming in salt water/chlorinated pools
- Avoid powders, creams, deodorant, medicated patches, and Band-aids
- Avoid shaving hair in treatment area
- Avoid exposure to the sun

Interventions for Dermatologic Reactions Caused By Chemotherapy

- Area should be kept clean and dry
- Area should be protected from direct sunlight exposure; suggest light-cotton clothing
- Important to apply topical moisturizers

Interventions for Radiation-Related Esophagitis

- Use antacids
- Use milk products (sour cream, yogurt, cottage cheese)
- Use a straw for liquids
- Use liquid Tylenol
- Eat foods high in calories and proteins
- Small frequent meals
- Avoid hot/spicy foods

Interventions for Chemotherapy-Related Mucositis, Stomatitis, Esophagitis

- Analgesics and anesthetics can be used. Xylocaine is a local anesthetic available as a gel or spray that can be used specifically on the site to decrease pain.
- Protective agents can also be used to provide a protective coating over ulcers and decrease their irritation. Examples of these agents are Maalox and Mylanta.
- A basic solution referred to as Miracle or Magic Mouthwash consists of a combination of agents (analgesic/lidocaine, antacid/Maalox or Mylanta, and an antihistamine/Benadryl) is commonly used to prevent and/or relieve discomfort of mucosa caused by ulcers.
- Sucralfate (Carafate) is available by prescription to coat the mucosa and relieve discomfort.
- Another agent, an antifungal, can be added or used in the presence of oral fungal infections (*Candida*). It can be either clotrimazole (Mycelex lozenges) or nystatin suspension (swish and swallow).
- Xylocaine or lidocaine solution should not be used before meals because of the threat of choking.
- Avoid the use of hydrogen peroxide because it may worsen or irritate ulcers.
- Topical steroids should not be used because they can facilitate infections.
- Patients should be advised not to eat spicy, hot, acidic, or course foods or beverages. Food selections should be steered toward moist, soft foods, such as mashed potatoes and soft scrambled eggs.

Interventions for Radiation-Related Mucositis

- Force fluids
- Use a systematic, consistent mouth care regime
- Avoid the use of tobacco
- Avoid alcoholic beverages
- Avoid foods that are thermally very hot or cold
- Avoid citrus fruits
- Avoid foods that are hard or coarse
- Avoid use of dental floss and water piks

Interventions for Radiation or Chemo-Related Nausea/Vomiting

- Encourage an intervention that helped relieve nausea or vomiting in the past, such as with a pregnancy, an illness, or times of stress.
- Eat cold foods or those served at room temperature, such as a deli sandwich, cereal, or saltine crackers. These foods are usually better tolerated than warm or hot foods. The odor of hot foods often aggravates the feeling of nausea.
- Clear liquid diets assist to reduce nausea. Liquids such as fruit ades, Gatorade, ginger ale, 7-Up, gelatin, and tea are usually well tolerated. These liquids should be served cold and sipped slowly.
- Bland foods such as mashed potatoes, applesauce, toast, and cottage cheese are also well tolerated.
- Sour foods, such as lemons, sour pickles, hard sour candy, or lemon sherbet, can also aid to reduce nausea.
- Avoid sweet, fatty, highly salted and spicy foods as well as those with strong odors.
- Minimize stimuli such as sights, sounds, and smells that can initiate nausea such as unpleasant odors, perfume/cologne/body sprays, and other people who are nauseated and vomiting.
- Avoid eating or drinking for 1 to 2 hours before and after chemotherapy or radiation therapy.
- Eat frequent small meals throughout the day.
- Avoid lying down flat at least 30 minutes after eating.
- Get fresh air by sitting near an open window or go out doors.
- Rest in a comfortable position in a quiet environment.
- Provide distractions such as listening to soft relaxing music, reading, or watching television.
- Use relaxation techniques with or without visual imagery. Seek services of a professional provider if unable to achieve relaxation alone.
- Use antiemetic

Interventions for Radiation or Chemo-Related Diarrhea:

- Anti-diarrheal therapy is the primary treatment. The following medications have been shown to be effective in the treatment of diarrhea:
- Loperamide (Imodium) two dosages (capsule or liquid) initially followed by one dose after each loose stool, up to eight doses a day. Side effects from this medication are sedation and drowsiness.
- Lomotil 1 or 2 tablets three to four times a day. Side effects include nervousness and drowsiness.
- The primary goal with episodes of diarrhea is prevention of dehydration. Therefore adequate fluid intake is critical. At least 3000 mL (12.5 cups) of fluid each day is recommended.
- Recommended fluids would include water, broth, soup, noncaffeinated beverages, and Gatorade.
- When diarrhea is occurring in severe amounts, intravenous fluid support may be required on a short-term basis.
- Additional options would include:
- Low-residue diet, high in protein and calories (Box 8-1)
- Eliminate foods and beverages that may be irritating or stimulating to the gastrointestinal (GI) tract (Box 8-2).
- Adding nutmeg to foods may decrease the motility of the GI tract.
- Foods high in potassium are recommended if the patient exhibits signs of fatigue or weakness or if the potassium level is low.

BOX 8-1 Low-Residue Diet

Cottage cheese, mild processed cheese, eggs, low fat milk, yogurt, rice, pudding, custard, tapioca, buttermilk
Broth, bouillon, gelatin, apple juice, grape juice
Fish, poultry, ground beef, broiled roast
Cooked cereals (i.e., cream of wheat), crackers, white bread, macaroni, noodles
Bananas, applesauce, peeled apples (apples contain pectin an antidiarrhea agent), avocados
Baked, boiled, or mashed potatoes
Smooth peanut butter
Cooked, mild vegetables (i.e., asparagus tips, beets, green or waxed beans, peas, carrots, spinach, squash, cream vegetable soups)

BOX 8-2 Foods Irritating or Stimulating to the GI Tract

Whole-grain bread and cereal, nuts, seeds, coconut, fried, greasy foods (i.e., pork)
Fresh and dried fruits
Raw vegetables, rich pastries, popcorn, potato chips, pretzels
Strong spices and herbs (i.e., chili powder, licorice, pepper, curry, garlic, horseradish, olives, pickles, relishes)
Flatus forming food, such as broccoli, onions, cabbage
Food and beverages containing caffeine such as chocolate, coffee, tea, and soft drinks
Alcohol beverages including strong liquor, beer, wine
Tobacco products

- High potassium foods include baked potato, halibut, and asparagus tips.
- Encourage eating small, frequent meals.
- Avoid extremely hot or cold foods. Extremes in temperature may aggravate the diarrhea.

Interventions for Chemo-Related and Analgesic-Related Constipation

- Increase dietary fiber amount in food choices (Box 8-3).
- Drink warm or hot beverages, especially upon arising.
- Drink 3000 mL (12.5 cups) of fluid daily (unless contraindicated).
- Increase physical activity level.
- Use prophylactic stool softener daily, such as Colace 200 mg twice a day.
- If a patient does not experience a bowel movement in 3 days or longer, use of a laxative is necessary.
- Common laxatives include the following:
- Senokot: 2 tablets daily until regular bowel function, then 1 tablet daily
- Dulcolax: 1 to 2 tablets daily until regular bowel function, then 1 tablet daily
- If over-the-counter laxatives are ineffective, a prescription can be obtained.
- Lactulose solution is a common prescriptive laxative. With excessive use/doses, diarrhea and flatulence can be the result.

BOX 8-3 High Fiber Foods

Fresh raw fruit with skin and seeds, prunes, dates, raisins
Fresh raw vegetables
Nuts, coconut, corn, popcorn, whole grain products, bran
Fresh fruit and vegetable juices

Interventions for Radiation-Related or Chemo-Related Fatigue

- Conserve energy
- Rest when fatigue is experienced
- Force fluids
- Maintain nutrition
- Seek help with child care and household duties
- Explore alternative means of transportation

Interventions for Radiation or Chemo-Related Xerostomia

- Encourage the patient to drink (sip) fluid frequently throughout the day
- Suck ice chips
- Suck hard candy
- Chew gum
- A gentle soothing, alcohol free oral mouthwash referred to as Biotene is a common solution used by patients and is available over-the-counter.
- Patients should stay away from solutions containing alcohol or glycerin bases because they can irritate or aggravate dryness.

Interventions for Radiation or Chemo-Related Myelosuppression

- Table 8-2 lists interventions for radiation or chemotherapy-related myelosuppression; Figure 8-1 depicts the calculation of absolute neutrophil count (ANC).

Latent Effects from Radiation and Chemotherapy

- Table 8-3 includes radiation- and chemotherapy-related late effects.

Routine Assessments

Normal Patient Vital Signs

- Table 8-4 lists normal vital signs by age.

Normal Blood Count

- RBC: Ref. range 4.20 to 5.70 million/cc^3
- WBC: Ref. range 3900 to 10,000/cc^3
- HGB: Ref. range 13.2 to 16.9/cc^3
- HCT: Ref. range 38.5% to 49.0%
- Platelets: Ref. range 140,000 to 390,000/ cc^3

TABLE 8-2 Interventions for Radiation or Chemotherapy-Related Myelosuppression

Neutropenia	Anemia	Thrombocytopenia
ANC = 1500 *Avoid crowds, wash hands often* *Neupogen or Neulasta: subcutaneous injection (causes bone pain)* **ANC = 1000** *Above precautions and heightened housecleaning* **ANC = 500** *Above precautions and wear mask in public, limit visitors, no fresh fruit or vegetables; no fresh or artificial flowers, no raw foods*	**HGB <9.0 or HCT <30** ***Procrit or Aranesp:*** *subcutaneous injection (causes increased blood pressure)* **HGB <8.0** *Transfusion*	**PLT <50,000** *Soft toothbrush, limit fall potential and bruising hazards* **PLT <20,000** *Transfusion or subcutaneous Neumega: subcutaneous injection; interleukin (blood activating factor)*

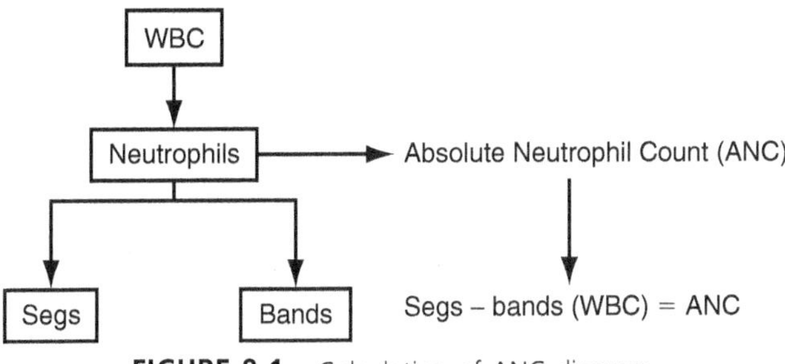

FIGURE 8-1 Calculation of ANC diagram.

TABLE 8-3 Sample Radiation and Chemotherapy-Related Late Effects

Radiation-Related Late Effects	Chemotherapy-Related Late Effects
Second cancers	Cardiomyopathy
Genetic mutations	Renal failure
Organ failure	Kidney failure
Tissue necrosis	Arrested development of bone and mental capacity
Chronic bowel irritability	Delayed, impaired memory (chemo brain)
Pneumonitis	Tissue necrosis
Decreased tissue elasticity	
Hyperpigmentation	

Performance Scales

- Karnofsky performance scale uses 0 to 100; describes patient's ability to care for himself and complete normal activities.
- Performance is related to patient's ability to endure aggressive therapies, such as radiation and chemotherapy.
- (ECOG) Eastern Cooperative Oncology Group performance scale assesses how a patient's disease is progressing, and assesses how the disease affects daily living using scale from 0 to 5.

  0—Fully active, able to carry on all predisease performance without restriction
  5—Dead
- Glasgow Coma scale uses range 3 to 15; assesses patient neurologic and cognitive function; good assessment tool when patient consciousness level changes.

Pain Assessment and Management

- Pain levels should be evaluated at regular intervals for all patients.
- Pain scales may take on many forms; when evaluating gather information about the frequency, nature, location, sensation, and duration.
- Simple pain scales may use numerical values 0 to 10; 0 indicating no pain and 10 indicating the worst pain.
- Pain assessment tools should allow the patient to independently express their level, frequency, nature, location, sensation, and duration of pain.
- Management of pain can include:

  a. Medication
  b. Meditation, visualization
  c. Conditioning

Nutritional Assessment and Education

- Patient's nutritional status is critical in fighting disease, cell building, and tolerance of therapy

Anorexia

- The causes of anorexia in a patient can occur due to:
- Fatigue
- Dry mouth, esophagitis, nausea, vomiting,
- Presence of pain
- Presence of an infection
- Presence of stress, anxiety, depression
- Change in usual life style patterns

TABLE 8-4 A Quick Reference to Normal Vital Signs By Age

Age	Temperature (Oral)	Temperature (Rectal)	Pulse	Respirations	Blood Pressure (Systolic)
Premature newborn		99.6 °F (37.5 °C)	140	<60	50-60
Full-term newborn		99.6 °F (37.5 °C)	125	<60	70
6 months		99.6 °F (37.5 °C)	120	24-36	90
1 year		99.6 °F (37.5 °C)	120	22-30	96
3 years		99.6 °F (37.5 °C)	110	20-26	100
5 years	98.6 °F (37 °C)	99.6 °F (37.5 °C)	100	20-24	100
6 years	98.6 °F (37 °C)	99.6 °F (37.5 °C)	100	20-24	100
8 years	98.6 ° F (37 °C)	99.6 °F (37.5 °C)	90	18-22	105
12 years	98.6 °F (37 °C)	99.6 °F (37.5 °C)	85-90	16-22	115
16 years	98.6 °F (37 °C)	99.6 °F (37.5 °C)	75-80	14-20	Below 120
Adult female	98.6 °F (37 °C)	99.6 °F (37.5 °C)	60-100	12-20	Below 120
Adult male	98.6 °F (37 °C)	99.6 °F (37.5 °C)	60-100	12-20	Below 120

From Ehrlich RA, Daly JA: Patient care in radiography: with an introduction to medical imaging, ed 7, St Louis, 2009, Mosby/Elsevier.

Ways to Prevent/Minimize Anorexia

- Serve all food attractively and in a pleasant environment
- Avoid eating three large meals; instead eat several small meals at frequent intervals throughout the day
- Consider protein-calorie intake
- Avoid drinking fluids with meals
- Remove all unpleasant smells
- Use nutritional supplements

Nausea, vomiting, and diarrhea lead to loss of electrolytes, vitamins, and nutrients. Therapists can recommend the following:

- Increase your fluid intake by drinking plenty of water each day.
- Eliminate milk and milk products until diarrhea is under control.
- Eat smaller, more frequent meals (example: five smaller meals as compared to three large ones).
- Avoid raw vegetables and fruits. Avoid foods with high roughage content (salads, corn, etc.).
- All vegetables should be cooked.
- Add nutmeg to foods. This spice may decrease stomach irritability.
- Reduce alcohol consumption.
- Avoid tobacco products.
- Avoid extremely hot or cold foods. Foods served warm or at room temperature are more easily tolerated.
- Avoid items that can produce gas or cause cramps, such as carbonated drinks, chewing gum, beans, cabbage, highly spiced foods, skipping meals and swallowing air while talking and eating.
- Include foods high in potassium—bananas, potatoes, red meat, apricot nectar, and vegetable juices.
- Eliminate caffeine from your diet (coffee, tea, cocoa, soda).

Nutritional Supplements

- Ensure
- Sustacal Plus
- Carnation Instant Breakfast Bars
- Vitamins
- Feeding tube

SAFE PRACTICES

Body Mechanics

- Body mechanics is the use of the correct muscles to complete a task safely and efficiently, without undue strain on any muscles or joints.
- Principles of body mechanics
- Maintain a stable center of gravity
- Keep your back straight
- Bend at the knees and hips
- Techniques of body mechanics
- Use leg muscles for lifting
- Avoid twisting or stretching
- Avoid bending at the waist

Assisting Patients with Medical Equipment

Patients with IVs

- Keep IV above injection site
- Keep IV free from tangles
- Keep pump plugged in

- If leakage is spotted, do not clean until verification of liquid is identified
- Handle with gloves

Chest Tubes

- Keep lower than injection site
- Keep hemostat available to shut off
- Keep upright, never lay down
- Always handle with two hands

Urinary Catheter

- Keep catheter line below site of origin
- Check for leakage
- Never pull out
- Keep untangled

Oxygen Administration

- *Do not* use around flames or sparks
- *Do not* stand oxygen cylinder upright unless it is secured
- *Do not* carry cylinder by regulator or valve

MANAGING MEDICAL EMERGENCIES

Anaphylactic Shock

- Life-threatening condition due to a severe allergic reaction causing bronchial airway to constrict

Symptoms of Anaphylactic Shock

- Difficulty breathing
- Swollen or tingling lips
- Drop in blood pressure
- Vomiting
- Metallic taste in the mouth
- Itching skin
- Hives
- Dizziness
- Temporary loss of consciousness

Treatment of Anaphylactic Shock

- Epinephrine

Cardiac Arrest

- Sudden abrupt loss of heart function

ABCs of CPR

A. Check airway
   - Open airway by lifting the chin with one hand and push down on the forehead with the other hand
   - Tilt head back
   - Listen for the sound of breathing
   - Feel for breath on your cheek

B. Breathing:
   - Pinch nose shut and keep head tilted
   - Airtight seal; give two full breaths

C. Circulation:
   - After giving two full breaths, locate the carotid artery pulse to see if heart is still beating
   - If no pulse, ratio 30 chest compressions to 2 breaths

Respiratory Arrest

- Caused by airway obstruction
- Obstruction may be partial or complete

Signs of Respiratory Distress

- Complaining of difficulty in breathing
- Tachypnea
- Abnormal breathing sounds
- Cyanosis

Signs of Respiratory Arrest

- Absence of breathing
- No chest rise and fall
- Progressive color change caused by lack of oxygen

Seizures

- Sudden change of behavior due to abnormal electrical activity in the brain
- Do not try to restrain the patient
- Do not try to move the patient
- Move dangerous objects away from the patient
- Do not place anything in the patient's mouth or try to move the tongue

After Seizure

- Do check breathing
- Do stay and talk to the patient
- Do not offer the patient something to drink or eat

Fainting

- Syncope is the temporary loss of consciousness
- Help person who has fainted to the ground
- Shake and call patient's name
- Check for pulse

Stroke

- Cerebral vascular accident (CVA) occurs when blood supply to part of the brain is disrupted, causing the brain cells to die.

Signs of a Stroke

- Sudden numbness or weakness of the face, arm, or leg on one side
- Sudden confusion or trouble speaking
- Sudden trouble seeing in one or both eyes
- Sudden trouble walking, loss of balance
- Sudden severe headache with no known cause

Choking

- Universal sign of choking is a patient clutching his throat with both hands
- Encourage patient to continue coughing
- Do not assist unless the patient is no longer able to cough or speak
- Clear obstruction-Heimlich Maneuver-abdominal thrust or back thrust for infants

INFECTION CONTROL

Important Terms

Asepsis

- Absence of disease producing microorganism called pathogens

Medical Asepsis

- Refers to the practice that helps to reduce the number and hinder the transfer of disease producing microorganisms.
- Also called clean technique

Surgical Asepsis

- Practices that render and keep objects and areas free from *all* microorganisms
- Also called sterile technique

Contamination

- Process by which something is rendered unclean or unsterile

Disinfection

- Process by which pathogenic organisms, but generally spores, are destroyed

Antiseptic

- Inhibits the growth of bacteria

Sterilization

- Process by which *all* microorganisms are destroyed

In order for an infection to manifest:

1. A germ must be present.

Examples include:

- Virus
- Fungus
- Bacterium
- Parasite

2. The germ must have a place to live and multiply such as:

- People
- Plants
- Food
- Soil
- Water

3. A susceptible host, specifically a person who does not have immunity to the germ.
4. A way for the germ to enter the host, such as:

- Direct contact
- Touch, sexual contact, kissing, etc.
- Indirect contact
- Through contaminated food, water, feces
- Water droplets
- Particles in the air

Removing any one of these four conditions breaks the chain of infection, thus preventing the infection from spreading.

- Breaking the chain of infection
- Practice good personal hygiene
- Treat all bodily fluids as potentially infectious
- Use protective barriers
- Gloves, mask
- Maintain a clean environment
- Hand hygiene (soap and water, antiseptic hand wash, alcohol-based rubs)

- Alcohol-based rubs are quick and effective before and after each patient contact, and before and after using gloves, as long as hands are not visibly soiled or contaminated; if hands are visibly soiled, soap and water is best.

Standard Precautions

- Universal precaution
- Designed to prevent the transmission of HIV, hepatitis, and other pathogens that are spread through contact with body fluids
- Requires the use of protective barriers
- Gloves, aprons, masks, and protective eyewear

Hospital Isolation

- Barriers in place to stop the spread of infection

Types of Hospital Isolation

Strict isolation

- Designed to prevent transmission of highly contagious infections that can be spread by air or contact
- Gowns
- Mask
- Gloves
- Hand washing after leaving room
- Contaminated articles from the room should be labeled and bagged.

Reverse isolation

- Designed to protect immunosuppressed patients from infection
- Patient should be isolated with minimum dust, dirt, and wet areas.
- Sterile glove
- Gown
- Mask
- Hand washed before entering the room

Contact isolation

- Designed to prevent transmission of infections that do not warrant strict isolation (disease usually spread by direct contact)
- Mask
- Gloves
- Gowns
- Hand washing after touching patient
- Contaminated articles from the room should be labeled and bagged.

Respiratory isolation

- Designed to prevent transmission of infection through the air
- Mask
- Hand washed after touching patient
- Contaminated articles from the room should be labeled and bagged.
- Patient in negative pressure and isolated air-flow room

DRUG ADMINISTRATION

Five Rights of Drug Safety

- Right patient
- Right time and frequency of administration
- Right dose
- Right route of administration

  Oral
  IV
  Subdural
  Intramuscular
  Topical
  Rectal
- Right drug

Drugs Commonly Used in Radiation Oncology

Antiemetics

- Drugs used to prevent or stop nausea and vomiting
- Can be given by mouth, injection, or suppository
- Reglan
- Compazine

Antidiarrheals

- Drugs used to treat persistent diarrhea
- Work in various ways to thicken the stool or slow spasms that occur in the intestines
- Lomotil
- Imodium

Antibiotics

- Drugs used to fight bacterial infections
- Penicillin
- Keflex

Pain Medication/Analgesics

- Drugs used to relieve pain
- Opioids

Short acting opioids

- Morphine
- Codeine
- Hydrocodone
- Oxycodone
- Fentanyl

Long-acting opioids

- MS-Contin
- Methadone
- Oxymorphone

Nonsteroidal Antiinflammatory Drugs

- Drugs with analgesic, antipyretic, and antiinflammatory effects that reduce pain, fever, and inflammation
- Naproxen
- Ibuprofen
- Sulindac

BIBLIOGRAPHY

Ehrlich RA, Daly JA: *Patient care in radiography: with an introduction to medical imaging*, ed 7, St Louis, 2009, Mosby.

Gates RA, Fink RM: *Oncology nursing secrets*, ed 3, St Louis, 2008, Mosby.

Hall JK: *Law and ethics for clinicians*, 2002, Jackhal Books.

Mahon S: *Study guide for the core curriculum for oncology nursing*, ed 4, St Louis, 2005, Mosby.

Torres LS, Dutton AG, Linn-Watson TA: *Patient care in imaging technology*, ed 6, Philadelphia, 2009, Lippincott Williams & Wilkins.

Varricchio CG: *A cancer source book for nurses*, ed 8, Sudbury, 2004, Jones and Bartlett.

Washington CM, Leaver D: *Principles and practice of radiation therapy*, ed 3, St Louis, 2010, Mosby.

REVIEW EXERCISES

1. The cycle of infection can be broken by the:

   1. Destruction of the infectious organism
   2. Removal of the source of infection
   3. Preventing the means of transmission

   a. a and b
   b. a and c
   c. b and c
   d. a, b, and c

2. The normal platelet count for an adult is approximately:

   a. 20,000/cc
   b. 80,000/cc
   c. 120,000/cc
   d. 250,000/cc

3. The normal adult resting respiration is about ______ .

4. The practice that helps reduce the spread of microorganisms is termed ______ .

5. The most common means by which infections are spread is by:

   a. Airborne particulates
   b. Indirect contact
   c. Direct contact
   d. Endogenous contact

6. The loss of hair after exposure to radiation is termed ____________.

7. Please list five important components of a low residual diet.

   a. ____________
   b. ____________
   c. ____________
   d. ____________
   e. ____________

8. For an infection to spread, a germ must have a way of entering the host such as through:

   a. ____________
   b. ____________
   c. ____________
   d. ____________
   e. ____________

9. Write definitions for each of the following:

   a. Asepsis

   b. Medical asepsis

c. Surgical asepsis

d. Contamination

e. Disinfection

f. Antiseptic

g. Sterilization

10. Match the following conditions in Column A with the recommended diets in Column B. Responses may be used more than once.

COLUMN A	COLUMN B
_____ diarrhea	A. regular diet
_____ nausea	B. clear fluids
_____ vomiting	C. liquids only
_____ mucositis	D. soft liquids
_____ dysphagia	E. low residue

11. The normal adult value for an oral temperature is ____________F.

12. The ABCs of CPR are__________, __________, and __________.

13. The ________________artery is the point where the pulse is often measured.

True or False (circle the correct answer).

14. After assisting with an IV, the therapist must cap the needle before disposing of it.

True or False

15. A pulse rate of 35 beats/min would be called tachycardia.

True or False

16. Match the following terms with the correct definition.

_____ bluish discoloration of skin	A. Syncope
_____ stroke	B. CVA
_____ fainting	C. Cyanosis
_____ profuse sweating	D. Diaphoresis
_____ tube used to pass fluids, gases into/out of body	E. Tachypnea
_____ an aggregation of blood	F. Thrombus
	G. Parenteral
	H. Cannula

17. For what reason is anaphylactic shock the type of shock most often seen in diagnostic imaging?

a. Patients who come for diagnostic imaging procedures are weak and debilitated
b. Iodinated contrast agents are frequently used
c. Patients here have more allergies
d. X-radiation causes this problem

18. Symptoms of a partially obstructed airway may include:

a. Cold, clammy skin; pallor; weakness; anxiety
b. Flushed, hot skin; hyperactivity; confusion
c. Labored, noisy, breathing, wheezing
d. Acetone breath, irregular pulse, noisy respiration

19. Alopecia, nausea, vomiting, stomatitis, and skin reactions are all possible side effects of radiotherapy. The correct response to someone asking whether he will experience them would be:

a. "Yes, but they'll subside once treatment ceases."
b. "No, they rarely occur."
c. "The type of side effects that will occur is dependent on the specific treatment site and dose."
d. "You'll have to ask your doctor."

20. Radiation recall:

a. The recurrence of the radiation skin reaction when given certain chemotherapy drugs

b. Can occur years after radiation
c. The recurrence of all radiation toxicities when given certain drugs
d. a and b only
e. All of the above

21. A patient with lung cancer has shortness of breath, a cough, facial and arm edema, and neck distention. The therapist suspects that the patient has developed:

a. Cardiac tamponade
b. Superior vena cava syndrome
c. Pleural effusion
d. Tumor lysis syndrome

22. The care plan for a patient receiving narcotics around the clock for pain control should include which of the following daily measures to prevent constipation?

a. Digital examination for impaction
b. Use of suppositories
c. Regular administration of mild laxatives
d. Fluid intake of approximately 1500 cc/day

23. A patient receiving treatment for lymphoma reports experiencing numbness and tingling in the feet, weakness when ambulating, and dribbling of urine. The therapist should suspect:

a. Development of diabetes mellitus
b. Development of spinal cord compression
c. Peripheral neuropathy
d. Production of ectopic hormone

24. The most common clinical manifestation of infection in patients with cancer who are neutropenic is:

a. Fever
b. Positive blood cultures
c. Dysuria
d. Redness at the catheter site

25. Match the types of shock in Column A with the causes in Column B

________	**low volume of circulating blood**	A. Anaphylactic
________	**systemic infection and bacteremia**	B. Hypovolemic
________	**injury or emotional trauma**	C. Cardiogenic
________	**hypoglycemia**	D. Septic
________	**heart failure**	E. Neurogenic
________	**severe allergic reaction**	F. Diabetic

26. Match the drugs with symptoms or conditions

____	**allergies**	A. Benadryl
____	**heart arrhythmia**	B. Lidocaine
____	**hypertension**	C. Inderal
____	**cardiogenic shock**	D. Lanoxin

27. If an area must be kept completely free of pathogens, you should follow:

a. Surgical asepsis
b. Gloved technique
c. Medical asepsis
d. Clean technique

28. If a patient appears to be fainting, the first thing that you should do is:

a. Assist the patient to a safe position and call for help
b. Give smelling salt
c. Get crash cart
d. Prepare to administer oxygen

29. All drugs given by parenteral routes are given by:

a. Medical aseptic techniques
b. Surgical aseptic techniques

30. The range for normal respiration for adults is:

a. 20 to 30
b. 80 to 90
c. 10 to 20
d. 8 to 10

31. The normal adult value for an oral temperature is ________C.

32. The process by which all forms of microorganisms are destroyed is called ________.

33. The best means of preventing the spread of microorganisms is ________.

34. A nosocomial infection is one that the patient has acquired at home.
True or False

35. Within 30 minutes of receiving the first dose of asparaginase, a patient with acute lymphatic leukemia experience tightness of the chest, dyspnea, and nausea. These symptoms suggest that the patient is experiencing:

a. An anaphylactic reaction
b. Cardiac toxicity
c. Pulmonary fibrosis
d. Anxiety

36. The practice that helps reduce the spread of microorganisms is termed:

a. Lethargy
b. Contracture
c. Asepsis
d. Isolation

37. In general, the best method for a therapist to maintain medical asepsis and prevent the spread of infection is by frequent and proper:

a. Mask usage
b. Hand washing
c. Isolation usage
d. Personal hygiene

38. The patient has the right to:

a. Refuse medical treatment
b. Know the qualifications of the medical personnel
c. Confidential treatment of his or her records

a. a and b
b. a and c
c. b and c
d. a, b, and c

39. A patient that is said to be experiencing dyspnea has:

a. Breathing difficulties
b. High blood pressure
c. A fever
d. A urinary problem

40. The loss of hair after exposure to radiation is termed:

a. Epistaxis
b. Epilation
c. Erythema
d. Elation

41. A drug used to relieve symptoms of nausea and vomiting due to irradiation is a/an:

a. Laxative
b. Analgesic
c. Antiemetic
d. Antidiarrheal

42. List the five Rights of Drug Safety.

a. ____________
b. ____________
c. ____________
d. ____________
e. ____________

43. Name three routes of administering drugs.

a. ____________
b. ____________
c. ____________

44. List three important facts regarding oxygen therapy.

a. ____________
b. ____________
c. ____________

45. List five things you would tell a patient to avoid during treatment regarding their skin care.

a. ____________
b. ____________
c. ____________
d. ____________
e. ____________

46-55. Complete the chart of common radiation side effects to include anticipated onset dose and appropriate interventions.

	Onset Dose	Intervention
Skin Reaction		
Diarrhea		
Fatigue		
Pain		
Nausea		
Weight Loss		
Mucositis		
Alopecia		
Cystitis		
Esophagitis		

56-65. Complete the chart of medical emergencies, related symptoms, likely causes, and appropriate interventions.

Emergency	Symptoms	Likely Cause	Intervention
Anaphylactic Shock			
Cardiogenic Shock			
Hypovolemic Shock			
Pulmonary Embolism			
Hypoglycemia			
Hyperglycemia			
Respiratory distress			
Cardiac distress			
Seizure			
Syncope			

Think About It

66. Review the code of ethics for radiation therapists and identify the language supportive of each of the seven ethical principles.

67. How might you prevent negligence or malpractice as you practice professionally?

68. What is the rationale for formulating and publicizing a code of ethics?

69. How might you prevent being accused of "invading the privacy" of patients in the clinical setting?

70. You observe an error during a procedure. The error causes the patient to require an extended stay in the hospital. The clinician does not share the nature of the error. The patient asks *you* what happened. How do you respond? What ethical principle(s) support your response?

71. You have a part-time job as a file clerk in the hospital. You recognize the name on a chart as that of a family friend who was recently admitted and you see the initials HIV in the chart. You assume that these familiar initials mean that your family friend has the virus associated with AIDS. You feel concerned and go home and call your mother and father with the news and plan a visit to console him. What are the ethical and legal considerations in this case?

72. What acute side effects do you anticipate your patient will experience during radiation therapy for brain metastases? How will you assist your patient in managing those symptoms?

73. An adult patient who has tachycardia would have a pulse higher than:

a. 60 beats/min
b. 90 beats/min
c. 80 beats/min
d. 100 beats/min

74. A drug that would increase the flow of urine is a:

a. Derivative
b. Diuretic
c. Diarrheal
d. Antiemetic

75. Refusing to care for a patient who has different religious beliefs from your own would be violation of:

a. Criminal law
b. Ethical code
c. Administrative law
d. Personal law

76. Professional ethics are:

a. A set of principles that govern a course of action
b. Values of any professional person
c. The same as federal law
d. A set of rules and regulations made up by the facility manager

77. Information about a patient's condition:

a. May be discussed with close relatives only
b. Must always remain confidential
c. Is open for discussion if their condition is discussed in medical rounds
d. Can be shared with other medical professionals only

78. If your manager asks you to perform a duty outside of your scope of practice, the best course of action would be to:

a. Proceed as best as you can
b. Ask a colleague for directions and then proceed
c. Explain that you do not have the education required and feel uncomfortable
d. State that you are ill and retreat

79. A persistent threat for HIV or HBV infection for the health care provider is:

a. The water supply
b. Careless patients who do not reveal their status
c. Needle-stick injuries
d. Tuberculosis exposure

80. An example of a potential source of infection would be:

a. A co-worker with a cold
b. A visitor with a "fever blister" on the mouth
c. A patient with pneumonia
d. All of the above

81. The method by which all health care providers can control the transmission of blood-borne disease transmission is:

a. Enteric precautions
b. Universal precautions
c. Strict isolation
d. Reverse isolation

82. The "scope of practice" for the radiation therapist

a. Could never be used in a court of law
b. Describes the responsibilities of the therapist
c. Can be used to defend the actions of a nurse
d. Can be used to defend the actions of a physician

83. In Latin, fide means:

a. Half contract
b. On the face of
c. Do no harm
d. To be faithful

84. A patient undergoing chemoradiation may complain of:

a. Fatigue
b. Hyperpigmentation
c. Bone and joint pain
d. Any of the above

85. A patient experiencing constipation should be advised to:

a. Eat fresh fruits and vegetables
b. Drink liquids only
c. Begin a clear liquid diet
d. Decrease dietary fiber

86. Mismanagement of an acute side effect such as oral mucositis may result in:

a. Painful ulcerations and bleeding in the mouth
b. Compromised ability to speak
c. Compromised ability to take oral medications
d. All of the above

87. Those patients treated with radiation therapy alone at moderate to high risk for radiation induced nausea and vomiting would be those receiving radiation to the:

1. Extremities
2. Oropharynx
3. Upper abdomen
4. Total body

 a. 1, 2
 b. 2, 3
 c. 3, 4
 d. 2, 3, 4

88. Complementary measures for managing nausea and vomiting include all of the following, *except*:

a. Imagery
b. Ginger root tables, tea
c. Increasing intake of greasy food
d. Exercise

89. Cancer cachexia is:

a. An increase in appetite
b. An inflammatory response to disease
c. Progressive, involuntary weight loss
d. The result of low fiber dieting

90. Radiation therapy to the pelvis may cause acute:

a. Proctitis
b. Mucositis
c. Nausea and vomiting
d. Xerostomia

CHAPTER 9

Clinical Applications in Radiation Therapy

Leia Levy and Beverly K. Coker

FOCUS QUESTIONS

- What epidemiologic and etiologic information is pertinent to each anatomic site?
- How are basic anatomy, physiology, and lymphatic nodal drainage related to disease spread and radiation therapy management?
- Describe the observable clinical presentation of disease associated with each site.
- Compare the detection and diagnosis mechanisms used to classify various neoplastic diseases.
- What is the pathology associated with certain malignancies?
- Apply the appropriate grading and/or staging system associated with each disease site.
- Describe the spread patterns of disease.
- Analyze the principle and practice of simulation, treatment, and appropriate billing as they apply to each disease site.
- Describe the treatment regimens and fractionation schemes used in disease management.
- Interpret acute and chronic side effects and/or complications encountered during and after a course of therapy.

HEAD AND NECK CANCERS

GENERAL FACTS, EPIDEMIOLOGY, AND ETIOLOGY

- Represents about 4% of cancers
- Depending on size, site, and pattern of spread they can cause varying degrees of structural deformities and functional disabilities
- Tobacco and alcohol use are recognized risk factors.
- Epstein-Barr virus (EBV) associated with cancers of the nasopharynx
- Recent study of human papillomavirus (HPV) and associations with carcinomas of the tongue, floor of the mouth, and tonsils
- Prognosis is good for those compliant to aggressive treatment regimens and high dose chemotherapy and radiation
- Prevention of regional recurrence has long been a challenge due to dose-limiting factors.
- Anatomic subdivisions of the upper aerodigestive tract include:

Oral Cavity

- Anterior two thirds of the tongue, lip, buccal mucosa, retromolar trigone, floor of the mouth, hard palate

Nasopharynx

- Posterosuperior pharyngeal wall and lateral pharyngeal wall, eustachian tube orifice, and the adenoids

Oropharynx

- Base of tongue, tonsils (fossa and pillars), soft palate, and oropharyngeal walls

Hypopharynx

- Pyriform sinuses, postcricoid, and lower posterior pharyngeal walls below base of tongue

Larynx

- Glottis, supraglottis, subglottis

ORAL CAVITY

Extends from the skin-vermilion junction of the lip to the posterior border of the hard palate superiorly and to the circumvallate papillae inferiorly

Clinical Presentation

- Poor oral and dental hygiene
- Plummer-Vinson syndrome (iron deficiency in females)
- Leukoplakia/erythroplasia (severe dysplastic changes)
- Nonhealing ulcers
- Squamous cell carcinoma common

Detection and Diagnosis

- Oral inspection and palpation
- Biopsy
- CT/MRI

Lymphatic Drainage By Site

- Lips to submandibular, preauricular, and facial nodes
- Buccal mucosa to the submaxillary and submental nodes
- Gingiva to the submaxillary and jugular nodes
- Retromolar trigone to the submaxillary and jugulodigastric nodes
- Hard palate to the submaxillary and upper jugular nodes
- Floor of mouth to the submaxillary and jugular (middle and upper nodes)
- Anterior two thirds of the tongue to the submaxillary and upper jugular nodes

Treatment

- Surgical removal when tumors are small (<1 to 1.5 cm)
- Radiation (dependent upon area of oral cavity involved)—5000 to 7000 cGy with opposed laterals and boost fields.
- Hyperfractionation radiation therapy and use of radiosensitizers or radioprotectors
- Chemotherapy drugs often used in combination and may be given in sequence or concurrent with radiation
- High precision radiation using IMRT and IGRT techniques to escalate dose

Radiation Treatment Borders

- Anterior—anterior portion of mandible (excluding lower lip)
- Posterior—behind vertebral bodies or spinous processes
- Superior—1.5 cm above the tongue
- Inferior—thyroid notch

NASOPHARYNX

Cuboidal structure lying on a line from the zygomatic arch to the EAM, extending inferiorly to the mastoid tip. Nasopharynx is located behind the nose and extends from the posterior nares to the level of the soft palate.

Clinical Presentation

- Bloody discharge
- Auditory dysfunction
- Respiratory dysfunction
- Cranial nerve involvement (III, V, VI, IX, XII)
- Squamous cell carcinoma common

Detection and Diagnosis

- History and Physical
- Inspection—indirect mirror examination
- Palpation
- Biopsy
- Fiber optic endoscopy
- CT/MRI
- Chest x-ray
- EBV—specific serologic tests
- Liver function test/bone scans with advanced disease

Lymphatic Drainage

- Retropharyngeal nodes into the superior jugular and posterior cervical nodes
- Lateral retropharyngeal node (node of Rouvière)

Treatment

- Opposing lateral fields to cover tumor and possible pathways of spread
- Supraclavicular area treated
- IMRT replacing most conventional treatment

- 50 to 70 Gy with electron boost, and special consideration to spinal cord, optic nerve, pituitary, and brainstem

Radiation Treatment Borders

- Superior—2 cm beyond tumor (seen on CT) to include base of skull and sphenoid sinuses
- Posterior—2 cm margin beyond mastoid process, or posterior margin may extend further to allow a 1.5 cm margin on enlarged nodes
- Anterior—to include the posterior third of the maxillary sinus and nasal cavity, careful attention to adequate margin (2 cm) for more anterior tumors
- Inferior—thyroid notch to allow sparing of larynx
- Lower neck—anterior supraclavicular field with larynx block

OROPHARYNX (TONSILS)

Clinical Presentation

- Sore throat
- Pain on swallowing
- Upper spinal nodal swelling
- Referred otalgia
- Squamous cell carcinoma common

Detection and Diagnosis

- Direct inspection
- Palpation
- Biopsy

Lymphatic Drainage

- Base of tongue into jugulodigastric, low cervical, and retropharyngeal nodes
- Tonsillar fossa into jugulodigastric and submaxillary nodes
- Soft palate into jugulodigastric; submaxillary, and spinal accessory nodes
- Pharyngeal walls into retropharyngeal nodes, pharyngeal nodes, and jugulodigastric nodes

Treatment

- T1-T2 soft palate, tonsil, pharyngeal wall, tongue; Conventional 66-70 Gy
- T3-T4 oropharyngeal and T2 base of tongue; 70-81.6 Gy
- Hyperfractionation—70 Gy
- Clinically negative nodes—50-54 Gy
- With node dissection—60 Gy
- IMRT (major salivary glands and oral mucosa are spared, less trismus and xerostomia)
- Spinal cord block at 45 Gy

Radiation Treatment Borders

- Anterior—2 cm from known tumor
- Superior—1.5 to 2.0 cm superior to the soft palate
- Posterior—posterior spinous processes
- Inferior—level of the hyoid

HYPOPHARYNX (PYRIFORM SINUSES)

Clinical Presentation

- Sore throat
- Odynophagia
- Neck mass
- Dysphagia (hallmark of postcricoid carcinoma)
- Weight loss
- Squamous cell carcinoma common

Detection and Diagnosis

- Inspection
- Palpation
- Biopsy
- Fiber optic endoscopy
- CT/MRI

Lymphatic Drainage

- Superior deep, middle, and low jugular nodes
- Rouvière (lateral retropharyngeal lymph nodes at base of skull)

Treatment

- T1-2 (rare) could be treated with radiation or surgery
- T2-4 surgery and large radiation fields
- Large fields treated to 45 Gy; reduced off cord then continued to 70 Gy

Radiation Treatment Borders

- Superior—inferior border of mandible and mastoid process, to the base of skull

- Inferior—lower border of the cricoid cartilage; 1.5 to 2.0 cm margin
- Anterior—in front of the thyroid cartilage "shine off" (fall off) if larynx involved
- Posterior—behind the spinous processes

LARYNX

- Glottis
- Supraglottis
- Subglottis

Clinical Presentation

- Persistent sore throat
- Hoarseness and stridor
- Cervical lymph node—supraglottic lesions
- Squamous cell carcinoma common

Detection and Diagnosis

- Palpation
- Direct inspection
- Biopsy

Lymphatic Drainage

- Glottis—extremely rare for nodal involvement
- Subglottis—into the peritracheal and low cervical nodes
- Supraglottis—into the peritracheal, cervical, submental, and submaxillary nodes

Treatment

- Early lesions—surgery or radiation
- Advanced lesions—surgery and postoperative radiation
- Helophytic lesions—more responsive to radiation than infiltrative lesions
- Poorly differentiated carcinoma—radiation alone or concurrent with chemotherapy
- Veracious carcinoma—conservative surgery

Radiation Treatment Borders

Glottis

- Superior—upper thyroid notch
- Inferior—cricoids cartilage (lower border of C6)
- Anterior—1 to 1.5 cm shine over (flash) over the skin surface at the level of the vocal cords
- Posterior—just anterior to the vertebral body, including the anterior portion of the posterior pharyngeal wall

Supraglottic and Subglottis

- Often much larger fields
- Fields should include jugulodigastric, anterior and posterior cervical and supraclavicular lymph nodes

SALIVARY GLANDS—PAROTID

- Play a role in digestion and tooth protection
- Parotid gland is the largest of all salivary glands and located superficial to and partly behind the ramus, covering the masseter muscle
- Two thirds of tumors are benign; salivary gland malignancies are rare.
- Majority of salivary gland malignancies occur in the parotid gland

Clinical Presentation

- Asymptomatic parotid mass lasting 4 to 8 months
- Pathology-adenoid cystic, mucoepidermoid and adenocarcinoma
- Extensive lymphatic capillary plexus
- Localized swelling of face, pain, facial palsy
- Rapidly growing
- Facial nerve involvement—causing paralysis

Treatment

- Surgery
- Radiation postoperatively for residual, recurrent, or inoperable lesions

Radiation Treatment Borders

- Superiorly-zygomatic arch or higher
- Anteriorly-anterior edge of the masseter muscle
- Inferior-thyroid notch
- Posterior-just behind mastoid

Treatment Delivery

- Treatment delivered by wedged field technique superior and inferior oblique combination; opposed lateral field if target extends beyond midline
- Doses: postoperative case-60-63 Gy; 70-75 Gy if gross residual disease
- Target volume will include local invasion and lymphatics involved
- Concern—preservation of salivary function by sparing at least one parotid gland has been a primary objective of head and neck IMRT

- *Submandibular and sublingual* only account for 2% to 3% of all head and neck cancers

MAXILLARY SINUS

General Facts and Epidemiology

- Pyramid-shaped cavity lined by ciliated epithelium
- Carcinomas arise from the ciliated epithelium or mucous glands
- Roof of maxillary sinus is the floor of the orbit
- Alveolar process and hard palate separate the maxillary sinus from the oral cavity
- Maxillary sinus disease accounts for 80% of all sinus cancer with 2:1 male prevalence
- Older than 40 years average age
- Although lymphatics are in the region, maxillary sinus tumors rarely involve regional lymphatics.

Etiology

- Adenocarcinoma of nasal cavity and ethmoid sinus has been associated with *wood dust exposure.*
- Squamous cell carcinomas of the maxillary sinus and nasal cavity are associated with *chemical agents found in nickel refinery and leather tanning.*

Clinical Presentation and Workup

- Tumors may involve the trigeminal branches of the cranial nerves.
- Displacement of the eye
- Most useful studies—CT to define early cortical bone erosion and MRI delineates soft tissue and can differentiate among opacification of the sinuses due to fluid, inflammation, or tumor. MRI can also demonstrate subtle perineural spread and involvement of the cranial nerve foramen and canals.

Treatment

- Surgery—only for small lesions of nasal septum or those limited to the infrastructure of the maxillary sinus
- Surgery and *postoperative* radiation—advanced stages
- Radiation may be used when a massive tumor exists that involves the nasopharynx, base of skull, sphenoidal sinuses, brain, or optic chiasm.
- Postoperative radiation (Figure 9-1)—60 to 63 Gy (1.8 to 2.0 per fraction), external beam, wedged pair technique with coned down boost; 70 Gy recommended for unresectable tumors; orbit block if not involved; care taken in order to miss the cord and contralateral lens; intensity modulated radiation therapy (IMRT) offers a more therapeutic ratio for tumor over conventional treatment

Treatment Delivery and Considerations for Head and Neck

- Table 9-1 lists typical curative radiation doses for head and neck lesions; Table 9-2 includes an approximate dose-tissue response schedule.
- Periodontal disease and caries—Teeth extractions should be done before radiation treatment.
- Maintaining adequate nutrition is a major problem for these patients.

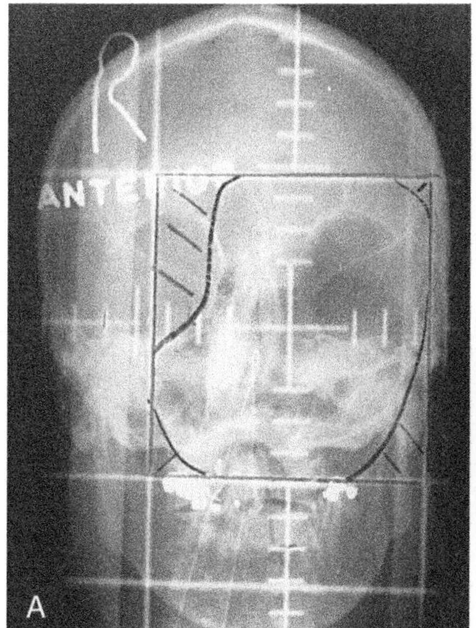

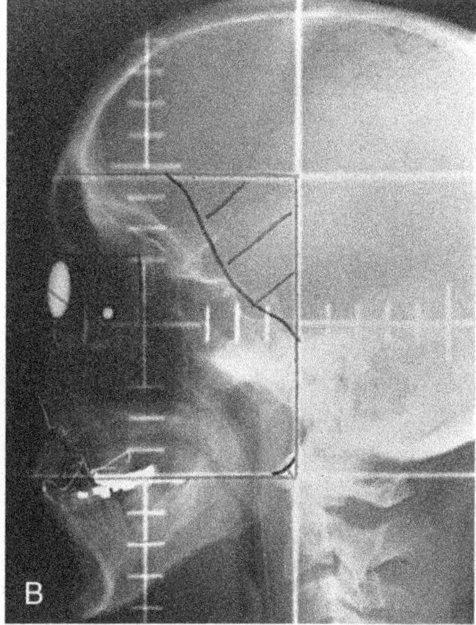

FIGURE 9-1 **A**, Anterior left maxillary sinus portal. **B**, Left lateral maxillary sinus portal.

TABLE 9-1 Typical Curative Radiation Doses for Head and Neck Lesions

5000 cGy	Nodes
5000 cGy	Any subclinical disease
6000-6500 cGy	T1 lesions
6500-7000 cGy	T2 lesions
7000-7500 cGy	T3-4 lesions

From Washington CM, Leaver D: *Principles and practice of radiation therapy*, ed 3, St Louis, 2010, Mosby.

TABLE 9-2 Approximate Dose-Tissue Response Schedule for a Conventional Fractionation Scheme

Response	Dose (cGy)
Dry mouth	2000
Erythema	2000
Brachial plexus	5500
Spinal cord	4500
Lhermitte sign	2000-3000
Mandible, teeth and gums	5000-6000
Mucositis	3000
Ears	4000
Cataracts	500-1000
Dry eye	4000
Optic nerve	5000
Retina	5000
Trismus	6000
Laryngitis	5000

From Washington CM, Leaver D: *Principles and practice of radiation therapy*, ed 3, St Louis, 2010, Mosby.

- Mucositis/stomatitis—inflammation of the oral mucous membranes with edema and tenderness (3000 cGy)
- Xerostomia—dry mouth may be seen after 1000 to 2000 cGy and may be permanent after 4000 cGy. Poses risk for dental caries and oral infections.
- Cataract formation if lens is treated; doses as low as 1000 cGy
- Lacrimal glands—dry painful eye (severe dry eye syndrome reported in 100% of patients receiving more than 5700 cGy)
- Taste changes—taste buds are radiosensitive and atrophy and degeneration are noted at 1000 cGy
- Skin reactions—usually acute and depending upon dose, energy of beam, and use of radiosensitizing chemotherapy drugs
- Box 9-1 describes an oral hygiene program; Box 9-2 lists a skin-care program.

BOX 9-1 Recommended Oral-Hygiene Program

- Clean teeth and brush gums after meals.
- Use fluoride toothpaste or fluoride rinses daily.
- Floss daily.
- Rinse the mouth with salt and a baking-soda solution (1 qt water, 1/2 Tsp salt, 1/2 Tsp baking soda).
- See a dentist regularly during treatment for a teeth and gum examination.
- To reduce the severity of any head and neck complication, the patient should be encouraged to avoid the following:
  - Spicy hot foods, coarse or raw vegetables, dry crackers, chips, and nuts
  - Smoking, chewing tobacco, and alcohol
  - Sugary snacks
  - Commercial mouthwash that contains alcohol because it dries the mouth
  - Cold foods and drinks

From Washington CM, Leaver D: *Principles and practice of radiation therapy*, ed 3, St Louis, 2010, Mosby.

BOX 9-2 Recommended Skin Care Program

- Wash the skin with lukewarm water, pat dry, and do not wash off marks.
- Use mild soaps (e.g., Basis, Neutrogena).
- Use water-based lotions or creams (e.g., Aquaphor, Eucerin).
- Avoid lotions with perfume and deodorants.
- Avoid direct sunlight.
- Do not use straight razors.
- Avoid tight-fitting collars and hat brims.
- Do not use aftershave lotions or perfumes.
- Apply only nonadherent, hydrophilic dressings to wounds.

From Washington CM, Leaver D: *Principles and practice of radiation therapy*, ed 3, St Louis, 2010, Mosby.

- Many head and neck protocols incorporate the use of radioprotectors and/or concurrent chemotherapy; be mindful of treatment delivery time.
- It is important to be mindful of specific protocol instructions regarding documentation of daily treatments, portal verification, monitoring of progress, and side effects.
- Standard fractionation schemes may be used but hyperfractionation schemes are not uncommon.
- High total doses require extensive treatment planning and application of IMRT, PET/CT image fusion planning, complex immobilization systems, and use of accessories such as wedges, bolus, and/or compensators.
- Simulation, planning, and daily treatment billing should be at the complex level.

HEAD AND NECK REVIEW EXERCISES

1. List clinical detection for each of the following sites.
   a. Oral cavity
   b. Oropharynx
   c. Hypopharynx
   d. Nasopharynx
   e. Larynx
   f. Maxillary sinus

2. Label Figure 9-2. (12 answers)
3. Match the landmark to the description.

____ **Superior orbital margin (SOM)**
____ **Inferior orbital margin (IOM)**
____ **External occipital protuberance (EOP)**
____ **Mastoid process**
____ **Zygomatic arch**
____ **Glabella**
____ **Nasion**
____ **Inner canthus (IC)**
____ **Outer canthus (OC)**
____ **Tragus**
____ **Commissure of the mouth**
____ **C1**
____ **C2**
____ **C3**
____ **C4**
____ **C6**
____ **C7**
____ **Sternocleidomastoid muscle**

a. Located at the outer aspect of the eye where the upper and lower eyelids meet
b. Lies inferior to the mastoid process
c. The depression at the base of the nose
d. The first prominent process of the cervical vertebrae
e. Located at the level of the angle of the mandible
f. The roof of the orbit
g. A thick band attached to the mastoid and occipital bones superiorly and sterna and clavicular heads inferiorly
h. Corresponds to the level of the thyroid cartilage
i. The bony prominence of the cheek
j. Located between the orbits
k. Located at the junction of the upper and lower lip

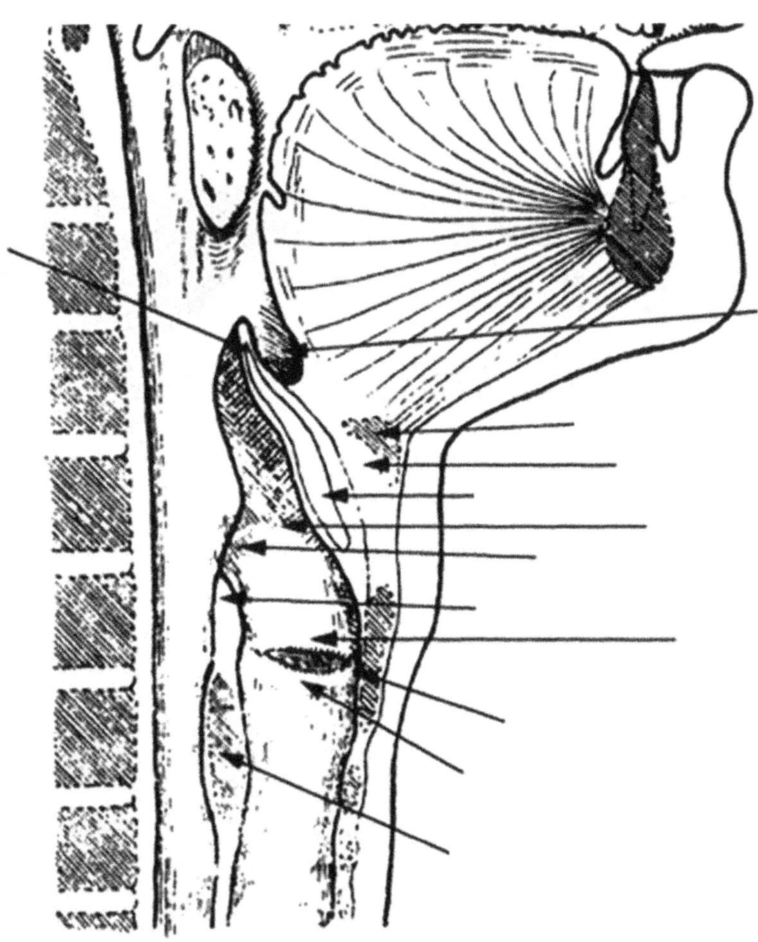

FIGURE 9-2

l. Located at the level of the cricoid cartilage
m. Lies at the level of the hyoid bone
n. Forms the lateral margin of the bony orbit
o. Located at the medial aspect of the eye where the upper and lower eyelids meet
p. The central prominence in the occipital bone
q. Located near the external auditory meatus
r. The most lateral and inferior extension of the temporal bone

4. Unscramble the following words associated with head and neck cancers, and then unscramble the letters in the parentheses of each word and fill in the blank to answer question 5.

UAGSPHSOE ______( )__

NAYRLX ( )_____

IOCCDIR ____( )__

YRITODH ( )______

TCEAARH ( )______

PIEGTOLTSI __( )_______

VASLAIYR ( )_______

5. This area accounts for 65% of all the larynx cancers. Lesions in this area are well to moderately differentiated. Most of these lesions appear on the anterior two thirds of one of the cords. It contains the true vocal cords. Lymphatic involvement is very rare in this area. ______

6. Fill in the function of each of the cranial nerves:

Olfactory	I	______
Optic	II	______
Oculomotor	III	______
Trochlear	IV	______
Trigeminal	V	______
Abducens	VI	______
Facial (masticator)	VII	______
Acoustic	VIII	______
Glossopharyngeal	IX	______
Vagus	X	______
Spinal accessory	XI	______
Hypoglossal	XII	______

7. About ______ of the body's lymph nodes are located in the head and neck area.

a. one fourth
b. one third
c. two thirds
d. one half

8. How many cartilages make up the larynx?

a. 3 pair
b. 6 pair
c. 9
d. 12

9. What muscle divides the neck into anterior and posterior triangles?

a. Trapezius
b. Pterygoid
c. Longissimus dorsi
d. Sternocleidomastoid

10. The ______ nodal group, below the mastoid tip, receives nearly all of the lymph from the head and neck area and is often included in the treated area.

a. Submandibular nodes
b. Carotid nodes
c. Jugulodigastric nodes
d. Rouvière nodes

11. What is the function of the hyoid bone?

a. Acts as an attachment site for muscles associated with swallowing
b. Prevents food from entering the trachea
c. Protects the delicate vocal cords
d. Acts as a base for the laryngeal cartilages to rest on

12. Which of the following is typically the largest vascular structure located in the neck?

a. Common carotid artery
b. Internal jugular vein
c. Internal carotid artery
d. External carotid artery

13. The jugulodigastric node may also be referred to as:

a. Node of Rouvière
b. Subdigastric node
c. Retropharyngeal nodes
d. Circle of Willis

14. Postcricoid and pyriform sinuses are located in which of the following?

   a. Oropharynx
   b. Hypopharynx
   c. Ethmoid sinuses
   d. Maxillary sinuses

15. Which of the following is not considered part of the oral cavity?

   a. Buccal mucosa
   b. Hard palate
   c. Floor of the tongue
   d. Soft palate

16. The tonsils are the most common site of disease in which of the following area?

   a. Oral cavity
   b. Oropharynx
   c. Nasopharynx
   d. Hypopharynx

17. In treating the oropharynx area with conformal treatment (IMRT), all of the following structures can be avoided, except:

   a. Temporomandibular joint
   b. Part of the pterygoid muscles
   c. Salivary glands
   d. Tonsils

18. Many structures and soft tissue of the aerodigestive track within the facial/cervical regions can be directly examined by means of:

   1. Palpation
   2. Direct inspection
   3. Biopsy

      a. 1, 2
      b. 1, 3
      c. 2, 3
      d. 1, 2, 3

19. Which of the following lymph node area is a very high risk for dissemination of disease, is inaccessible for surgery, and therefore must be included as the minimum target volume when treating the nasopharyngeal area?

   a. Waldeyer ring
   b. Rouvière nodes
   c. Circle of Willis
   d. Jugulodigastric nodes

***Define* the following symptoms often indicated in specific areas of head and neck cancers. *List* the specific areas where they often occur.**

20. Otalgia

21. Dysphagia

22. Stridor

23. Diplopia

24. Erythroplasia

25. Leukoplakia

26. Keratosis

27. Dysplasia

28. Odynophagia

29. Explain the relationship in the use of smokeless tobacco and cancer that is now being seen at an increased rate among young Americans.

30. Explain the relationship of the evidence suggesting a connection of head and neck cancers to human papilloma virus (HPV).

31. Discuss and define the Epstein-Barr virus in connection to head and neck cancers.

32. The majority of the head and neck cancers arise from epithelial surfaces and mucosal linings of the upper digestive tract and are mostly:

a. Adenocarcinoma
b. Squamous cell carcinoma
c. Lymphomas
d. Keratinized carcinoma

33. The two most common etiologic factors contributing to head and neck cancers are:

1. Smoking
2. Heredity
3. Alcohol
4. Environmental

a. 1, 2
b. 1, 3
c. 2, 3
d. 2, 4

34. The main goals in treating head and neck cancers and determining the best modality of treatment are:

1. Eradication of disease
2. Maintenance of physiologic function
3. Preservation of social cosmesis

a. 1, 2
b. 1, 3
c. 2, 3
d. 1, 2, 3

35. Plummer-Vinson syndrome (iron deficiency anemia), often seen in females, is considered an important etiologic factor in which of the following cancers?

a. Oral cavity
b. Oropharynx
c. Nasopharynx
d. Hypopharynx

36. In some head and neck cancers, the supraclavicular area is often treated if there is advanced disease or lower involved nodes. The normal dosage of irradiation to this area:

a. 2500 cGy
b. 3000 cGy
c. 5000 cGy
d. 6500 cGy

37. Which of the following is found at the base of the tongue?

a. Uvula
b. Vallecula
c. Tonsillar fossa
d. Posterior pillar

38. The treatment field for a primary tumor in the hypopharynx includes the node of Rouvière. A sharp field edge is necessary to avoid and protect the:

a. Spinal cord
b. Base of the brain
c. Larynx
d. Epiglottis

Define each of the following areas of the pharynx:

39. Nasopharynx

40. Oropharynx

41. Hypopharynx

42. The highest rate of nodal metastases in all head and neck cancers is found with cancers in the:

a. Oropharynx
b. Hypopharynx
c. Nasopharynx
d. Maxillary sinus

43. Tumors of the head and neck may involve the cranial nerves that control our major senses. This may lead to signs and symptoms that can point to a possible location of the tumor. Which area would be the most common for involvement of cranial nerves?

a. Oral cavity
b. Oropharynx
c. Hypopharynx
d. Nasopharynx

44. A mouth stent or tongue blade may serve more than one purpose in use during irradiation treatments to head and neck cancers. They may serve to separate or ______ the palate.

a. moisten
b. displace
c. keep still
d. keep patient from swallowing

45. Which of the following is considered at the most risk when treating the maxillary antrum with radiation?

a. Brain
b. Eye
c. Skin
d. Pituitary

46. The most common site of distant metastatic disease from the head and neck area is the:

a. Brain
b. Bone
c. Lungs
d. Liver

47. More than 80% of head and neck cancers arise from the surface epithelium of the mucosal linings of the upper digestive tract and are:

a. Adenocarcinomas
b. Squamous cell carcinomas
c. Transitional cell carcinomas
d. Seminoma cancer

48. The usual wedge-pair technique often used in treatment of the parotid gland is:

a. Superior/inferior oblique combination
b. Anterior/posterior oblique combination
c. Anterior/posterior combination
d. Anterior/inferior oblique combination

49. The most commonly involved site for malignancy of the sinuses would be:

a. Ethmoid
b. Maxillary
c. Sphenoid
d. Frontal

LUNG

GENERAL FACTS AND EPIDEMIOLOGY

- American Cancer Society statistics for 2008 report lung cancer as the number one killer in men and women in the United States.
- Five-year survival rates are low
- Men have slightly higher incidence than women
- Mortality rates have increased greatly in women over the past half century
- More cigarettes consumed daily increases risk
- Average age for onset is 60 years
- Smoking cessation decreases risk over time

Etiology

- Smoking
- Exposure to combustion by-products
- Asbestos
- Pollution
- Pitchblende
- Chemicals
- Metals
- Ionizing radiation

Clinical Presentation

Signs and Symptoms

- History of smoking
- Persistent, unproductive cough
- Hoarseness
- Hemoptysis
- Weight loss
- Dyspnea
- Unresolved pneumonitis
- Chest wall pain
- Apical tumors: weakness in arm, swelling in neck
- Atelectasis
- Pleural effusion

Histology

- Small cell/oat cell-high mortality; very aggressive
- Non-small cell

- Squamous cell
- Adenocarcinoma
- Adenosquamous
- Mesothelioma
- Carcinosarcomas
- Carcinoid

Lymphatic Drainage and Spread Patterns

- Mediastinal and supraclavicular lymph nodes (Figure 9-3) are regional drainage.
- Paratracheal, subcarinal, interlobar, paraesophageal, upper aortic are mediastinal nodes.
- Regional spread may be to adjacent lobe (considered metastatic).
- Blood metastasis to liver, brain, bone, bone marrow
- Small cell cancer has high risk for brain metastasis early.

Workup

- Physical examination
- Chest x-ray

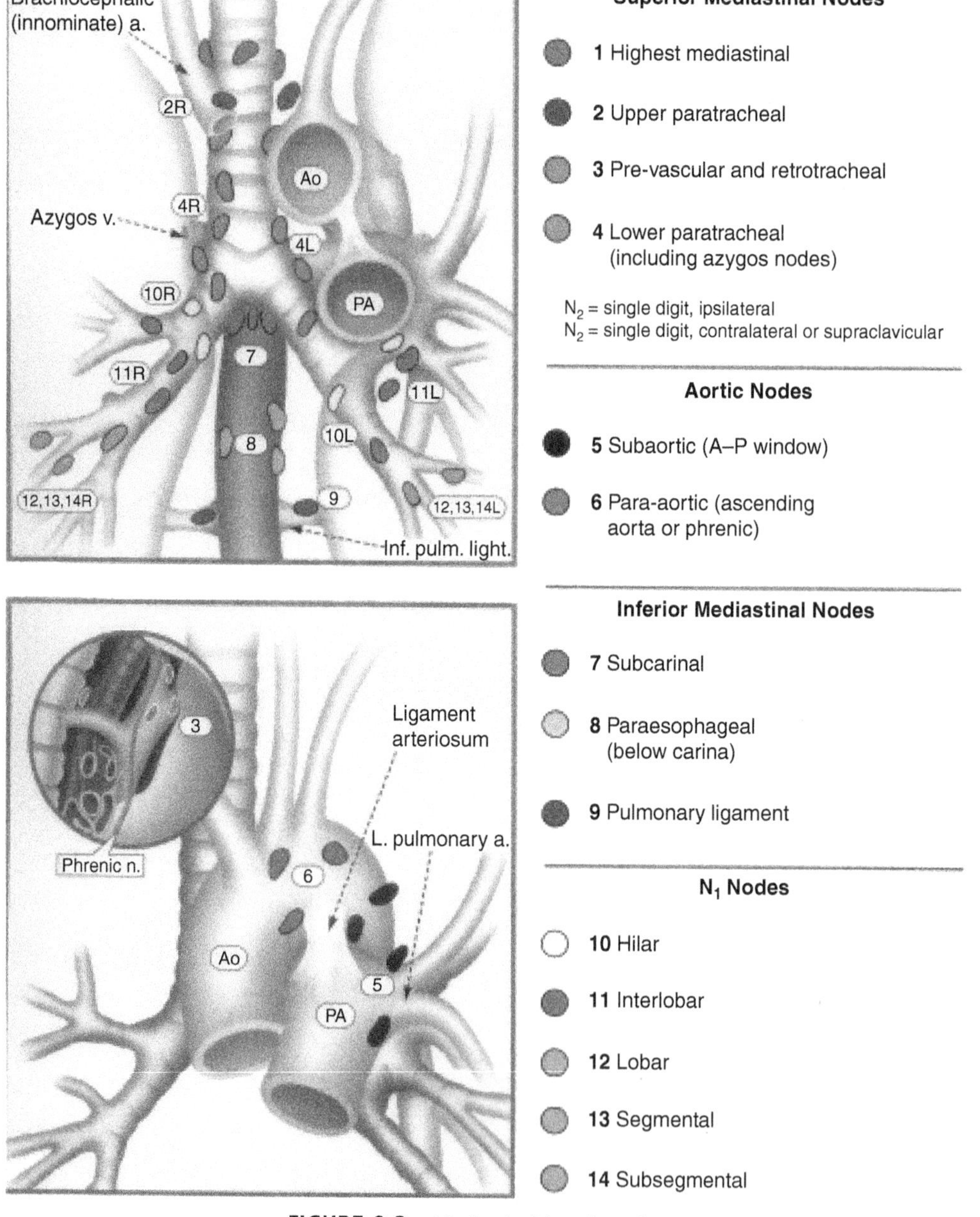

FIGURE 9-3 Mediastinal lymph nodes.

- CT thorax and abdomen
- Needle biopsy
- Sputum cytology
- Bronchoscopy with biopsy
- Bone and liver scan to rule out metastasis
- CT brain if small cell
- Blood markers: Carcinoembryonic antigen (CEA), neuron-specific enolase (NSE) for small cell especially

Staging

- TNM

Treatment

- Patient performance must be evaluated using a tool such as Karnofsky scale.
- Surgery is the treatment of choice for early disease with a lobectomy or segmentectomy.
- Unresectables include confirmed distant metastasis, pleural effusion, superior vena cava obstruction, tracheal wall invasion, and small cell histology.
- Radiation may be used definitively if unresectable or adjuvant to surgery and chemotherapy; for recurrent disease; emergently for relief of superior vena cava syndrome (SVC) or prophylactic to CNS in small cell carcinoma; palliatively
- Chemotherapy under investigation for more substantial adjuvant role in management of non-small cell carcinomas
- Chemotherapy primary treatment for small cell carcinomas
- Small cell carcinomas very sensitive to chemotherapy

Radiation Treatment Borders

- Radiation treatment fields should include lesion and margin and regional lymph nodes.
- Upper lobe lesions—tumor and margin, along with mediastinal and supraclavicular nodes
- Middle and lower lobe lesions—tumor and margin, along with mediastinal nodes
- Prophylactic cranial fields for small cell include the entire brain with sufficient margin on the fourth ventricle.
- PET/CT fusion helpful in defining region of interest

Treatment Delivery

- Total dose to lung lesion and margin typically 50 Gy if radiation is adjuvant to surgery or chemotherapy
- Total dose to lung for palliative intent typically 45 Gy
- Total dose to lung and margin typically 60 Gy if radiation used alone
- Positive lymph nodes should receive maximum of total dose when possible
- Negative lymph nodes should receive 45 Gy
- Daily fraction size 180 cGy
- Protocols for small cell lung carcinomas may require hyperfractionation; 1.5 Gy fractions twice daily to 24 Gy, then 2 week break before receiving an additional 24 Gy.
- Critical organs in thorax have low tolerance to radiation, so complex strategies are used; often oblique off-cord and boost fields incorporated.
- Patient should be positioned to accommodate complex portal arrangements; arms elevated in reliable positioning and immobilization device.
- Prone position for posterior, middle/lower lobe lung lesions facilitates easy daily setup for off-cord and boost fields.
- Wing boards, prone pillows are intermediate positioning aids
- Use of alpha cradle or vac lock for daily positioning and immobilization are complex aids
- Advanced internal volume localization such as breath-hold, respiratory gating, and CT simulation at full inspiration and full expiration are helpful in planning.
- As tissue densities vary greatly in the thorax, modifiers will likely be used such as wedges or tissue compensators *or* unequal beam weighting techniques.
- Small localized lesions may be treated with dynamic therapy such as IMRT, and stereotactic or tomotherapy.
- Prophylactic cranial irradiation (PCI) for small cell lung carcinoma typically given in 18 fractions to 36 Gy.
- Emergency treatment of superior vena cava typically in 300 to 400 cGy per fraction; three or four consecutive treatments for quick response then complete workup is needed
- Slight incline helps facilitate easier breathing for short course treatment plans such as SVC syndrome palliation.
- Remind patient of the importance of nutrition despite esophagitis/mucositis caused by radiation or chemotherapy; avoid alcohol, smoking, and acidic and spicy foods that would further irritate the trachea and esophagus
- Skin care: keep area clean and dry, no deodorants if axillary areas treated, no commercial lotions or creams on irritated areas; protect chest from sun exposure and extreme temperatures

LUNG REVIEW EXERCISES

1. Define the following:

   Odynophagia

   Hemoptysis

   Dyspnea

   Atelectasis

2. List all mediastinal lymph nodes.

3. Using the cross-sectional images in Figure 9-4 below, complete the following:

   a. Outline the gross tumor volume.

   b. Outline the critical structures and list tolerance doses for each.

   c. Diagram possible directions for off-cord and boost treatment fields.

4. List four etiologic factors for lung cancer.

5. Note common anatomic locations and physical characteristics for the manifestations of the following lung tumors:

   Adenocarcinoma:

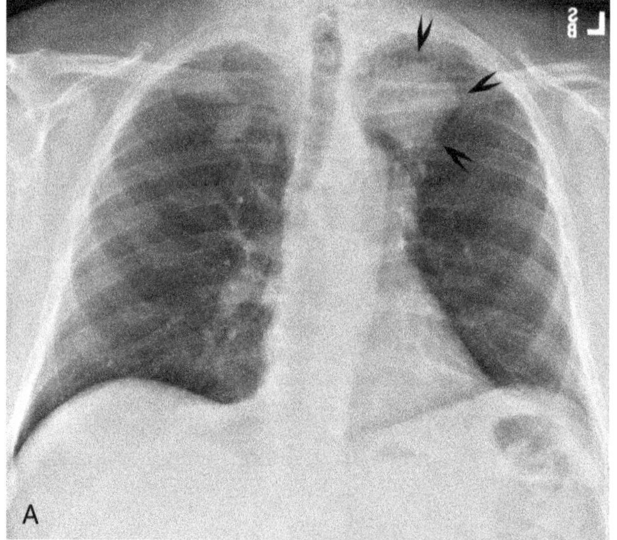

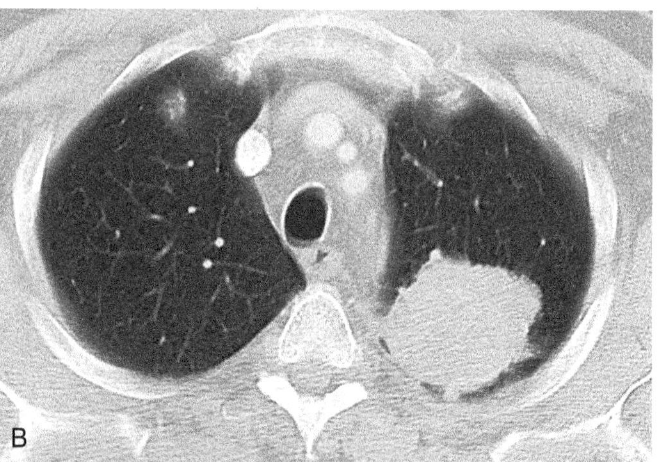

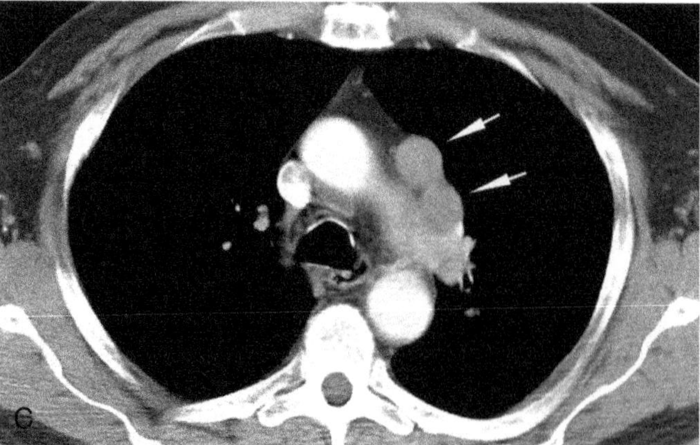

FIGURE 9-4 **A**, Anterior chest x-ray. **B**, CT lung window axial. **C**, CT axial chest.

Squamous cell carcinoma:

Pancoast tumor:

Mesothelioma:

Large cell carcinoma:

6. Briefly explain the situations in which high dose rate (HDR) brachytherapy would be an appropriate management for lung cancer.

7. The histologic type of lung cancer seen in patients with no history of smoking is:
   a. Adenocarcinoma
   b. Small cell carcinoma
   c. Large cell carcinoma
   d. Squamous cell carcinoma

8. "Clubbing" of the fingers is one physical symptom of:
   a. Chronic obstructive pulmonary disease
   b. Pleurisy
   c. Atelectasis
   d. Pneumonitis

9. The histologic type assumed to indicate that there is already distant disease at the time of diagnosis is:
   a. Oat cell carcinoma of the lung
   b. Squamous cell carcinoma of the lung
   c. Adenocarcinoma of the lung
   d. Large cell lung carcinoma

10. A patient with a middle lobe posterior lung tumor may be positioned prone to facilitate:
    a. Easier breathing
    b. Clinical verification of spinal alignment
    c. Easier alignment of off-cord obliques and boost fields directed posteriorly
    d. Easier alignment of off-cord obliques and boost fields directed anteriorly

11. Initial AP/PA fields for lung cancer may require an anterior wedge to:
    a. Compensate for the natural slope of the chest
    b. Compensate for excessive boney structures in the chest
    c. Push the dose lines further toward the vertebral bodies
    d. Bring the dose lines closer to the skin surface

12. Using Figure 9-5, draw the likely emergency treatment field for the patient diagnosed with superior vena cava syndrome caused by right Pancoast tumor.

13. Using Figure 9-6, draw the likely initial treatment field for the above patient who after workup was diagnosed with T2, N0, M0 squamous cell lung carcinoma.

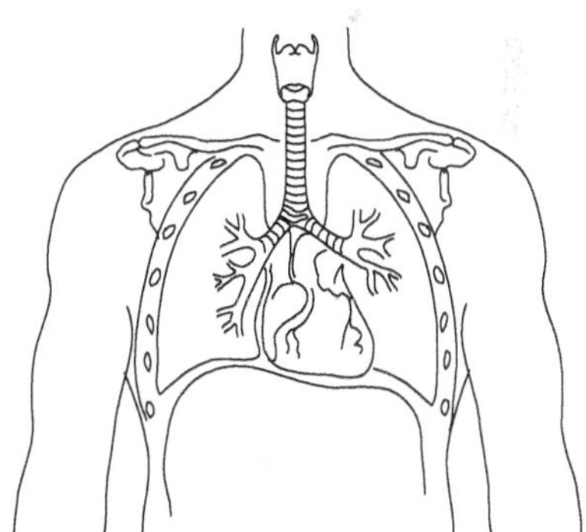

FIGURE 9-5 Anterior chest.

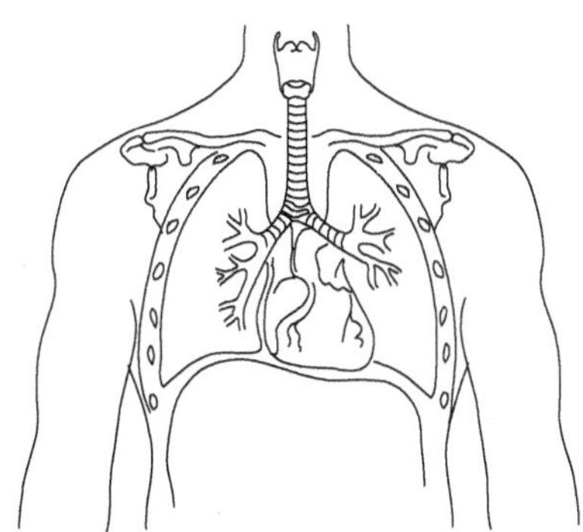

FIGURE 9-6 Anterior chest.

14. Total dose for prophylactic cranial irradiation is typically:

a. 2000 cGy
b. 3000 cGy
c. 3600 cGy
d. 4500 cGy

15. To verify the histology of a suspected lung cancer, all of the following could be helpful except:

a. Excisional biopsy
b. CT scan
c. Bronchoscopy with biopsy
d. Sputum cytology

16. How many lobes does the right lung have?

a. 2
b. 3
c. 4
d. 5

17. Target volume delineation for lung tumors may involve cardiac or respiratory gating procedures. The rationale for this is that lung tumors:

a. Are often metastatic
b. Are difficult to image
c. Move with cardiac and respiratory motion
d. Change shape with cardiac and respiratory motion

18. The histologic type of lung cancer most closely associated with asbestos exposure is:

a. Adenocarcinoma
b. Mesothelioma
c. Squamous cell carcinoma
d. Oat cell carcinoma

19. The natural slope of the chest may cause high dose regions in the upper mediastinum. This area of increased dose may be managed by the use of a:

a. Bolus
b. Custom compensator
c. Bite block
d. Wing board

20. A radiation treatment field with an upper border above both clavicles and lower border approximately 5 cm below the carina, including mediastinal lymphatics and blocking most of the left lung would likely be:

a. An initial field for treatment of an upper lobe right lung tumor
b. An off-cord field for the treatment of a middle lobe right lung tumor
c. Emergency treatment field for right superior vena cava syndrome
d. Palliative treatment for Hodgkin lymphoma

ALIMENTARY CANAL: ESOPHAGUS, STOMACH, SMALL BOWEL, COLON, ANUS

GENERAL FACTS AND EPIDEMIOLOGY

- Cancer of the digestive tract is very common.
- Most common location is the colorectal area.
- Men affected more frequently than women for all areas except small bowel, then incidence is 1:1.
- These tumors often present late due to vague symptoms. Symptoms may mimic several benign conditions of the digestive tract. By the time there is a palpable mass in the abdomen or there is hemorrhaging, the tumor is quite large.
- Grow from inner layers of the organ to the outside; from mucosa out to the serosa
- Incidence for esophageal cancer is higher in African Americans; China, Japan, Finland, Iran are high risk locations; average age of onset is 60
- Incidence for stomach cancer is higher in African Americans and Native Americans; higher risk in low socioeconomic groups; Japan, Chile, Costa Rica are high risk areas; average age of onset is 55
- Remarkable decrease in the past 50 years for stomach cancers in the United States but is still quite prevalent in other countries; worldwide it is considered a leading cancer killer.
- Occurrence by location in the stomach→Antrum or distal stomach 40%; body 25%; fundus, cardia, esophagogastric junction 35% together
- Small bowel cancer is very rare; only make up 5% of gastrointestinal cancer cases; average age is 59
- Colon/rectum cancers are second in incidence for men and women in the United States.
- Risk increases with age, male sex, family history, and increased body mass index for colon/rectum. The risk is strongly related to diet. Adenomas and polyps are precursors; average age is 50.

- The anus is generally a rare site for cancer; however, there has been an increased incidence in the past 30 to 40 years.
- Etiology is unknown for anal cancers. It is associated with a variety of chronic colorectal conditions. Most cases are non-Hispanic whites, with incidence higher in urban areas; may have an association with HIV; average age is 62.

ESOPHAGUS

The esophagus can be divided into two, three, or four divisions (Table 9-3)

Etiology

Direct causes unknown

Associated conditions:

- Chronic consumption of hot, highly seasoned foods
- Alcohol, tobacco
- Chemical exposure
- Short esophagus
- Tylosis (genetic disorder involving hyperkeratosis of palms and soles of the feet)
- Barrett disease

Clinical Presentation

Signs and Symptoms

- Dysphagia and weight loss most common
- Chest pain
- Odynophagia
- Hoarseness if laryngeal nerve compressed
- Superior vena cava syndrome
- Hematemesis

Histology

- Squamous cell found mostly in proximal and midesophagus
- Adenocarcinoma found in distal esophagus and gastroesophageal junction

TABLE 9-3 Divisions of the Esophagus

2 divisions	3 divisions	4 divisions
Cervical	Upper 1/3	Cervical: C6-SSN
Thoracic	Middle 1/3	Upper thoracic: SSN-carina
	Lower 1/3	Mid thoracic: carina-esophagogastric junction
		Lower thoracic: at the cardia

- Three fourths of those diagnosed in the United States will have adenocarcinoma of the distal esophagus.

Workup

- History and physical
- Barium swallow under fluoroscopy
- Esophagoscopy with biopsy
- Ultrasound shows depth of invasion through organ layers
- CT of chest and abdomen
- CBC and liver function

Spread Patterns

- Rarely localized at the time of diagnosis
- High incidence of local and distant spread
  - Local → trachea, mediastinum, lung, pleura, aorta, heart
  - Distant → liver 53%, lung 35%, bone 11%, adrenals 8%, brain 4%
  - Lymph node drainage (Figure 9-7) to cervical, supraclavicular, paraesophageal, celiac axis, and perigastric

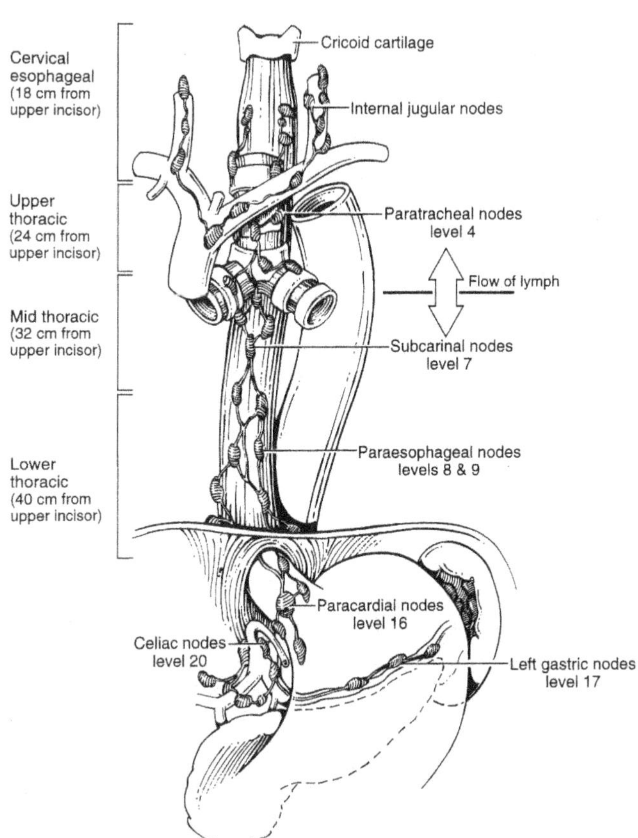

FIGURE 9-7 Esophagus with divisions and lymphatics.

Staging

- AJCC staging system using TNM

Treatment

- Surgery is standard whenever possible with anastomosis (reconstruction).
- Complications from surgery include anastomosis leak, respiratory failure, motility disorders, and reflux.
- Local control and survival improves with radiation and concurrent chemotherapy.
- Upper esophagus lesions best managed with chemoradiation due to high mortality with surgery.
- Pre-op or post-op radiation dose to 45 to 50 Gy
- Radiation dose to 50 to 70 Gy depending on whether previous surgery or concurrent chemotherapy
- Radiation alone total dose 60 to 70 Gy
- Intraluminal HDR controversial
- Chemotherapy drugs may include 5-FU, cisplatin, bleomycin, methotrexate, mitomycin, ifosfamide, VP-16, and several others.
- Complications from chemotherapy depend on the combination of drugs.

Radiation Treatment Borders

- AP/PA treatment fields to include GTV, plus generous margin of about 5 cm above and below tumor plus regional lymph nodes to 40 Gy
- Remainder of dose given using obliques, opposed laterals, or AP and posterior obliques to spare spinal cord
- Field may be reduced after 45 Gy to decrease margin to 2.5 cm

Treatment Delivery

- After surgery, enteral nutrition may be necessary via feeding tubes.
- Nutritional support very important as nutritional status was likely marginal before the start of therapy. Offer the patient hyperalimentation products if still taking food orally.
- Take care not to dislodge feeding tubes when transferring/transporting patients.
- Patient may be positioned supine or prone; slight displacement of esophagus away from the thoracic spine in the prone position
- Arms should be raised to accommodate lateral or posterior oblique fields for spinal cord sparing.
- Prone position is accomplished with a prone pillow or Duncan mask with arms up around pillow or mask.
- Supine with both arms up on a wing board, alpha cradle, or vac lock system
- All treatment fields will need beam shaping to spare lung, heart, spinal cord
- Positioning aids such as prone pillow, Duncan mask, and wing board are billable as simple treatment devices; vac lock is complex.
- Daily delivery is complex due to field shaping and the use of modifiers such as wedges on oblique/lateral fields.
- May have special protocols, stay abreast of required documentation if participating in protocol
- Acute reaction to radiation is mainly dysphagia; onset at about 20 Gy
- Educate patient on starting a soft, bland diet for dysphagia; esophagitis cocktails
- Chemoradiation intensifies dysphagia and lowers onset dose
- Late complications from radiation therapy include perforation, hemorrhage from tumor dissolution, stricture, lung necrosis, and pneumonitis.

STOMACH

Sections of the stomach:

- Cardia
- Fundus
- Body
- Greater curvature
- Lesser curvature
- Pylorus

Etiology

- Diet (red meat, spices, fish, smoked foods, heavily salted)
- Coal mining
- Rubber working
- Asbestos exposure
- Gastric ulcers/polyps
- Alcohol/tobacco
- Poor nutrition
- Inadequate sanitation of consumables
- *Helicobacter pylori* infection (*H. pylori*)

Clinical Presentation

Signs and Symptoms

- Vague epigastric discomfort is the No. 1 symptom
- Loss of appetite
- Weight loss
- Nausea, vomiting
- Palpable, epigastric mass
- Ascites
- Jaundice, left supraclavicular adenopathy (Virchow node)
- Left axillary adenopathy (Irish node)

Histology

- Adenocarcinoma 90% to 95%
- Leiomyosarcomas and lymphomas 5% to 8%

Workup

- CBC (most have anemia)
- Guaiac stool test
- Upper gastrointestinal series with contrast
- Endoscopy with biopsy
- CT scan of abdomen and chest
- Laparoscopy

Spread Patterns

- One third have distant metastasis at diagnosis
- May spread through lymph, blood, or direct to any organ
- More than likely spread to bowel, omenta, pancreas, colon, regional nodes
- Will take the blood route to the liver and lung since the portal system is in close proximity
- Peritoneum is a likely site for metastasis too; invasion is often diffuse.
- There are abundant lymphatic channels within the layers of submucosa and subserosa.
- Initial drainage is to the nodes along the greater and lesser curvatures (channels present in the layers of the gastric wall), then splenic, celiac and hepatic nodes

Staging

- TNM system used or modified Astler-Coller

Treatment

- Surgery is always in order; the only mode capable of cure is if tumor remains at submucosa
- Radical distal subtotal gastrectomy is common; removes 80% of stomach
- Radiation therapy is used adjuvantly along with multiagent chemotherapy; intraoperative investigational
- Postoperative or preoperative radiation dose 45 to 50 Gy; radiation alone totals 60 Gy
- Chemotherapy-hopeful
- Drugs may include: etoposide, 5-FU, methotrexate, cisplatin, Adriamycin, leucovorin, biologic modifier-interferon

Radiation Treatment Borders

- Unresectable disease or tumor bed plus regional lymphatics: lesser and greater curvature, celiac axis, pancreatic, splenic, and porta hepatis
- Paraesophageal nodes and lower third of the esophagus should be included if disease was in the proximal portion of the stomach
- Dose limiting organs are kidneys, liver, and bowel
- Field shaping to spare as much liver, kidney, and bowel as possible; some portion of the left kidney cannot be avoided

Treatment Delivery

- Could use four field box technique with beam shaping on all fields
- IMRT produces the best dose distributions
- Pay close attention to nutritional support, especially in postoperative patients
- Most will not be able to manage three full meals a day; advise patients to eat small meals more frequently
- Those on chemoradiation may also have feeding tubes
- Multiple fields will incur complex daily treatment charges

SMALL BOWEL

Divisions of the small bowel:

- Duodenum
- Jejunum
- Ileum

Etiology

- May be inherited connected to disorders such as polyposis, Crohn disease, Gardner syndrome

Clinical Presentation

Signs and Symptoms

- Abdominal pain, cramping
- Abdominal hemorrhage
- Weight loss
- Abdominal mass, usually movable
- Occult or gross rectal bleeding
- Watery diarrhea

Histology

- Adenocarcinoma (in duodenum and jejunum)
- Sarcomas
- Lymphomas (mucosa associated lymphoid type-MALT)
- Carcinoid (No. 1 in ileum)

Workup

- Upper gastrointestinal series with small bowel follow-through
- Small bowel enema
- Flexible endoscopy with biopsy
- CBC for anemia, liver function (bilirubin, amylase)
- CT scan of abdomen, pelvis
- CT-guided biopsy

Spread Patterns

- Regional lymph node review
- Neighboring organs are possibility

Staging

- Classification of these tumors correlates to the histologic type. TNM system is also used.
- Grading is a good indicator for prognosis and guides treatment.

Treatment

- Surgery is standard.
- Postsurgical complications would include anastomosis leak, adhesions, and obstructions.
- Generally recognized as radio-resistant; sarcomas respond
- If unresectable, radiation and chemotherapy will be considered.
- Radiation can be given preoperatively or concomitant to chemotherapy.
- Chemotherapy is 5-FU or cisplatin-based.

Radiation Treatment Borders

- Irradiation of whole abdomen for lymphomas, carcinoids that are unresectable or partially resected
- Total abdominal radiation puts low tolerance organs at risk such as the kidneys
- Adjuvant radiation for the tumor bed plus nodal areas can be considered following complete resection of most histologies.

Treatment Delivery

- Whole abdomen RT postoperatively to dose of 20 to 25 Gy in 1 to 1.25 Gy fractions
- This low dose limits the risk of low tolerance tissues in the abdomen
- Bowel irradiation will lead to acute nausea, vomiting, diarrhea; late effects may include perforation
- For nausea and vomiting recommend clear liquids, no strong odiferous foods, drink plenty of fluids to prevent dehydration; keep ice chips available
- For diarrhea recommend low fiber diet and plenty of fluids
- Beam shaping for the whole abdomen using AP/PA fields will incur complex billing charges.

COLON/RECTUM

Divisions include:

- Cecum
- Ascending colon
- Transverse colon
- Descending colon
- Sigmoid
- Rectum

Etiology

Associated Risk Factors

- Diet (red meat, processed meats, low fiber, high fat)
- Alcohol
- Genetic polyposis
- Crohn disease
- Diverticulosis

Clinical Presentation

Signs and Symptoms

- Blood in stool (microscopic or visible)
- Diarrhea
- Palpable mass in right lower quadrant
- Rectal bleeding
- Pencil stools

Histology

- Adenocarcinomas 90%
- Leiomyosarcomas
- Lymphomas
- Carcinoids

Workup

- Liver function, CBC
- Renal function
- CEA tumor marker
- Digital rectal examination
- Sigmoidoscopy; colonoscopy with biopsy
- Barium enema
- Endorectal ultrasound or coil MRI
- CT of pelvis and abdomen

Spread Patterns

- Local invasion out through the mucosal walls, then pelvic lymph nodes (Figure 9-8) and finally distant metastasis to lung, liver, bone, ovaries, adrenal
- There is very little propensity for colon cancers to creep longitudinally in contrast to esophageal and gastric cancers.

Staging

- Three staging systems are Dukes, TNM, modified Astler-Coller (Table 9-4)
- Grading is important: G1—2 55% 5-year survival, G3—4 30% 5-year survival

Treatment

- Early lesions should have total resection
- Surgical complication include fistula, abscess, hemorrhage, stomal issues, obstruction
- Beginning of the colon not routinely treated with radiation
- Surgery and multiagent chemotherapy used for colon above sigmoid
- Pelvic floor needs reconstruction after lower bowel resection to minimize small bowel within the true pelvis.

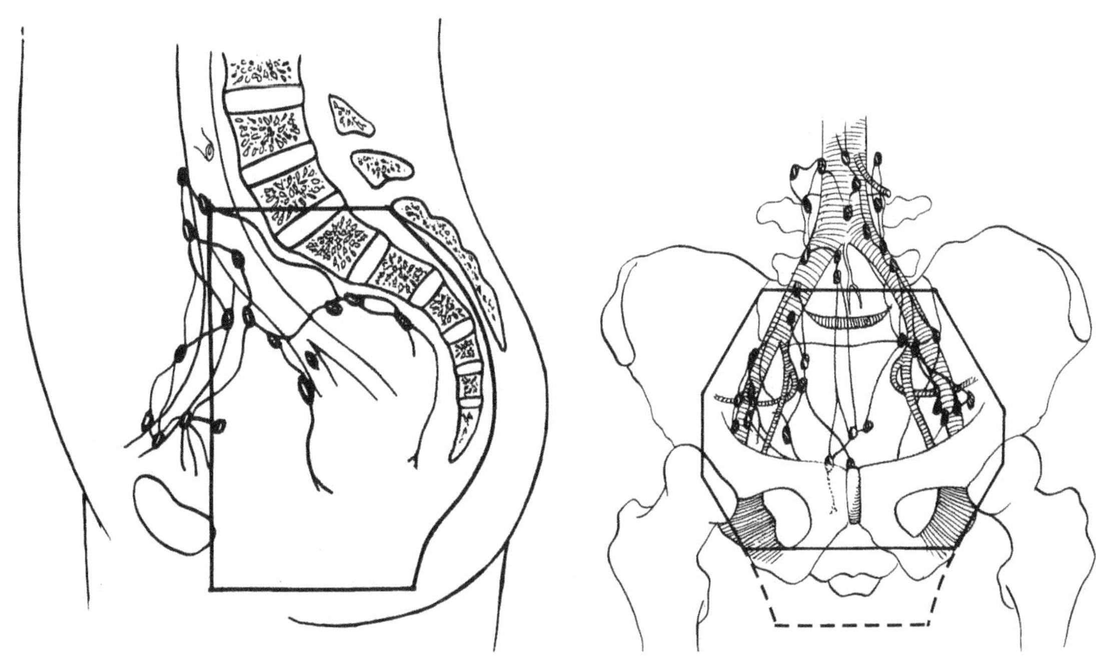

FIGURE 9-8 Pelvic lymph nodes.

TABLE 9-4 Comparison of Staging Systems for Colorectal

AJCC TNM	Dukes	Modified Astler-Coller
I	A	
Tis, N0, M0		A
T1-2, N0, M0		B1
II	B	
T3-4, N0, M0		B2
T4b, N0, M0		B3
III	C	
T1-2, N1-2, M0		C1
T3-4a, N1-2,M0		C2
T4b, N1-2, M0		C3
IV	D	
Any T, Any N, M1		D

- Abdomino-perineal resection (APR) removes the terminal end of the colon and inserts an abdominal colostomy.
- A reanastomosis (reverse of colostomy) can be safely performed after moderate doses of radiation 45-50 Gy. An unirradiated section of bowel can be used for this.
- Radiation may be used without APR for rectal cancers to preserve the sphincter.
- Adjuvant radiation therapy doses 50 to 54 Gy; up to 60 Gy if late stage
- Colorectal cancer traditionally regarded as chemoresistant
- 5-FU and gemcitabine may be used as radiosensitizers.

Radiation Treatment Borders

- Pelvic lymph nodes should be included in treatment fields for the rectum.
- Lymphatic drainage follows the inferior mesenteric vein in the upper rectum, whereas the middle and lower third rectal lymphatic drains to the internal iliac and presacral nodes.
- AP/PA fields should cover the pelvic inlet with margin on the pelvic nodes up to the common iliac.
- Lower border has to leave 2.0 cm margin on the tumor; attempt to spare the anus if sphincter preserved

Treatment Delivery

- Patient may be positioned supine or prone.
- Prone allows positional shift of small bowel up and away from the pelvis; also allows gluteal fold to decrease; belly board may help avoid small bowel on lateral fields.
- Three field technique common PA/RT/LT for rectum sparing the bowel anteriorly
- Field shaping to protect remaining bowel, bladder, bone marrow
- Positioning aids and immobilization devices may range from the simplest block between the feet with Velcro to complex lower pelvis and extremity vac-lock or Aquaplast systems
- Beam shaping and modifiers on the lateral fields will incur complex daily treatment charges.
- Desquamation in the gluteal fold probable; advise patient to keep fold clean and dry, pat after toilet, avoid extreme temperatures during bathing
- Radiosensitizing chemotherapeutic agents intensive desquamation
- If diarrhea, advise patient to begin low residue diet with plenty of fluids

ANUS

Etiology

- Exact cause unknown
- Associated with human papilloma virus (HPV)
- Associated with fissures, leukoplakia, and Bowen disease
- Chronic genital infections and smoking risk factors
- Incidence higher in homosexual males
- Also high incidence in men and women with AIDS

Clinical Presentation

Signs and Symptoms

- Bleeding
- Rectal pain
- Palpable mass
- Rectal discharge

Histology

- Most true anal cancers are squamous cell.
- Adenocarcinomas are likely rectal tumors that have extended.

Workup

- Digital anorectal examination
- Proctoscopy with biopsy
- Colonoscopy

- Transluminal ultrasound
- CBC, creatinine, liver function
- CT of pelvis and abdomen

Spread Patterns

- Local spread is common; this is considered a locoregional disease.
- There can be lymphatic involvement in superficial inguinal nodes, perirectal, internal iliac, and inferior mesenteric nodes.
- Invasion through the rectum into the prostate or vaginal space

Staging

- TNM system works—T categories are quantified by the size (diameter) of the tumor and depth of invasion

Treatment

- Early disease can be managed with surgery APR.
- RT can be used when disease is bulky as definitive or when no surgery.
- Chemotherapy can also be used; chemoradiation has become the standard of care using radiosensitizing 5-FU and/or mitomycin C.

Radiation Treatment Borders

- Pelvis treated with upper border up to internal iliac
- Lower border margin on anal sphincter/tumor
- Width must be wide enough for margin on internal iliac and include superficial inguinal lymph nodes

Treatment Delivery

- Radiation without previous surgery dose ranges from 45 to 65 Gy
- Radiation along with chemotherapy dose ranges from 45 to 65 Gy
- 45 Gy administered to the large pelvic fields; AP/PA to start with inguinal nodes included
- Fields reduced and anal canal boosted to total 65 Gy; PA/RT/LT fields; final anal boost possible with electron beam with patient in lithotomy position
- Positive inguinal nodes may also need to be boosted using electron beams.
- If inguinal node boost anticipated, supine position is desired.
- If no inguinal node boost, patient may be positioned prone to open the gluteal fold and decrease skin reaction in the area; facilitates final anal boost with electron beam if elected
- Desquamation may also be realized in the genital area.
- Advise patients to keep skin clean and dry; pat after toilet and no extreme temperatures during bath
- If diarrhea, low fiber diet with plenty of fluids
- Treatment fields with beam shaping, electron boosts incur complex treatment charges.

ALIMENTARY CANAL SECTION REVIEW EXERCISES

1. The esophagus is located ____ to the trachea.
2. The junction of the transverse and descending colon takes place at the _______.
3. An out pouching or weakening of the intestinal wall most commonly seen in the large intestine is termed:
   a. Diverticulum
   b. Aneurysm
   c. Calculus
   d. Fistula
4. The first portion of the small intestine, which is about 25 cm long, is the _______.
5. The longest segment of the normal human intestinal tract is the _______.
6. Using Figure 9-9, draw typical AP/PA fields for upper one third esophagus squamous cell carcinoma.
7. Complete Table 9-5:
8. The most common histologic type for small bowel cancer is:
   a. Squamous cell
   b. Hepatic sarcoma
   c. Adenocarcinoma
   d. Small cell carcinoma
9. The most common histologic type for cancer of the stomach is:
   a. Squamous cell
   b. Adenocarcinoma
   c. Lymphoma
   d. Transitional cell

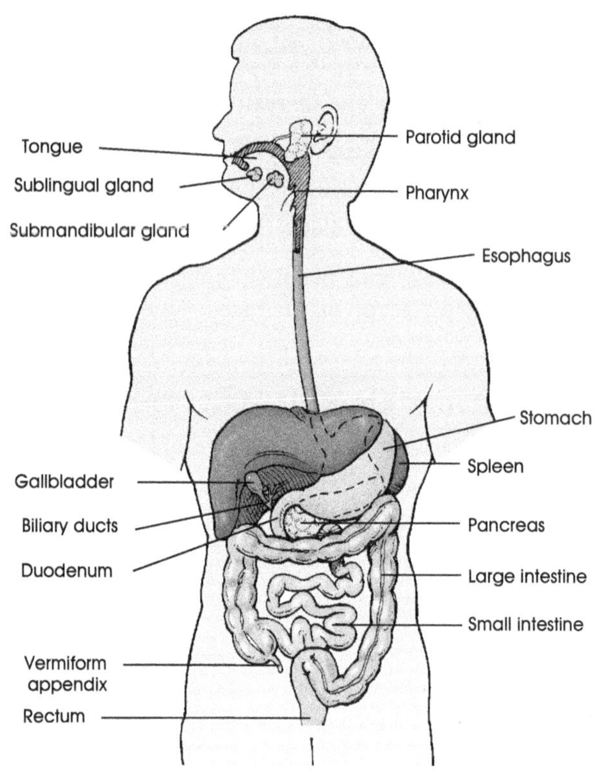

FIGURE 9-9 Alimentary canal.

TABLE 9-5 Alimentary Canal Review

Treatment Site	Anatomy Included in Typical Treatment Fields	Critical Tissues in the Area	Optimal Position/ Immobilization
Rectum			
Anus			

10. The curative treatment of choice for gastric carcinomas is:

a. Chemotherapy
b. Radiation therapy
c. Surgery
d. Cryotherapy

11. The most common presenting symptom of cancer of the stomach among the following is:

a. Severe pain
b. Hematemesis
c. Vague epigastric discomfort
d. Palpable mass

12. Define the following:

Cachexia:

Hematemesis:

Dysphagia:

For questions 13-16, indicate whether the statement is true or false.

13. Dysphasia is a common complaint of patients with esophageal carcinoma. ______

14. Surgery is used more for tumors located in the upper one third of the esophagus. ______

15. Adenocarcinomas of the esophagus are more frequently found in the lower one third of the esophagus. ______

16. The surgical procedure in which an incision is made through the abdominal wall to examine lymph nodes and establish disease extent is called an APR. ______

17. Common sites of metastasis for colon cancer are:

1. Liver
2. Lung
3. Peritoneum
4. Bone

a. 1, 3
b. 2, 3
c. 2, 3, 4
d. 1, 2, 3

18. Dietary factors associated with increased risk of gastric cancers are:

a. Low consumption of fruits and vegetables
b. Low consumption of salted and smoked foods
c. High consumption of salted and smoked foods
d. a and c

19. Radiation treatment fields for cancer of the ______ should include inguinal lymph nodes.

a. Small bowel
b. Anus
c. Sigmoid colon
d. Rectum

20. Three field technique for treatment of the rectum are weighted 2:1:1-PA:RT:LT. Total prescribed dose is 50 Gy. The posterior field contribution will be:

a. 12.5 Gy
b. 20 Gy
c. 25 Gy
d. 40 Gy

21. Intense desquamation may occur in the gluteal fold during radiation therapy to the lower pelvis. Patients should be advised to:

a. Use cold packs in the folds twice daily
b. Take hot baths daily
c. Apply Vaseline every other day
d. Gently pat the area dry after each toilet

22. A risk factor associated with colon cancer is:

a. Exposure to ultraviolet radiation
b. Diet high in salty foods
c. History of colon polyps
d. Human papilloma virus

23. Patients scheduled for radiation therapy to the lower esophagus will likely experience:

a. Diarrhea
b. Diplopia
c. Diverticulitis
d. Nausea

24. Patients scheduled for radiation therapy to the upper esophagus will likely experience:

a. Diarrhea
b. Dysphagia
c. Abdominal distention
d. Nausea

25. Intestinal tumors grow progressively through the layers of the intestines in the following order:

a. Serosa, submucosa, mucosa, muscularis
b. Muscularis, serosa, submucosa, mucosa
c. Mucosa, submucosa, muscularis, serosa
d. Submucosa, mucosa, serosa, muscularis

26. In an anal cancer case, an electron boost will be required for the superficial inguinal nodes determined to be approximately 5 cm deep from the anterior surface. The appropriate electron energy beam would be:

a. 5 MeV
b. 9 MeV
c. 15 MeV
d. 30 MeV

27. Which patient position helps reduce the volume of small bowel in the pelvis?

a. Supine
b. Prone
c. Lateral
d. Lithotomy

28. To avoid exceeding the dose limits of the kidneys, the ______ technique is often employed when treating the pancreas.

a. Three field
b. Four field
c. Posterior oblique
d. Wedged pair

29. Which histologic type of small bowel cancer has the best prognosis?

a. Adenocarcinoma
b. Sarcoma
c. Lymphoma
d. Carcinoid

30. MAC stage A for colorectal cancer correlates to the TNM system stage ______:

a. 0
b. I
c. II
d. III

PANCREAS, LIVER, AND GALLBLADDER

PANCREAS

General Facts and Epidemiology

- Tenth most common cancer; slightly higher risk in women
- Most (75%) occur in the head, neck, or uncinate process-periampullary region
- Fourth and fifth cause of cancer death in men and women, respectively
- Prognosis depends on resectability; only 5% to 25% are resectable

- Rarely localized at the time of diagnosis
- Surgery is the best chance for cure.
- Two-year survival with surgery alone is 20% to 40%.
- Despite surgery, local recurrence is 80% to 90%
- Relapse occurs in the liver, regional nodes and tissues, peritoneum and lung
- If there is metastasis to the liver, lung, or peritoneum, median survival is 3 to 6 months (majority have subclinical disease in the liver at the time of diagnosis).
- Increased incidence in Western and industrialized countries
- In the United States, Japanese-Americans have a lower incidence
- TP16 tumor suppressor has been found to be inactivated in 95% of cases
- Average age at onset is the late 60s

Etiology

- Smoking is the strongest factor
- High fat diet increases risk
- Diabetes increases risk
- Chronic pancreatitis increases risk
- Previous radiation therapy to the abdomen increases risk
- Ten percent may be familial with first degree relatives diagnosed with pancreas, ovarian, or breast carcinoma

Clinical Presentation

- Symptoms depend on location (Table 9-6)

Histology

- Infiltrating ductal adenocarcinoma No. 1
- Adenosquamous carcinoma
- Acinar cell carcinoma (associated with subcutaneous pathways and fat necrosis, usually tumors are large and occur in the head mostly)

TABLE 9-6 Pancreatic Cancer Symptoms

Head, Neck, Uncinate Process	Body and Tail
Obstructive jaundice	Back pain
Dark urine, clay colored stools	Upper gastrointestinal bleeding
Abdominal pain	Splenomegaly
New diagnosis of diabetes	Jaundice (late)

- Giant cell carcinoma (present large; very aggressive, there are no 5-year survivors)
- Mucinous and serous cystic epithelial
- Intraductal papillary mucinous neoplasm (good prognosis)
- Pancreatoblastoma (occurs in childhood)
- Lymphoma

Lymphatic Drainage and Spread Patterns

- Area lymph nodes include pancreaticoduodenal, superior pancreatic, inferior pancreatic, porta hepatic nodes, paraaortic nodes
- Venous drainage of the pancreas is to the liver through the portal vein; easy metastasis to the liver
- Local metastasis to the peritoneum and neighboring abdominal tissues
- If liver is positive for metastasis, distant metastasis is assumed
- Lung is the most likely extraabdominal site for metastasis

Workup

- History and physical
- CBC
- Blood chemistry
- Chest x-ray
- CT/MRI abdomen
- Endoscopic ultrasound
- CA 19-9 (elevation may also indicate a benign condition)

Staging

- TNM system is used, although system slightly different for ampulla of Vater

Treatment

- Surgery is the mainstay—pancreaticoduodenectomy, also known as the Whipple procedure, is classic for pancreatic cancer located in the head
- With Whipple, you must consider possibility of leaks, infections, delayed gastric emptying, pancreatic fistula
- Chemoradiation versus surgery alone still under investigation (recall that most are unresectable)

- Debate regarding preoperative chemoradiation because after surgery there is devascularization of the area leading to low oxygen concentration
- Intraoperative RT has been attempted, but no advantage found over chemoradiation
- Brachytherapy is another possibility with I^{125} and Pd^{103}
- Radiation therapy can be split course or continuous to a total of 40 to 60 Gy. Fractions are at 160 to 180 for continuous or split course. The University of Michigan has reported split course therapy that may begin with 160 cGy/day up to 24 Gy then 280 cGy/day for additional 42 Gy.
- Locally advanced cancers may use radiation + 5 FU (radio-sensitizer).

Radiation Treatment Borders

- Radiation treatment fields are typically 3-4 fields (AP/RT/LT or AP/PA/RT/LT with wedges on the lateral fields) to include tumor bed, peripancreatic lymph nodes, paraaortic lymph nodes between T11 and L3 (be careful of kidney tolerance).
- Upper border—T 10
- Lower border—L3
- Anterior lateral borders give margin on tumor and include paraaortic nodes (Figure 9-10); may extend more into the left abdomen if tumor in the body
- For lateral fields, posterior border should be anterior to the kidneys and anterior border margin on the tumor

HEPATOBILIARY TUMORS

General Facts and Epidemiology

- Linked to hepatitis B, hepatitis C, liver cirrhosis, aflatoxin ingestion
- Gallbladder and biliary cancers related to cholelithiasis
- Primary therapy is surgical resection
- Resected hepatocellular cancer has a median survival of 2 years; 5-year survival is 30%.
- Gallbladder 10% to 30% 5-year survival
- Radiation via external beam is challenging because high doses to whole liver will cause radiation induced liver disease. The advanced treatment planning in RT is opening doors for volume control.
- Hepatocellular carcinoma (HCC) is increasing in incidence in the United States as result of hepatitis C epidemic, although it is still rare in relation to other cancer types.
- Currently no accepted standard for the management of these but may combine systemic and/or regional chemotherapy—chemoembolization, immunotherapy
- Histologic types include hepatocellular carcinoma (HCC), intrahepatic cholangiocarcinoma (IHCC), extrahepatic cholangiocarcinoma (EHCC), adenocarcinoma, and mucinous carcinoma of the gallbladder
- Disease of the elderly

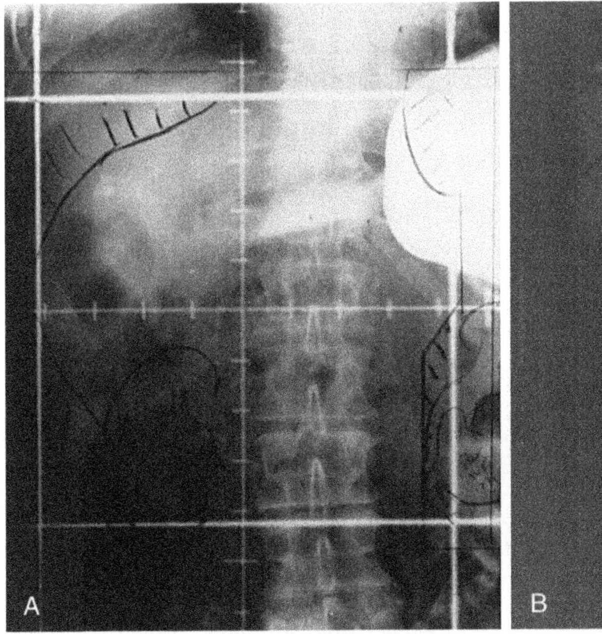

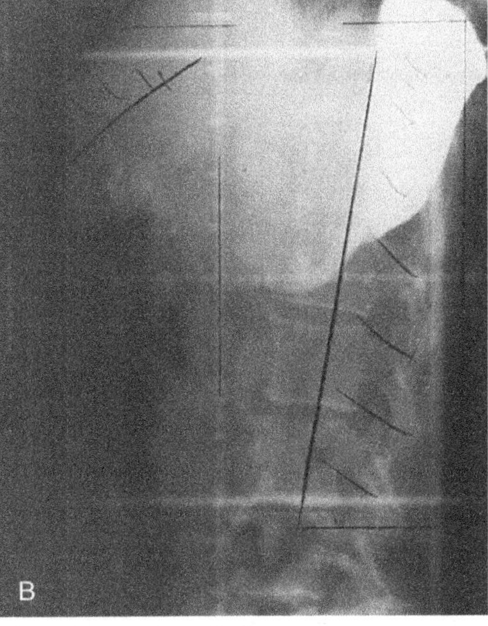

FIGURE 9-10 AP and lateral fields for pancreas radiation.

- HCC 3:1 men: women; high incidence in black men versus white women; high incidence in Asia and Africa due to high incidence of hepatitis B
- IHCC 3:1 men: women; Southeast Asia high incidence
- EHCC 1:1 men: women
- Gallbladder 1:3 men: women; high incidence in Northeastern Europe

Etiology

Liver
- Hepatitis B
- Hepatitis C
- Cirrhosis
- Aflatoxin B (toxic metabolite of fungi that can grow in stored grain and peanuts)

Gallbladder
- Cholelithiasis (stones irritate or bile acid is carcinogenic)

Cholangiocarcinoma
- Liver fluke infestation
- Hepatolithiasis
- Congenital bile duct cysts
- Ulcerative colitis

Clinical Presentation

- Symptoms depends on location (Table 9-7)

Histology

Liver
- Hepatocellular No. 1
- Carcinoid
- Hepatoblastoma
- Angiosarcoma
- Leiomyosarcoma

TABLE 9-7 Symptoms for Hepatobiliary Cancers

HCC/IHCC	EH/Cholangiocarcinoma	Gallbladder
Right upper abdomen pain	Jaundice	Jaundice
Sharp or dull pain	Abdominal pain	Abdominal pain
Abdominal mass	Weight loss	Weight loss
Jaundice (rare)	Fatigue, fever, night sweats	Fatigue

Gallbladder
- Adenocarcinoma No. 1
- Mucinous carcinoma

Lymphatic Drainage and Spread Patterns

- Regional lymph nodes include porta hepatic, celiac, cystic, pericholeductal and hilar nodes
- HCC can appear spreading or show multiple tumors scattered throughout the liver; may invade the portal vein, hepatic vein, or diaphragm
- One third of HCC have regional spread at diagnosis, then spread to regional nodes and then to lung, brain, or muscle tissue in abdomen
- Forty percent to 50 percent of gallbladder carcinomas have distant spread at diagnosis; usually to liver or peritoneum

Workup

- History and physical
- CBC
- Blood chemistry; liver function, coagulation studies
- CA 19-9
- AFP (hepatocellular)
- CEA
- Hepatitis testing
- Ultrasound
- Abdomen CT/MRI
- Transhepatic or endoscopic cholangiography (if bile duct blockage)

Staging and Grading
- Grading is used 1 to 2 low grade 3 to 4 high grade
- There are several systems for staging recommended; most are surgical relying on the surgeon/pathologist to evaluate invasion quite extensively. The T categories vary for liver, IHCC, EHC, and gallbladder.

Treatment

- Surgery is always in order.
- Adjuvant therapies have been attempted but efficacy not yet established.
- Liver transplant for patients with cirrhosis
- Most advocate chemotherapy via chemoembolization, percutaneous ablation, or combination of these

- Ablation with chemicals such as ethanol or acetic acid or by extreme temperatures via radiofrequency, microwave, laser, or cryoablation (this can occur percutaneously or laparoscopically)
- IHCC needs complete resection, right or left hepatectomy
- Gallbladder cancers need resections; can be quite radical taking the gallbladder, nodes plus head of pancreas, part of the liver, and bile duct
- Chemoembolization, known as transcatheter arterial chemoembolization (TACE) for unresectables studies show:

Median Survival	
1. TACE + 50.4 Gy RT	23 months
2. TACE + 36-60 Gy RT	20 months
3. TACE + 48.2-79 Gy RT	10 months
4. TACE + 25-55 Gy RT	18 months

Hepatocellular and IHC

- Surgery is No. 1 choice but most are not candidates (Figure 9-11)

Cholangiocarcinoma and Gallbladder

- Surgery is No. 1 choice but most are not candidates (Figure 9-12)

Treatment Delivery

- Need support for nausea, weight loss, malabsorption, pancreatic enzyme insufficiency, lactose intolerance, hyperglycemia, dehydration, electrolyte imbalance, pain, depression, jaundice, anxiety, constipation, anemia
- Pancreas typically treated with three field technique (AP/RT/LT) to avoid exceeding kidney tolerance
- Lateral fields usually have wedges to compensate for external curvature of the abdomen
- Gallbladder and liver fields usually limited since normal liver has very low tolerance to radiation, and surgery and chemotherapy take on definitive roles
- Ninety-degree wedged pair for liver, gallbladder
- Position patient supine with both arms elevated on simple wing board or complex vac or alpha cradle
- Use of complex immobilization, wedges, and multiple fields with field shaping to protect kidneys and small bowel incur complex daily treatment charges

PANCREAS, LIVER, AND GALLBLADDER SECTION REVIEW EXERCISES

1. The pancreas is a retroperitoneal organ. What is its anatomic relationship to the:

   Stomach ______
   Duodenum ______
   Liver ______
   Spleen ______

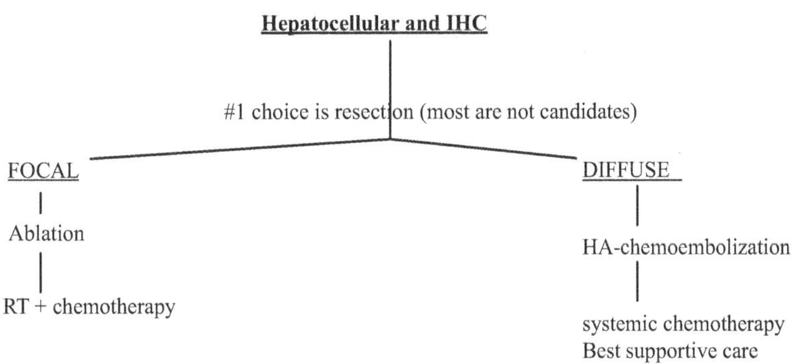

FIGURE 9-11 Hepatocellular and IHC management diagram.

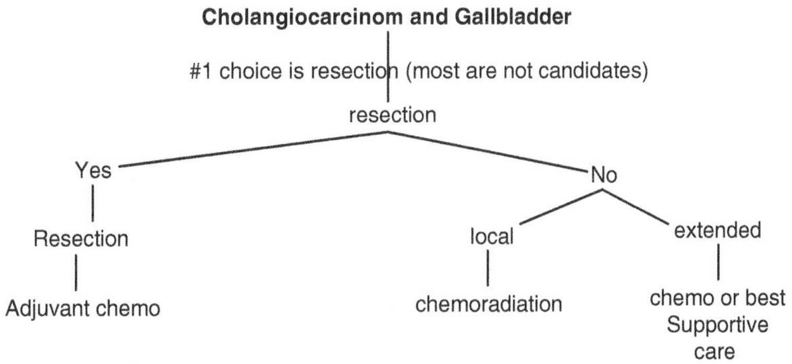

FIGURE 9-12 Cholangiocarcinoma and gallbladder management diagram.

2. What is the function of the pancreas?

3. The liver is the largest abdominal organ. What is its anatomical relationship to the:

Stomach ________
Gallbladder ________
Aorta ________
Inferior vena cava ________
Diaphragm ________

4. What is the function of the liver?

5. The gallbladder is a small organ tucked under the right lobe of the ________.

6. What is the function of the gallbladder?

7. The celiac axis is the first branch of the abdominal aorta, which serves to supply arterial blood to the:

1. Spleen
2. Pancreas
3. Stomach

a. 1, 2
b. 1, 3
c. 2, 3
d. 1, 2, 3

8. Cirrhosis of the liver is often associated with the excessive intake of toxic ________:

a. Cholesterol
b. Heparin
c. Renin
d. Alcohol

9. The failure of the liver to absorb bilirubin will often lead to a yellowish discoloration of the skin and eyes known as:

a. Cyanosis
b. Xanthosis
c. Jaundice
d. Chlorosis

10. The highest portion of the normal adult stomach sitting just below the left diaphragm is the:

a. Pylorus
b. Cardiac orifice
c. Fundus
d. Greater curvature

11. The biliary ducts are principally concerned with the transport of bile and digestive enzymes into the:

a. Colon
b. Stomach
c. Small intestine
d. Lymphatic system

12. The gallbladder is normally found by its attachment to the ventral surface of the:

a. Right lobe of the liver
b. Left lobe of the liver
c. Spleen
d. Duodenum

13. The head of the pancreas will normally be located within the:

a. Lesser curvature of the stomach
b. Splenic flexure
c. Sweep of the duodenum
d. Falciform ligament

14. The release of bile by the gallbladder is triggered by the presence of ________ in the stomach.

1. carbohydrates
2. clear liquids
3. fats

a. 1
b. 2
c. 3
d. 1, 2, 3

15. The ascending and transverse colon join at an area under the right lobe of the liver called the:

a. Splenic flexure
b. Gastric flexure
c. Hepatic flexure
d. Duodenal flexure

16. A severe complication associated with excessive irradiation of the liver is:

   a. Thrombocytopenia
   b. Cholelithiasis
   c. Acute hepatitis
   d. Diabetes

17. A common sight for metastatic spread from the liver is the:

   1. Stomach
   2. Lung
   3. Brain

      a. 1, 2
      b. 1, 3
      c. 2, 3
      d. 1, 2, 3

18. The most common type of tumors found in the pancreas are:

   a. Sarcomas
   b. Anaplastic carcinomas
   c. Leiomyomas
   d. Adenocarcinomas

19. Define the following:

   Cholelithiasis:

   Barrett esophagus:

   Crohn disease:

20. List two symptoms of pancreatic cancer.

21. Complete Table 9-8:

22. Chemoembolization is:

   a. Systemic administration of chemotherapy with one bolus injection
   b. Systemic administration of chemotherapy using the enteral route
   c. Local administration of chemotherapy using proximal venous access
   d. Local administration of chemotherapy using the transdermal route

TABLE 9-8 Digestive Gland Review

Cancer Site	2 Signs/ Symptoms	3 Methods of Detection
Liver		
Stomach		
Esophagus		
Colon		

23. Hepatocellular carcinoma is increasing in incidence in the United States due to the rising cases of:

   a. Epstein-Barr virus
   b. Hepatitis C
   c. Cholelithiasis
   d. Diabetes

24. A pancreaticoduodenectomy is also known as:

   a. Whipple procedure
   b. Halsted technique
   c. Stanford technique
   d. Endoscopy biopsy

25. The best chance for cure in pancreatic carcinoma is:

   a. Intraoperative radiation
   b. Local radiation
   c. Surgery
   d. Chemoembolization

BREAST

GENERAL FACTS AND EPIDEMIOLOGY

- Most common malignancy in women in the United States
- One in eight women will be diagnosed with breast cancer.
- One percent of diagnosed cases will be men.
- Used to be first in mortality, now second to lung cancer

- Breast tissue made up of fat, glands, and ducts
- Location of growths may be referred according to breast quadrant
- Four quadrants: upper outer quadrant (UOQ), upper inner quadrant (UIQ), lower outer quadrant (LOQ), lower inner quadrant (LIQ)
- Most common location is upper outer quadrant
- Rare location is central
- Minimum size for a palpable lump is 1.0 cm
- Prognosis good overall even with positive lymph nodes

Etiology

- Direct cause unknown but there are some associated risk factors (Table 9-9)
- Some factors increase risk (high risk factors)
- Some factors decrease risk (low risk factors)
- Genetics have a strong influence
- Exposure to estrogen has strong influence

Clinical Presentation

Signs and Symptoms

- Painless lump (hard, nonmobile)
- Nipple discharge (bloody, watery)
- Changes in breast skin color or shape
- Swelling
- Dimpling
- Inverted nipple if unusual
- Crusting or scaling of the nipple or areola

Histology

Invasive/Infiltrating

- Ductal
- Lobular
- Tubular
- Medullary (usually well circumscribed)
- Papillary
- Mucinous
- Inflammatory

Noninvasive

- Lobular or ductal carcinoma in situ (LCIS or DCIS)
- Paget disease (from underlying in situ or invasive disease)

TABLE 9-9 Risk Factors Associated with Breast Cancer

High Risk Factors	Low Risk Factors
Female gender	Asian ancestry
Family history	Early pregnancy (by age 18)
History of benign breast disease	Early menopause
Early menarche	Late menarche
Late menopause	Oophorectomy by age 37
Nulliparity	
Children at late age	
Oral contraceptives	

Lymphatic Drainage and Spread Patterns

- Typically spreads by contiguous pattern through drainage lymph nodes (Figure 9-13) including: axillary, internal mammary, and supraclavicular
- Distant metastasis through the blood and Batson plexus to skin, bone (especially thoracic spine), liver, lung, and brain
- Axillary lymph nodes will be positive in about 55% to 70% of cases.

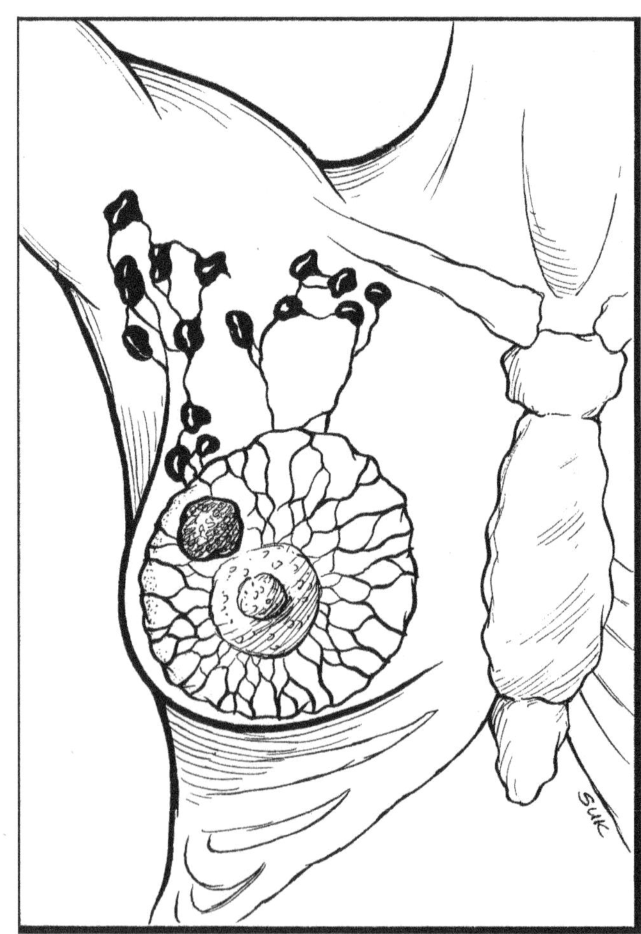

FIGURE 9-13 Breast with lymphatics.

- Axillary node dissections are common for staging.
- Internal mammary nodes positive depending on location of mass (central or inner quadrants)

Workup

- Physical examination
- History
- Needle-guided biopsy with mammogram, ultrasound, or CT
- Open biopsy (lumpectomy and node dissection)
- Sentinel node biopsy (removal of node(s) first containing metastasis using radioactive tracer and blue colored dye)
- Fresh tissue needs evaluation for estrogen and progesterone receptors (ER, PR)
- CT of chest and abdomen
- Bone scan and liver scan for suspected metastasis

Staging

- TNM; clinical staging in office, pathologic staging required; positive supraclavicular nodes classified as M1

Treatment

- Removal of primary tumor by surgery is preferred with lumpectomy
- Radical mastectomy (breast, pectoralis muscles and regional lymph nodes—three levels of axillary)
- Partial excision, also known as wide excision (removal of lump and axillary nodes dissected through separate incision)
- Total mastectomy (removes breast and axillary tail, leaving the pectoralis muscles behind)
- Modified radical mastectomy is a total mastectomy with axillary nodes dissected and pectoralis minor
- Consequence of removing too many lymph nodes is chronic lymphedema
- Local recurrence slightly lower for those with radical mastectomies versus total mastectomies
- Partial mastectomy/lumpectomy has psychological advantages.
- Surgery may be used for reconstruction (silicone implants, grafts using autologous tissue from abdomen and upper thigh for areola).
- Surgery may be used prophylactically for patients with a high risk for developing cancer in the opposite breast (family history, HER2neu, BRCA1 and 2).
- Radiation used definitively to irradiate the entire breast following lumpectomy or chest wall following mastectomy
- Chest wall radiation therapy for those who had large tumors, positive surgical margins, or at least four positive lymph nodes (en face electron fields or photon tangential fields)
- Local radiation, accelerated breast therapy with brachytherapy used following lumpectomy for low risk patients (older age, small tumors, negative nodes)
- Chemotherapy has role following surgery (cytotoxic and hormonal therapy)
- If ER and/or PR positive, hormonal therapy to maintain remission
- Common cytotoxic combinations are: CMF or CAF—cyclophosphamide, methotrexate, 5-FU, Adriamycin (doxorubicin)
- Adriamycin has increased cardiac toxicity so cardiac gating procedures may be employed for patients receiving radiation to the left breast, especially.
- Concomitant cytotoxic chemotherapy and radiation is the standard following surgery for candidates not suited for accelerated brachytherapy.
- Usually chemotherapy first then radiation

Radiation Treatment Borders

- Radiation treatment fields for the intact breast should have medial border at midline, lateral border beyond breast tissue, upper border above the superior tail of the breast (about the second intercostal space), lower border about 2 cm inferior to breast fold
- Therapy fields may be initially set clinically.
- Lymph nodes included as per disease stage
- At minimum first level axillary nodes are included in tangential fields.
- If third level axillary nodes (apical nodes) found positive or if no axillary dissection, or if tumor was extracapsular, another field may be added and treated AP/PA or posterior only with a posterior axillary boost (PAB).
- Supraclavicular nodes treated if positive with medial border at midline, lateral border about two thirds of the clavicle and upper border about 2 to 3 cm above the clavicle; lower border carefully matched to tangential fields

- Combination supraclavicular and apical nodes would show an extended field down to the second rib
- Internal mammary field may be treated in a wider tangential field or separate anterior field if tumor was located near midline
- Internal mammary nodes located lateral of sternum about 2.0 cm on each side and from the level of the third to eighth rib; border should be carefully matched to medial tangent and/or supraclavicular field

Treatment Delivery

- Total dose to intact breast of about 50 Gy in 5 to 6 weeks using tangents to avoid underlying lung
- Wedges or tissue compensators are used for uniform dose distribution within the breast
- Wedges and tissue compensators may be dynamic
- Shrinking fields may be used to decrease skin toxicity and eliminate high dose areas at the inferior portion of the breast
- Boost the lumpectomy site for an additional 10-20 Gy depending on tumor size and margins at surgery time; electron energy depending on depth of tumor bed
- Accelerated breast irradiation using iridium for 1 week using hyperfractionated twice daily; brachytherapy treatment for low recurrence risk cases instead of entire breast radiation
- Chest wall radiation following lumpectomy to about 45 to 60 Gy with photons; bolus scar or entire chest wall
- Chest wall radiation may be delivered with electrons
- Supraclavicular fields treated AP only to depth of 3.0 cm to 45 Gy at 2 Gy per day; Cerrobend or MLC beam shaping to protect the head of the humerus and larynx; gantry angle may facilitate sparing of the larynx
- Apical axillary fields (AP/PA or PAB) treated to midline to 45 Gy
- Matching tangential and supraclavicular fields will likely employ half-beam techniques and/or couch angles to prevent overlap at junction.
- Internal mammary fields treated with single anterior photon field or en face electrons or a combination; IM nodes at depth of 3.0 cm; careful dosimetric planning to avoid overdose at junction
- Patient position supine with affected arm or both arms up, chin turned away from the affected side
- Large breasted patients may be positioned prone to pull breast away from chest wall
- Breast boards used to decrease the slope of the chest
- Immobilization for the arms and upper torso
- Lung dose to be minimized, so watch match lines between tangents and supraclavicular fields
- Skin reactions are expected; patient education should include instructions about no razor shaving under the affected arm, protection from the sun, only radiation dermatitis creams should be used, prophylactic application of radiation dermatitis creams under strict instruction (application three times daily, avoid application 1 hour before treatment)
- Use of beam modifiers and multiple fields with use of beam shaping incur complex billing charges

BREAST REVIEW EXERCISES

1. The Posterior Axillary Boost (PAB) field is intended to irradiate:

   a. Level 1 axillary nodes
   b. Level 2 axillary nodes
   c. Level 3 axillary nodes
   d. Supraclavicular nodes

2. Lymphatic drainage of the breast is primarily to the:

   1. Axillary nodes
   2. Supraclavicular nodes
   3. Internal mammary nodes

   a. 1, 2
   b. 2, 3
   c. 1, 3
   d. 1, 2, 3

3. Using Figure 9-14 below, draw the location of all lymphatic drainage for the breast.
4. For estrogen receptor positive cases, an antiestrogen may be used to maintain remission known as:

   a. Taxol
   b. Tamoxifen
   c. Megace
   d. Prednisone

5. Two common cytotoxic drug combinations for the management of breast carcinoma are CMF and CAF. Complete Table 9-10 below:

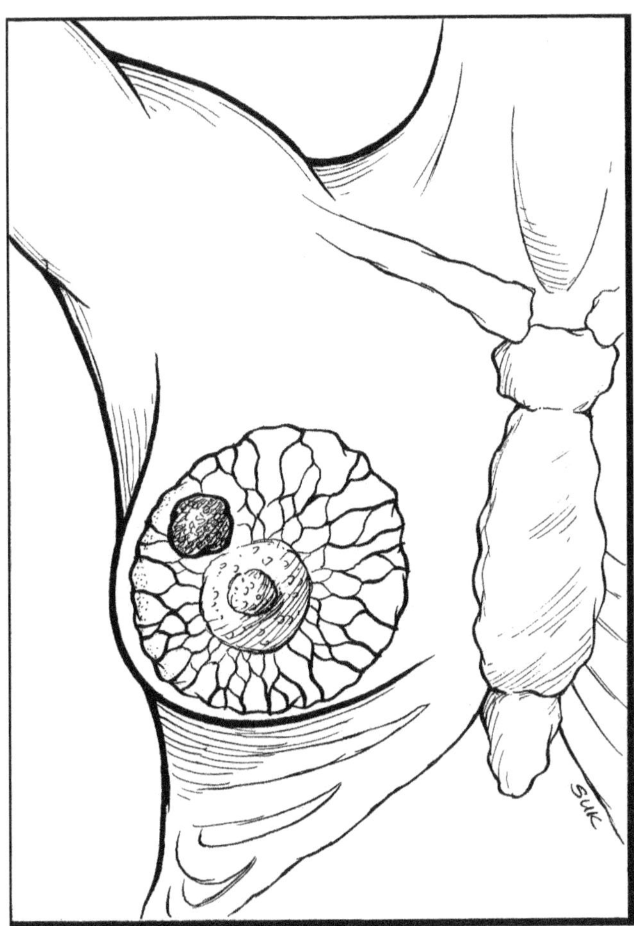

FIGURE 9-14 Right breast.

TABLE 9-10 Breast Review

Drug Name	Drug Class	Toxicities
C		
M		
F		
C		
A		
F		

Think About It

6. Special care must be taken to limit dose to the heart when treating left breast patients who have undergone CAF chemotherapy. Briefly explain.

7. Briefly describe the difference between clinical and pathologic staging for breast cancer.

8. The prescription for the lumpectomy bed boost calls for an enface electron field. The deepest aspect of the tumor bed is 5 cm beneath the skin. What is the most appropriate electron energy for 90% dose line coverage on the tumor bed?

9. In the figure for question 3, the lumpectomy bed is located in the right upper outer quadrant of the breast. What possible patient, table, and gantry position(s) would adequately deliver uniform dose distribution to the site?

10. The couch kick method will be used for tangential and supraclavicular fields in the management of a breast cancer case. The field size for the tangential fields is 8 × 24 cm. The SSD for both the medial and lateral tangents is 91 cm. A 100-cm SAD linear accelerator is used. The supraclavicular field size is 12 × 10 cm and will be treated at 97 cm SSD.

    a. What is the calculated couch angle?

    b. For which field(s) will the couch need to be angled?

11. Referring to the figure for question No. 3, draw the following treatment fields:

a. Tangential fields
b. AP supraclavicular field
c. Lumpectomy bed boost

12. Using the information given, calculate the monitor units required for each treatment field per fraction.

Prescription: * 5040 cGy to right breast 180 cGy per fraction-6 MV photons
* 4500 cGy to right supraclavicular fossa 180 cGy per fraction-6 MV photons
* 1000 cGy boost lumpectomy scar 200 cGy per fraction-12 MeV en face electrons
6 MV beam output = 1 cGy/MU 12 MeV beam output = 1 cGy/MU
Medial and lateral tangents
Field size = 8 × 24
SSD = 91 cm
Field size factor = 1.034
TAR @ 9 cm = 0.892

AP supraclavicular field
Field size = 12 × 10
Field size factor = 1.003
TAR@ 3 cm = 1.002

En face electron boost field
Cone factor = 1.02
Dose to 90% dose line

13. The most common symptom of breast cancer is:

a. Painless lump
b. Clear nipple discharge
c. Dimpling of the skin
d. Inverted nipple

14. Define the following:

Radical mastectomy:

HER2neu:

BRCA1:

Peau d'orange:

15. When using a breast board for positioning, the optimal incline angle is influenced by:

a. The angle of the elbow when it is raised
b. The ability of the patient to raise the arm(s)
c. The slope of the patient's chest
d. The gantry angle on the medial tangent

16. When the supraclavicular fossa is treated along with opposing tangents, the supraclavicular field is best treated using:

a. AP/PA ports
b. Wedged pair
c. Rotational beam
d. Half field technique

17. The total radiation dose received by the lumpectomy bed in standard whole breast irradiation followed by lumpectomy site boost is:

a. 40 to 50 Gy
b. 50 to 60 Gy
c. 60 to 70 Gy
d. 70 to 80 Gy

18. The most common histologic type of breast cancer is:

a. Infiltrating ductal
b. Lobular in situ
c. Paget disease
d. Medullary

19. The acceptable amount of lung tissue included in tangential breast fields is 2.0 cm in order to decrease the chance of latent:

a. Pneumonia
b. Lung fibrosis
c. Pleural effusion
d. Atelectasis

20. An en face electron boost to the lumpectomy bed is accidentally treated at 105 cm SSD instead of 100 cm SSD. The error in dose delivered is about:

a. 5% over dose
b. 5% under dose
c. 10% over dose
d. 10% under dose

21. Ductal carcinoma in situ (DCIS) is classified as:

a. Stage 0
b. Stage I
c. Stage II
d. Stage III

22. A breast cancer classified as T3 N1 M1 with the metastasis to the supraclavicular nodes only would be grouped as:

a. Stage I
b. Stage II
c. Stage III
d. Stage IV

23. A sentinel lymph node biopsy involves the injection of a blue dye and radioactive:

a. Iridium 192
b. Technetium 99m
c. Strontium 89
d. Samarium 137

24. The hinge angle between two half-beam tangential ports is 180 degrees. The medial tangent gantry angle is 310 degrees. What is the gantry angle for the lateral tangent?

a. 230 degrees
b. 140 degrees
c. 130 degrees
d. 50 degrees

GYNECOLOGIC TUMORS

- Table 9-11 lists gynecologic epidemiology figures in the United States; Figure 9-15 is a view of the female pelvis; Figure 9-16 portrays pelvic lymph node drainage.

GENERAL FACTS AND EPIDEMIOLOGY

- Deaths rates (calculated from ratio of deaths to new cases):
  - Ovarian 68%
  - Cervical 33%
  - Endometrial 19%
- Even with 24% more endometrial cancers, ovarian cancer deaths have 250% more incidences than endometrial due to:
  - Relatively nonspecific early symptoms, resulting in late stage disease
  - Endometrial cancer has higher cure rate due to early symptom of postmenopausal bleeding, resulting in physical evaluation at an early stage
- Cervical cancer more prevalent in younger women (intraepithelial neoplasia) and invasive cervical cancer peaks in women age 50 to 60
- Low socioeconomic status patients have a greater risk for cervical cancer, due to higher nonparticipation rate in cancer screening programs.
- Early sexual activity, multiple partners, and multiple pelvic infections (genital warts, HPVs, and herpes simplex type 2) are also related to increased risk of cervical cancer.
- Incidence higher among wives of men with penile cancer

TABLE 9-11 Gynecologic Epidemiology in the United States

Overall Yearly Incidence		78,490		
Endometrial	50%		Cervical	14%
Ovarian	29%		Others	7%
Overall Yearly Mortality		28,490		
Endometrial	27%		Cervical	14%
Ovarian	56%		Others	3%

Data from American Cancer Society: *Cancer facts and figures*: 2008, Atlanta, 2008, American Cancer Society.

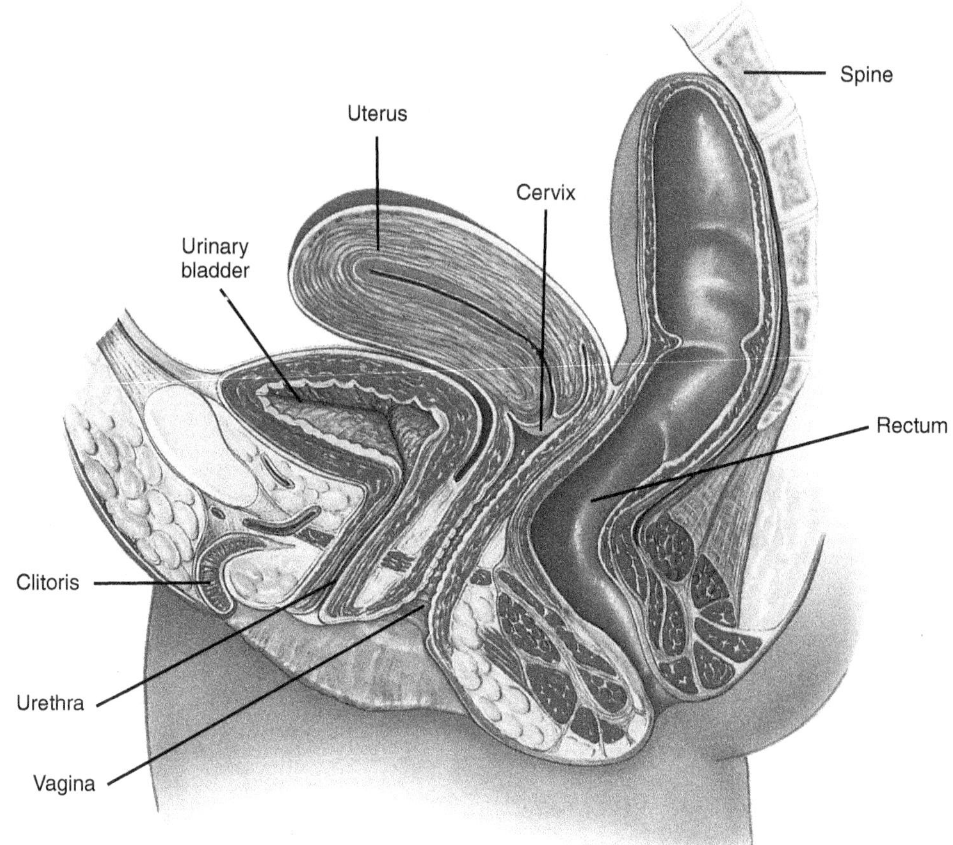

FIGURE 9-15 Sagittal view of female pelvis.

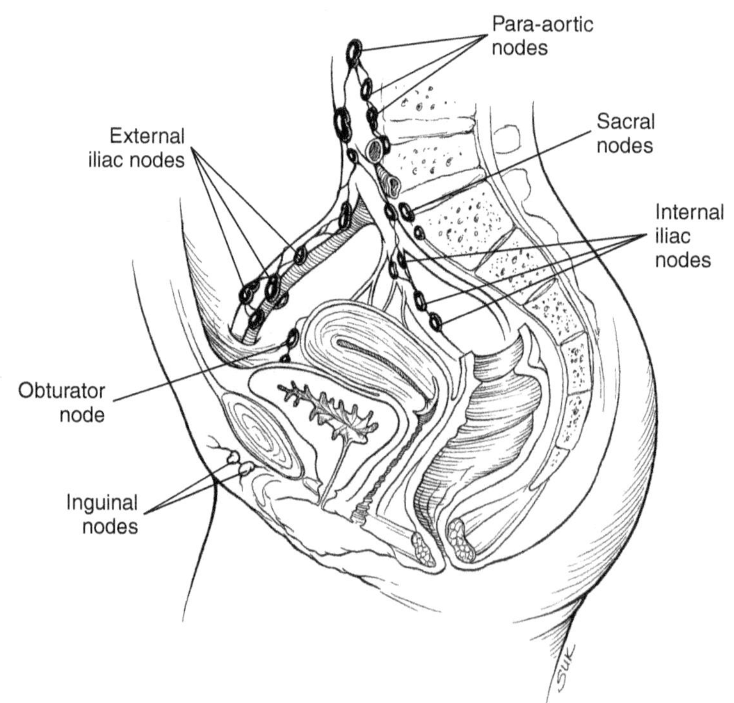

FIGURE 9-16 Pelvic lymph nodes.

- As with vagina cancer, the cervix is at increased risk of clear cell adenocarcinoma and women whose mothers were given diethylstilbestrol (DES) during pregnancy.
- Cervix—Due to the prevalence of Papanicolaou (PAP) smears, two thirds of cervical cancers are detected in the noninvasive stage and are highly curable with local therapy.
- Endometrial cancer has increased as a result of an aging population, high-calorie and high-fat diets, and estrogen use.
- Diabetes and hypertension increases the risk of endometrial cancer.
- Women—Patients who are 50 pounds overweight have a ninefold increased risk.
- Endometrial cancer risk with an increase in estrogen or the estrogen-to-progesterone ratio, as occurs with nulliparity, infertility secondary to anovulation, dysfunctional bleeding during menopause or prolonged hormone replacement therapy (HRT)
- Vagina and vulvar cancers are rare and usually occur in older women.
- Vulvar cancer is three times as common as vaginal and maybe associated with diabetes and sexually transmitted disease.
- Atrophic and dysplastic changes in vaginal lining, a loss of hormone stimulation, and poor hygiene may be associated with vulvar cancer
- Ovarian cancer primarily affects women between ages 50 and 70 and is the fifth leading cause of death in women following lung, breast, colon, and pancreatic cancer.
- Ovarian—screening tools are inadequate because the disease is only intermittently detectable during physical examinations, radiographic studies, and serologic tests; therefore it is generally found when in a late stage.
- International Federation of Gynecologists & Obstetricians (FIGO) staging as well as American Joint Committee on Cancer (AJCC) staging

VULVA

Anatomy

- Outermost portion of gynecologic tract
- Major parts—labia majora and labia minora
- Clitoris
- Area bound by these three—vestibule (triangular and located anterior to the vaginal opening), usually contains the urethral meatus
- Perineum—area between the vulvovaginal complex and anal verge

Etiology and Epidemiology

- Atrophic and dysplastic changes in normal vaginal lining
- Loss of hormone stimulation
- Poor hygiene
- Three times more common than vagina
- Diabetes
- Sexually transmitted diseases
- Melanoma may be associated
- Usually occurs in older women

Clinical Presentation

- Subcutaneous lump or mass
- Advanced disease—ulcerative exophytic mass
- Unifocal—labia majora is most common
- Patient usually has long history of local irritation

Lymphatic Spread Patterns

- Lymphatic spread predictable (increased in lymph involvement lowers the survival rate)
  - *Superficial inguinal* nodes first, followed by *deep femoral* nodes, and then *pelvic* nodes

Prognosis

- Prognostic factors include the size of the lesion, depth of invasion, and histologic subtype

Detection and Diagnosis

- Biopsy—with histologic examination
- History and physical
- CBC and chemistries
- Urinalysis
- Chest x-ray, IVP, CT (pelvic)
- Cystourethroscopy
- Liver and bone scans sigmoidoscopy

Pathology and Staging

- Squamous cell carcinomas—90%
- Staging—TNM
  - Stage I—tumor confined to vulva or vulva and perineum with a maximum diameter of 2 cm or less at greatest dimension
  - Stage II—Tumor confined to the vulva or vulva and perineum with maximum diameter greater than 2 cm in greatest dimension
  - Stage III—Tumor of any size with contiguous spread to the lower urethra and/or vagina or anus
  - Stage IVA—Tumor invades any of the following: upper urethra, bladder mucosa, rectal mucosa, or is fixed to the pelvic bone

Treatment Considerations

- Surgery—wide local excision first
- Radiation—(alone, or adjunctively with chemo)
  - Stage I and II—local excision and 50 Gy; simple vulvectomy with 60 Gy + 5 to 10 Gy boost
  - Stage III—Post op if tumor is >4 cm, margins + for tumor or less than 8 mm
  - Dose of 50 Gy with boosts up to 65 to 70 Gy for microscopic disease or clinically involved lymph nodes (fraction size 1.7 to 1.8 daily)
  - Vulva and perineum will develop moist desquamation, result of thinner tissue (40 Gy—patient may be put on break for severe vulvar skin reaction)
  - Vulva—survival rate
    - Overall 5-year about 70%
    - Surgically treated survival rate:
  - Stage I—100%
  - Stage II—86%
  - Stage III—59%
  - Stage IV 25%
  - Dependant on lymph node involvement

Treatment

- Field includes primary + inguinal region
- Pelvic fields include pelvic inlet
- Field wider at inguinal lymph nodes
- Patient maybe in "frog-leg" position
- Bolus may be placed over vulva and perineum
- Inguinal nodes best treated anteriorly (helps to minimize dose to femoral head and neck)

VAGINA

Anatomy

- A muscular tube that extends 6 to 8 inches superiorly from the vulva and is located anterior to the rectum and posterior to the bladder,
- Most commonly presents in the posterior upper third of vagina
- Lymphatic involvement greater with the depth of invasion
- Lower one third of vagina may involve the inguinal nodes

Etiology and Epidemiology

- Rare—2% of all gynecologic cancers
- Arising in vagina
- No definite etiologic factors
- Rare—Clear cell seen in 1 in 1000 women (mother exposed to DES while in utero); found mostly in women aged 15 to 27, median age is 19 years old)
- Squamous cell carcinoma occurs in older women (median age 65-years-old)

Presenting Symptoms

- Vaginal bleeding
- Painful intercourse

Detection and Diagnosis

- Biopsy
- Cytologic examination
- H & P
- CBC and chemistries
- Urinalysis
- Chest x-ray, IVP, abdominal-pelvic CT
- Cystourethroscopy
- Advanced disease—liver/bone scan
- Proctosigmoidoscopy

Pathology and Staging

- Squamous cell (80% to 90%); melanoma 5%; clear cell adenocarcinoma (rare)
- Staging:
  - I—Tumor confined to vagina
  - II—Tumor invades paravaginal tissue, but not pelvic wall.
  - III—Extends to pelvic wall (muscle, fascia, neurovascular structures, or skeletal portions of the bony pelvis)
  - IVA—invades the mucosa of the bladder or rectum and/or extends beyond true pelvis

Treatment Considerations

- Radiation therapy treatment of choice
- Surgery for recurrent or persistent squamous cell and young women with early clear cell
- Small superficial lesions—only vaginal tissues treated (local excision or brachytherapy)
- Invasive lesions—entire pelvis treated 45 to 50 Gy; more involved tumors 65 to 80 Gy
- Problems—early acute dermatitis

Treatment

- Brachytherapy—60 Gy with a vaginal cylinder, which is a canal-filling cylinder into which an isotope (usually Cs 137) is placed; HDR afterloaders may use Ir 192 isotope
- External therapy—Anterior/posterior fields or IMRT

CERVIX

Anatomy

- The part of the uterus that extends into the apex of the vagina
- A firm rounded structure from 1.3 to 3.0 cm in diameter
- Protrudes into the vagina, producing lateral spaces in the vaginal apex called the *fornices*
- A canal called the *cervical os* extends from the vagina, through the central cervix, and into the uterine cavity, or pelvic portion of the uterus

Etiology and Epidemiology

- Prevalent in younger women
- Invasive cervical cancer age 50 to 60
- Low socioeconomic status at greatest risk (less than average participation in cancer screening programs)
- Early sexual activity, multiple partners, and multiple pelvic infections (genital warts and HPVs), and herpes simplex type 2
- Risk higher in wives of men with penile cancer
- DES
- Screening should begin at age 18 or earlier in sexually active women

Signs and Symptoms

- Signs of invasive cervical cancer:
  - Postcoital bleeding
  - Increased menstrual bleeding
  - Discomfort with intercourse
  - A malodorous discharge, pelvic pain, and urinary or even rectal symptoms may indicate more advanced stage
  - Invasive cancer—friable, ulcerative, or exophytic mass (extension into vaginal canal and involve vagina sidewalls, or invade other organs and tissues such as parametrium, bladder, or rectum)

Lymphatic Spread Patterns

- Orderly spread
- Parametrial nodes, followed by pelvic, common iliac, periaortic, and supraclavicular spread
- When periaortics are involved—35% risk exists for s/c involved
- Survival rates and local control decrease as the stage and bulk tumor increase
- Uterine involvement drops 5-year survival rates from 92%—54%
- Bulky or barrel-shaped tumor is associated with a 22% chance of developing distant metastasis within 5 years
- Lymph node involvement results in 50% reduction in survival rates. (Hemoglobin levels are extremely important due to anemia, a common side effect from treatment.)

Detection and Diagnosis

- Pelvic examination and Pap smear
- Biopsy of suspicious lesions
- History; physical examination under anesthesia
- D & C (dilation and curettage-surgical procedure) to assess uterine involvement
- CBC and chemistries, urinalysis
- Chest x-ray, BE, IVP (CT)—used in staging
- Abdominopelvic CT and MRI
- Cystoscopy and proctoscopy
- PET
- Laparoscopic or CT directed biopsy (now PET)

Pathology and Staging

- Squamous cell—most common
- Staging Summary:
- Stage 0 carcinoma in situ
- Stage I confined to uterus, may further express layer invasion
- Stage II invasion beyond uterus but not pelvic sidewalls or lower third of vagina
- Stage III extends to pelvic wall or lower third of vagina
- Stage IV bladder or rectum involved or extension beyond true pelvis
- Staging is based on a clinical examination before the initiation of therapy and may be supplemented by diagnosing options
- Higher stages decrease survival rates

Treatment Considerations

- *Stage 0* (carcinoma in situ) and stage *Ia1* (invasive)—Treatment—total abdominal hysterectomy (TAH) with a small amount of vaginal tissue, known as the vaginal cuff
- Conization—limited to cervix for stage Ia1 for women who desire to have children
- Medically inoperable patients—tandem and ovoids with 45 to 55 Gy to point
- *Stage Ia2* (TAH), or more aggressive modified hysterectomy
- Medically inoperable—70 to 80 Gy cervix and parametrial tissues (LDR or HDR); cervix treatment considerations
- *Stage Ib1 or small IIa*—surgery/radiation (age dependent); doses 80 to 85 Gy
- *Stage IIb, III, and IVa*—radiation/chemo (brachytherapy very important aspect)
- 5-year survival rates
- 95% for stage Ia
- 85% for stage Ib
- 70% for stage II
- 50% for stage III
- Less than 10% for stage IV

Treatment

- Whole pelvis, four field allows for exclusion of bladder and rectum in patients whose external beam dose is 45 to 50 Gy
- Lower border—inferior aspect of obturator foramen (if vagina is involved, lower border would be 4 cm below the most inferior aspect of disease)
- Upper border—top or bottom of L5 (inclusion of L4-nodal dependent)
- Lateral—1.5 to 2.0 cm lateral to the pelvic sidewall in AP/PA plane
- Extended AP if periaortics are involved
- Anal markers, rectal barium, vaginal markers, and bladder contrast use for delineating critical structures during simulation process
- Prone positioning with belly board or dull bladder may allow the exclusion of the small bowel without jeopardizing tumor coverage
- Cervical implant instruments
- Intrauterine tandem (small, hollow, curved cylinder that fits through *cervical os* and into the uterus—**Point A**)
- Vaginal colpostats (two golf-club-shaped, hollow tubes placed laterally to the tandem into the vaginal *fornices*—**Point B**)
- Numerous dose, field, and sequencing arrangements are possible with external and brachytherapy radiation—Oncologist's call based on experience
- Central doses prescribed to:

- **Point A**—prescription point defined as 2 cm superior to the cervical os and 2 cm lateral to the endocervical canal
- **Point B**—is 3 cm lateral to point A (2 cm superior to the cervical os and 5 cm lateral to the endocervical canal)
- Tissue tolerance in cervix Treatment
- **Bladder**—Point tolerance is about 70 Gy: whole bladder treatment results in acute cystitis at doses as low as 30 Gy, which results in acute bladder irritation with dysuria, frequency and urgency but usually resolves; Chronic cystitis with doses above 50 to 60 Gy.
- **Rectum** (immediately posterior to the vagina and cervix)—Point tolerance is also 70 Gy; whole organ tolerance is about 50 Gy; at 30 to 40 Gy diarrhea, bleeding, urgency, and pain; late effects include stricture, bleeding, and perforation

ENDOMETRIUM

Anatomy

- Hollow muscular structure that extends at a right angle from the vagina to overlie the bladder
- Extending laterally from the superior uterus are the twin fallopian tubes
- Fallopian tubes—hollow structures designed to transfer the ova from the ovaries to the uterus
- Parametrium—the connective tissue lateral to the uterine cervix
- Endometrium:
- Increased risk for endometrial cancer in women taking tamoxifen
- 75% of women with endometrial cancer have vaginal bleeding and a putrid vaginal discharge
- About one third of these cases are postmenopausal bleeding cases
- About 70% of cases are stage I
- Poor prognostic factors: more involvement of area

Lymphatic Spread Patterns

- Initially to internal and external iliac
- Stage I—10% of patients have nodes positive for tumor
- Stage II—25% to 35% increase of nodal involvement, a poorly differentiated histology, or a deep myometrial invasion
- If pelvic nodes involved—60% chance periaortic nodes are too

Detection and Diagnosis

- Aspiration curettage/endometrial sampling (usually done in doctors office) is reported as having a 94% sensitivity rate
- H & P
- Chest x-ray
- Blood counts, chemistries, and urinalysis
- Pelvic sonogram
- Pelvic CT or MRI

Pathology and Staging

- Adenocarcinoma—most common
- Adenocarcinoma with squamous differentiation is a variant seen 20% of time and usually more advanced
- Papillary serous adenocarcinoma—extremely malignant and spreads rapidly
- Clear cell adenocarcinoma
- Sarcomas—also advanced
- Staging summary:
    - Stage I limited to endometrium up to myometrium
    - Stage II limited to glandular epithelium; no stromal invasion
    - Stage III serosa involvement or ascites positive for cancer cells
    - Stage IV invasion of bladder or bowel

Treatment Considerations

- Surgery and/or radiation therapy—depending on stage, grade, medical condition of patient
- Pre-op radiation for high grade and high clinical stages (before surgery)
- Post-op after surgery
- Definite radiation for nonoperative patients
- After TAH (total abdominal hysterectomy), stage Ia and grade 1—no post-op
- Stage Ib, grades 1 and 2, Ia and grade 2—postoperatively with brachytherapy
- Radiation alone used for inoperable patients and stage III and IV
- Doses vary with stage and grading:

- 60 to 70 Gy brachytherapy; 45 to 50 Gy for nodes and implants can bring total dose to 80 Gy

Treatment

- Brachytherapy—a vaginal cylinder or colpostats to treat the vaginal cuff
  - LDR (low dose rate)—60 to 70 Gy (2 sessions)
  - HDR (high dose rate)—5 to 7 Gy to a 0.5 cm depth (3 fractions)
  - Increased stage and grade—increases pelvic nodal involvement, then external radiation given to pelvis
  - Fields are similar to cervical fields with midline blocking used after brachytherapy
- Heyman capsule technique or an intrauterine tandem is used when uterus is still present
- Uterus may tolerate 75 to 90 Gy when brachytherapy is combined with external, but the bladder and rectum must be kept to 65 to 75 Gy or less and small bowel at 45 to 50 Gy. This is accomplished with parametrial blocking when using external beam.

OVARIAN CANCER

Clinical Presentation

- Most deadly of the gynecologic cancers—few symptoms until it is widely disseminated
- Mainly affect women ages 50 to 70
- Fifth leading cause of cancer death in women
- Risk factors
  - Older age, late or few pregnancies, late menopause, lack of oral contraceptive use, family history of ovarian, with a personal history of breast, colon, or endometrial, diets high in meat/animal fat, living in industrialized nations (except for Japan)
- Screening tools are inadequate because the disease is only intermittently detectable during physical examinations, radiographic studies, and serologic tests and then it is usually found to be in an advanced stage
- Early if contained only to the ovaries
- Progression occurs within pelvis, abdominal cavity, and lymph nodes
- 80% of women have abdominal cavity involvement at the time of presentation
- Spread occurs through lymphatic channel of peritoneal lining and the diaphragm and lymph nodes as the peritoneal fluid circulates

Detection and Diagnosis

- Diagnosis and staging are surgical (laparoscopy)
- H & P
- Liver and renal function blood work
- Chest x-ray
- Pelvic sonogram (transvaginal views)
- Abdominopelvic CT/MRI
- Serum CA-125
- BE, GI, upper/lower endoscopy
- Surgical evaluation includes:
  - Cytologic evaluation of peritoneal fluid
  - Intraoperative evaluation for ovarian, fallopian tube, or other masses
  - Examination and biopsy of peritoneal surfaces
  - Removal of as much of tumor

Pathology and Staging

- 90% are epithelial (from ovary surfaces)
- 7% are stromal
- 3% ovarian germ (these include dysgerminomas, which are treated as seminomas—male testicular cancer)

Staging

- **Stage I:** Tumor limited to the ovaries (one or both).
- **Stage II:** Tumor involves one or both ovaries with pelvic extension and/or implants.
- **Stage III:** Tumor involves one or both ovaries with microscopically confirmed peritoneal metastases outside the pelvis.

Treatment

- Initial—surgical evaluation and debulking
- Standard postoperatively
  - Chemo—single agent or combination (*platinum based*)
    - Phosphorus-32 (P-32)—colloidal solution placed into the peritoneal cavity may be used over single agent
  - Radiation—whole abdominal with pelvic boost

Survival Rates

- Early stage I—90%, 5-year
- Stage III—20%
- Stage IV—5%

Treatment

- Entire peritoneal cavity (whole abdomen)—extends from the diaphragm to the pelvic floor (Figure 9-17)
- Dose—25 to 28 Gy (1.0 to 1.2 Gy/fraction)
- No liver blocking necessary, but renal blocking needed at 18 to 20 Gy
- Pelvis boosted up to 50 Gy (1.8 Gy/fraction)

SIDE EFFECTS OF PELVIC IRRADIATION

Acute

- Fatigue—First week of treatment
  - Exacerbated or complicated by anemia and depression (coming to terms with having being diagnosed with cancer)—treated with rest, reassurance, adequate nutrition, and antidepressants

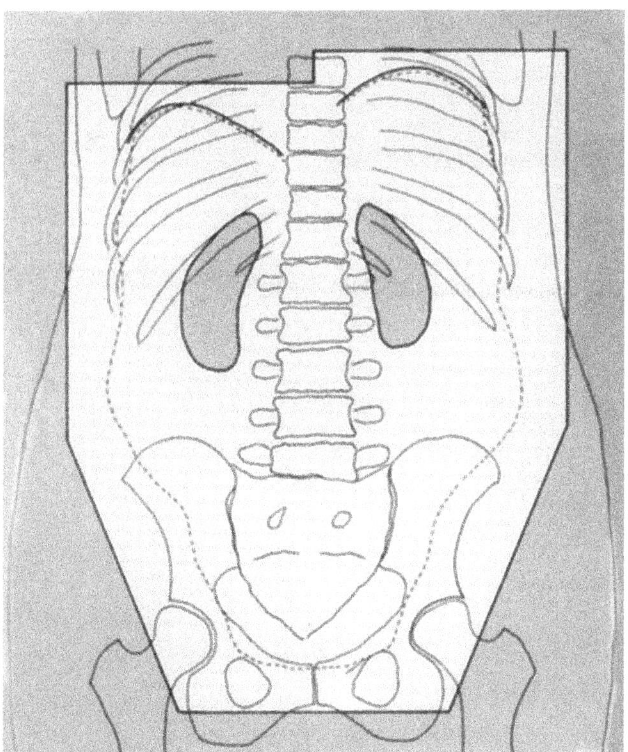

FIGURE 9-17 Whole abdomen radiation treatment field.

  - Anemia, secondary to blood loss should be corrected (hemoglobin level above 10 to 11* g/dL)
  - Diarrhea—second or third week of treatment (to large and small bowel);—patient advised—low-fiber diet; sucralfate (Carafate)-small bowel coating agent; diphenoxylate (Lomotil) and loperamide medication
  - Exclusion of small bowel helps by use of belly boards, prone position with full bladder, custom shielding, serial field-size reduction and IMRT
  - Addition of chemo heightens all side effects
  - Nausea and upper GI bleeding
- Dermatitis—more common with: low-energy beams, AP/PA fields only; perineal flash; use of bolus; concomitant chemo
- Treatment—Domeboro soaks, Aquaphor ointment, natural care gels (lessens severity and speeds healing); prevention and early treatment of local infection, correction of anemia and nutrition problems also helps skin heal
- Dysuria—third or fourth week of treatment; can be lessened by treatment with full bladder; partial bladder exclusion on lateral fields; maintenance of a partially full bladder during brachytherapy
  - Medications—Phenazopyridine (Pyridium), and Urised (anesthetize bladder). To relax bladder relieve urinary frequency-Ditropan, Levsin, and Hytrin. Infections should be treated early and completely.
- Bleeding
  - Anal irritation—Treated with hemorrhoidal preparations, steroids, topical anesthetic agents, and sitz baths
  - Bladder irritation
  - Hemorrhagic tumor

Chronic

- Menopause—HRT
- Vaginal dryness/narrowing/shortening—moisturizing agents
- Chronic cystitis—local meds (Trental)
- Proctosigmoiditis
- Enteritis
- Bowel obstruction—pain meds

GYNECOLOGIC REVIEW EXERCISES

1-18. Complete the crossword puzzle.

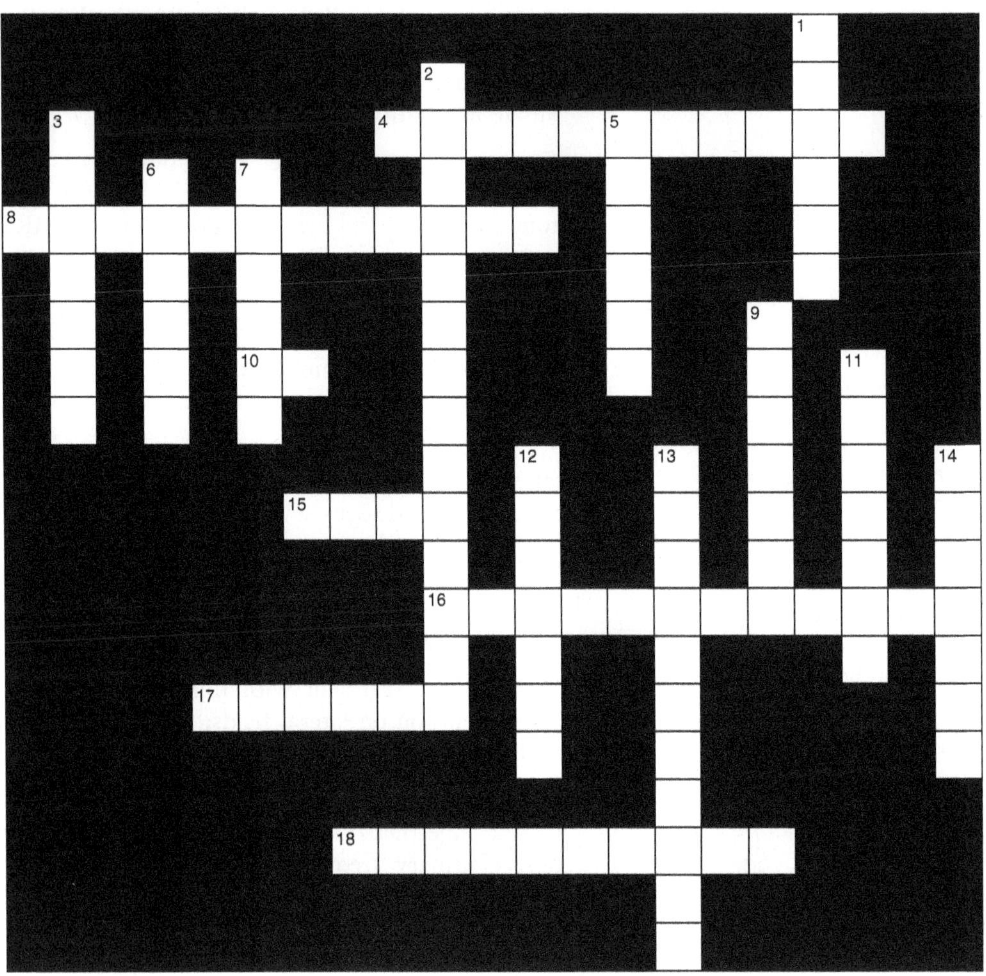

Across

4 The opening into the pelvis into which the baby's head enters

8 Name of the early screening techinque for cervical cancer

10 The posterior border of a lateral pelvic field

15 A treatment technique which would allow a lower dose to the femoral head and neck

16 Pathology for vulva, vagina and cervix cancers

17 Two golf-club-shaped hollow tubes placed laterally to the cervical os into the vaginal fornices

18 Pathlolgy for ovarian cancer

Down

1 The most common side effect from the radiation when treating cervix cancer

2 Fine superficial blood vessels caused from radiation in the areas of the vargina and cervix

3 Most lethal of all gynecologic tumors

5 A slow progressive disease, with the earliest phase (in situ) occuring approximately ten years earlier than invasive cancer

6 A small, hollow, curved cylinder that fits through the cervical os and into the uterus

7 Used to establish a precise diagnosis for cancer

9 The most radiosensitive gynecologic structure

11 Patient position for which a vulva field may be treated

12 Painful or difficulty urination

13 The most prevalent gynecologic malignancy

14 Shielding block used to eliminate dose to the bladder and rectum

19. In HDR implants, central doses are prescribed to *Point A* and *Point B*; define these points.

20. Bladder and rectal doses are very important to the gynecologic radiation therapy planning. The point tolerance for these organs is:

a. 2000 cGy
b. 3500 cGy
c. 5000 cGy
d. 7500 cGy

21. A recent study has warranted the research of endometrium cancer in women who take which of the following drugs:

a. Cisplatin
b. Methotrexate
c. Tamoxifen
d. Doxorubicin

22. The outermost portion of the gynecologic tract:

a. Vagina
b. Vulva
c. Cervix
d. Ovary

23. The connective tissue immediately lateral to the uterine cervix:

a. Parametrium
b. Parasagittal
c. Myometrium
d. Perineum

24. Which of the following cancers even at an early stage will often involve metastatic spread throughout the abdominal cavity?

a. Endometrium
b. Cervix
c. Ovarian
d. Fallopian tube

25. A patient having abdominal pain and distention, and/or nonspecific gastrointestinal symptoms (nausea, heartburn) could be symptomatic to which cancer:

a. Endometrium
b. Cervix
c. Ovarian
d. Vagina

26. Which of the following preoperative test might be used in detection of ovarian cancer?

a. PSA
b. BRCAI
c. BRCAII
d. Ca-125

27. Cervical cancer is more prevalent than other gynecologic cancers among younger women, this mainly stems from:

a. Intraepithelial neoplasia
b. Invasive cervical
c. Atrophic dysplasia
d. Low estrogen

28. The cervix often protrudes into the vagina, producing lateral spaces in the vaginal apex called:

a. Cervical os
b. Fornices
c. Paraaortics
d. Ovaries

29. According to the 2008 cancer estimates, which of the following is the fifth leading cause of death in women:

a. Cervix
b. Endometrium
c. Uterus
d. Ovarian

30. With vaginal and cervical cancers, there is an increased risk of clear cell adenocarcinoma and abnormalities of the stratified epithelium in women whose mothers (during pregnancy) used which of the following drugs:

a. Diethylstilbestrol (DES)
b. Dihydrotestosterone (DEET)
c. Dysmenorrheal (DMH)
d. Deoxyribonucleic acid (DNA)

31. Diabetes, hypertension, overweight and increased use of estrogen or the estrogen-to-progesterone ratio relate to which of the following cancers:

a. Cervix
b. Endometrium

c. Ovarian
d. Vagina

32. When treating ovarian cancer with radiation, often the abdominal cavity is involved with the disease; what is the tolerance dose to the kidneys?

a. 20 Gy
b. 30 Gy
c. 40 Gy
d. 50 Gy

33. Hemoglobin may often be affected when treating the cervix or ovaries for cancer, making anemia a major concern for the patient. What is the normal hemoglobin percentage range?

a. 10 to 11 g/dL
b. 12 to 16 g/dL
c. 14 to 18 g/dL
d. 36 to 47 g/dL

34. When treating pelvic tumors with a high radiation dose, a major side effect is diarrhea due to the small bowel in the field. It usually occurs the second or third week of treatment. Which of the following would be prescribed to alleviate this problem?

a. Sucralfate (Carafate)
b. Diphenoxylate (Lomotil)
c. Ibuprofen (Motrin)
d. Prochlorperazine (Compazine)

35. Which of the following isotopes may be used in treatment for ovarian cancer?

a. Iodine-131 (I-131)
b. Iridium-192 (Ir-192)
c. Cobalt-60 (Co-60)
d. Phosphorus-32 (P-32)

36. What type of contrast may be used in defining the rectum during simulation of treatment fields of the pelvis?

a. Diatrizoate meglumine
b. Iothalamate meglumine
c. Barium sulfate
d. Ioxaglate sodium

37. Ovarian cancer is the most deadly of all female cancers because:

1. Few symptoms
2. Widely disseminated
3. Usually found in one ovary

a. 1 and 2
b. 2 and 3
c. 1 and 3
d. 1, 2, and 3

38. If a patient with cervix cancer has periaortic nodal involvement, there is a 35% increase risk for spread to the:

a. Vulva area
b. Supraclavicular area
c. Lung
d. Brain

39. Dietary guidelines for patients receiving pelvic irradiation may include all of the following, except:

a. Whole-grain breads
b. Baked, broiled, or roasted meats
c. Cooked vegetables
d. Peeled apples and bananas

40. For carcinoma in situ and stage I well-differentiated cancer, the entire vagina may be treated with low dose rate brachytherapy using a vaginal cylinder, with cesium-137 to a dose of:

a. 1500 cGy
b. 2500 cGy
c. 4500 cGy
d. 6000 cGy

41. Upon completion of a radiotherapy course for cervix cancer, a patient experiences abdominal distention and hyperactive bowel sounds that could indicate:

a. Gastritis
b. Bowel obstruction
c. Chronic cystitis
d. Proctosigmoiditis

42. The most radiotolerant structure of the gynecologic organs is the:

a. Uterine canal
b. Cervix
c. Ovary
d. Bladder

43. Which of the following would be recommended for a patient that is having pelvic treatment concurrently with chemotherapy?

1. Rest
2. Reassurance
3. Antidepressants

a. 1 and 2
b. 1 and 3
c. 2 and 3
d. 1, 2, and 3

44. Inguinal nodes would most likely be treated when a cancer occurs in which area:

a. Cervix
b. Ovary
c. Endometrium
d. Vagina

45. If a patient is having a four-field pelvis treatment, calculate the diameter of the AP/PA and lateral using the following:

AP SSD readout is 85, PA SSD readout is 87.5; right lateral 81, left lateral 79.5

a. AP/PA diameter = ______
b. Rt/Lt lateral = ______

MALE GENITAL

- Prostate
- Testicular
- Penis

PROSTATE

General Facts and Epidemiology:

- Number one in cancer incidence in men in the United States
- Second in mortality in the United States
- African Americans present later stage and have worse prognosis than Caucasians
- Increased risk in Sweden, United States, and Europe
- Decreased risk in Japan, Taiwan, Jewish men, single men
- Overall, very slow-growing malignancy
- Early detection occurs often due to screening improvements
- Average age 60 years

Etiology

- Cause is unknown; maybe genetic
- Altered hormone levels possibility

Clinical Presentation

Signs and Symptoms

- Asymptomatic with digital rectal examination (DRE)
- Urinary tract obstruction
- Pain in back, pelvis
- Urinary incontinence
- Weight loss, fever, fatigue, anemia
- Bone pain associated with metastasis

Histology

- Adenocarcinoma 95% to 98%
- Transitional cell
- Squamous cell
- Sarcoma

Lymphatic Drainage and Spread Patterns

- Metastasis through nerve chains, lymph, and blood; external and internal iliacs, common iliac, obturator, periprostatic most commonly involved nodes; distant metastasis can occur without lymphatic involvement; liver, brain, lung, other soft tissue, bone are metastasis sites, with bone being number one site.
- Spread is influenced by grade; low grade stay local for a long time

Workup

- CT
- MRI
- Transurethral ultrasound (TRUS)
- Biopsy via transurethral resection of the prostrate (TURP)
- Cystoscopy
- PSA, PAP, SAP markers
- Bone scan for suspected mets

Staging/Grading

- AJCC TNM staging
- Gleason grading (Table 9-12) assesses differentiation of tissue sample

TABLE 9-12 Gleason Scoring

Gleason Score	Summary	Prognosis
2-4	Well differentiated	Good
5-7	Moderately differentiated	Fair
8-10	Poorly differentiated	Poor

- Grades 1-5 = well differentiated—poorly differentiated
- Two most predominant histologic patterns are identified by the pathologist and then added to give a score 2-10

Treatment

- Early lesions with no positive lymph nodes surgical resection; total prostatectomy
- Radiation therapy may be used curatively to tumor bed or to the unresected prostate
- Radiation doses 66 to 75 Gy in 180 cGy fractions external beam
- Permanent LDR brachytherapy using permanent, interstitial implant for local lesions and low grade
- Not chemo-responsive; hormonal therapy for larger lesions and metastatic lesions

Radiation Treatment Borders

- Radiation treatment fields may be simple four field box for larger lesions and positive lymph nodes
- AP/PA fields upper border at L5 down to obturator foramen, laterally 2 cm beyond the pelvic brim for coverage of external iliac nodes; opposing laterals should have anterior border to symphysis pubis and posterior border to S2 taking care to exclude as much rectum as possible
- Full bladder helps decrease bladder dose and displace small bowel in lateral fields
- Positioning patient prone for box field may decrease small bowel in lateral fields
- Belly board my help decrease bowel volume in lateral treatment fields
- Boost can be delivered using rotational arcs
- IMRT fields for small, local disease
- Modulation of dose to give adequate dose to gland and seminal vesicles; low dose to bladder and rectum

Treatment Delivery

- IMRT technique limited side effects
- IMRT fields should not be parallel opposed to limit skin dose
- Box field technique side effects include cystitis, proctitis, diarrhea, dysuria
- Pelvic immobilization and lower extremity immobilization with vac lock, alpha cradle, or block and Velcro for feet
- Internal fiducial markers or BAT used daily for IGRT since gland moves slightly
- Remember full bladder instructions as warranted
- Advise patient to eat low residue diet, drink plenty of fluids because urinary frequency may persist
- Box technique will require beam-shaping, IMRT and immobilization incur complex billing charges

TESTICULAR

General Facts and Epidemiology:

- Low occurrence overall but the most common male cancer for 15 to 35 year old males
- More common in Caucasians versus African Americans

Etiology

- Cryptorchidism
- Klinefelter syndrome
- Mumps orchitis

Clinical Presentation

Signs and Symptoms

- Painless, testicular mass
- Testicular swelling
- Gynecomastia
- Infertility
- Back pain

Histology

- Seminoma (classic, anaplastic, spermatocytic)
- Embryonal carcinoma
- Teratocarcinoma
- Choriocarcinoma
- Yolk sac tumors
- Teratomas

Lymphatic Drainage and Spread Patterns

- Local, then spreads to lymph nodes in orderly fashion; external and internal iliac, common iliac, para-aortic, paracaval, renal-hilar commonly involved;

inguinal, femoral nodes are rarely affected—previous surgeries may disrupt normal lymph flow patterns so contralateral nodes may be treated

- Distant spread to lungs

Workup

- CT of abdomen, pelvis
- Ultrasound of scrotum
- Lymphangiogram—traditional
- HCG, AFP, LDH serum markers
- Chest x-ray for metastasis

Staging

- Serum markers are strongly considered in staging using TNM

Treatment

- Radical inguinal orchiectomy and lymph node dissection for late stage
- Seminomas stage I, IIA, IIB radiation therapy follows orchiectomy
- Nonseminomas and beyond stage IIB treated with orchiectomy and nodal dissection then chemotherapy

Radiation Treatment Borders

- Inverted Y or hockey stick technique
- Upper border at T10, wide enough to include renal hilar nodes
- Lower border at top of symphysis pubis or margin on inguinal scar
- Wide enough to include bilateral paraaortic nodes and ipsilateral external iliac *or* bilateral external iliac if inverted Y preferred

Treatment Delivery

- Supine with arms at sides, elevated or high on chest (elevated makes it easy to use 3-point setup marks)
- Immobilization minimal
- AP/PA fields; field length may extend outside of collimator limits for tall males; SSD technique may be required in this instance
- Field will need beam shaping to protect kidneys, bowel, bladder, and bone marrow reserves in iliac crests
- Daily dose 125 to 180 cGy daily to total 25 to 30 Gy
- Total dose may go to 35 to 40 Gy for areas of gross nodal involvement
- Patient may experience some nausea so give antiemetic before treatment
- Advise patient to avoid heavy, greasy foods
- Some alopecia in the abdominal area may occur
- Opposite testicle needs shielding from internal scatter radiation; use absorbed dose detector (i.e., diode, TLD) to ensure integrity of shield
- Although AP/PA, beam shaping incurs complex billing charges

PENIS

General Facts and Epidemiology

- Rare in the United States
- Incidence higher in Asia, Africa, South America
- A disease of older men but age range is from 22 to 90 years old
- In the United States, 29% were younger than 30 years old

Etiology

- No circumcision at birth
- Phimosis
- Poor hygiene, smegma
- HPV
- Ultraviolet radiation
- Smoking

Clinical Presentation

Signs and Symptoms

- Mass
- Ulceration, bleeding, discharge
- Pain

Histology

- Queyrat and Bowen disease (shiny, red, velvety plaque on the prepuce or glans)
- Squamous cell
- Basal cell
- Melanoma

Lymphatic Drainage and Spread Patterns

- Penile and regional pelvic lymph nodes; metastatic deposits in the inguinal nodes, which may also ulcerate; distant spread to lung, liver, bone, and brain

Workup

- Physical examination of penis and inguinal nodes
- Tumor biopsy
- Chest x-ray
- CT of abdomen and pelvis
- Needle aspiration
- Sentinel node biopsy

Staging

- Jackson's staging or TNM; depth of invasion important; Mohs technique helpful

Treatment

- Radical surgery is the mainstay but consider function; partial or total penectomy
- Topical chemotherapy
- Laser ablation
- Mohs surgery
- Radiation with external beam or interstitial brachytherapy for those who refuse surgery or are low stage

Radiation Treatment Borders

- Should include the entire shaft and lower pelvic lymph nodes; inguinal nodes especially
- Uniform dose to shaft using special penile box

Treatment Delivery

- Prone on board or supine with penile box containing wax or water bath (Figure 9-18) and opposing lateral fields; 2 Gy daily up to 60 to 74 Gy total
- Inguinal nodes with electron therapy; unknown status of pelvic nodes should be treated
- If no penile box used, expect severe desquamation, stricture, fistula
- Take care to replace any wet desquamation coverings using sterile technique to prevent infection
- Lateral fields need no beam shaping and may incur simple charges

MALE GENITAL REVIEW EXERCISES

1. The most common cancer of germinal origin of the testis is:
   a. Teratocarcinoma
   b. Choriocarcinoma
   c. Seminoma
   d. Embryonal

2. Testicular cancers are most frequently diagnosed in men aged:
   a. 60 to 65 years
   b. 15 to 35 years
   c. 40 to 50 years
   d. 70 to 80 years

3. A blood serum marker used in determining extent of testicular cancer is:
   a. AFP
   b. CA 19-9
   c. CEA
   d. BRCA 1

4. The prostate gland lies _______ to the bladder and _______ to the rectum.

5. Gleason developed a grading system based on the degree of differentiation seen in tissue samples. His system uses _______ different histologic patterns.

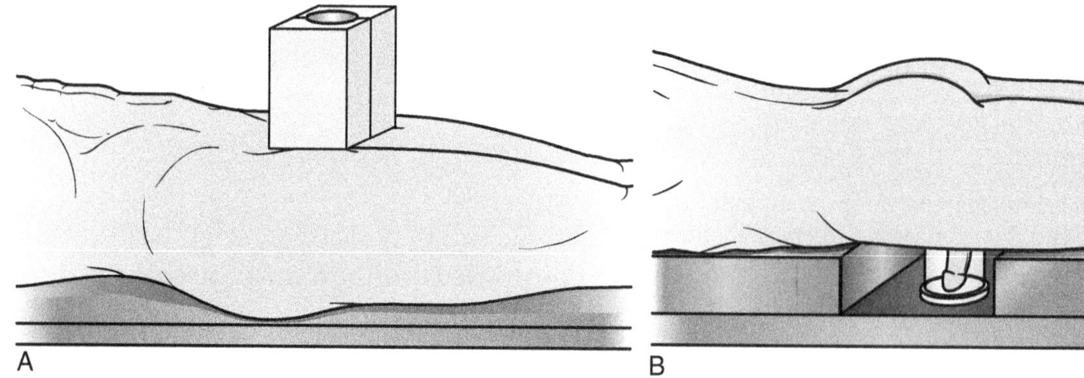

FIGURE 9-18 Penile box.

6. The seminal vesicles lie _______ to the prostate and _______ to the rectum.

7. Briefly define the following:

TURP

LDH

HCG

8. Of the following tumors, which would require the lowest dose to control disease?

a. Prostate
b. Testis
c. Penis
d. Breast

9. Of the following tumors, which would require the highest dose to control disease?

a. Prostate
b. Testis
c. Penis
d. Breast

10. When irradiating seminoma stages I, IA, IB, the following nodes should be included:

1. Paraaortic
2. Ipsilateral iliac
3. Mediastinal
4. Scalene

a. 1, 2
b. 3, 4
c. 1, 2, 3
d. 1, 2, 3, 4

11. The most common histologic type found in prostate cancer is:

a. Adenocarcinoma
b. Squamous cell
c. Transitional cell
d. Clear cell

12. Brachytherapy in the management of prostate cancer would be:

a. HDR interstitial
b. LDR interstitial
c. HDR intracavitary
d. HDR intraluminal

13. Hormonal therapy for prostate cancer may include the administration of:

a. Lupron
b. Tamoxifen
c. Megace
d. Taxol

14. Using Figure 9-19 below, identify the following:

a. Prostate gland
b. Seminal vesicles
c. Rectum

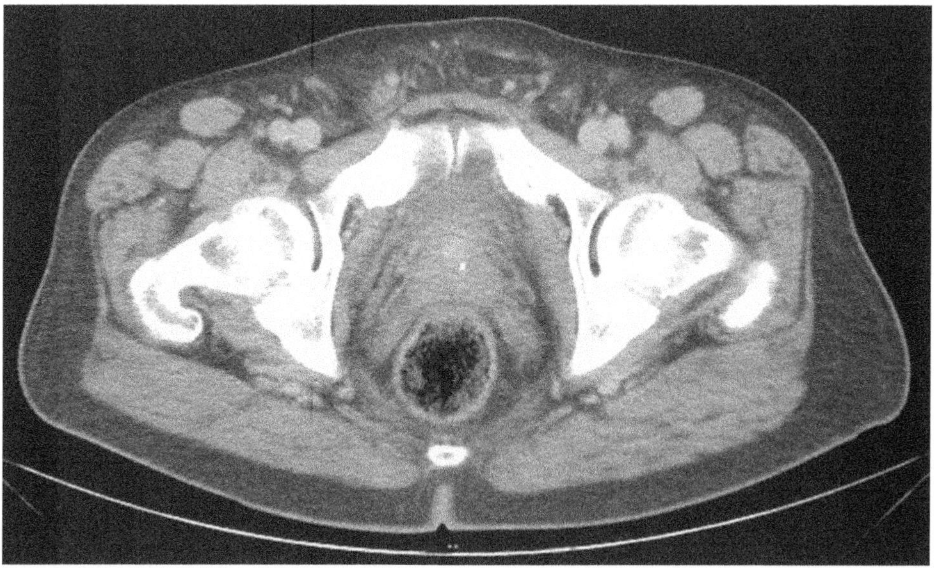

FIGURE 9-19 CT axial view pelvis.

15. The patient complaining of diarrhea should be advised to:

 a. Eat fresh fruit and vegetables
 b. Eat more starch and dairy products
 c. Avoid high fiber foods
 d. Consume liquids only

16. The appropriate treatment position for the patient treated with opposing hockey stick fields is:

 a. Supine with arms above head
 b. Supine with hands folded on abdomen
 c. Prone with arms up around pillow
 d. Lateral decubitus with elbows bent

17. Severe wet desquamation should be managed with:

 a. Applications using cold packs
 b. Hot baths with Epsom salts
 c. Applications for severe radiation dermatitis; open wounds
 d. Applications of petroleum jelly

18. A common location for distant metastasis from seminoma is:

 a. Brain
 b. Skin
 c. Liver
 d. Lung

19. The inguinal nodes should be included in radiation treatment fields for:

 1. Prostate
 2. Testicular
 3. Penile

 a. 1, 3
 b. 3
 c. 2
 d. 1, 2, 3

20. The four field box technique would likely be used in the management of ___ cancer:

 a. Prostate
 b. Testicular
 c. Penile

21. The upper border of the inverted Y field for the management of early-stage seminoma is at the level of:

 a. T 10
 b. T 12
 c. T 8
 d. L 1

22. The lower border of the inverted Y field for the management of early-stage seminoma is at the level of:

 a. The ischial tuberosity
 b. The symphysis pubis
 c. The lower edge of the SI joints
 d. The lesser trochanter

23. Total dose for irradiation of the prostate tumor bed is:

 a. 20 to 30 Gy
 b. 30 to 45 Gy
 c. 50 to 60 Gy
 d. 66 to 75 Gy

24. Inguinal node dose is to be delivered with the 80% dose line at a depth of 5 cm. The electron energy most appropriate would be:

 a. 5 MeV
 b. 10 MeV
 c. 12 MeV
 d. 15 MeV

Think About It

25. Our inverted Y for our 6-foot 7-inch patient requires a length of 45 cm. The 100-cm SAD linear accelerator field size limit is 40 × 40 cm. What extended distance is required?

26. The above patient will be treated with a 10 MV beam. Our manual calculation will require an inverse square factor correction. What is the inverse square factor?

27. If the treatment depth for the above case is 11.0 cm and the %DD is 76% for this depth and field size, what is the new %DD using the Mayneord F factor correction?

28. What if we elect to split the inverted Y fields for our tall patient into two fields? The upper field is 9 × 20 and the lower field is 15 × 25. The depth at which the fields will intersect is 11 cm. SSD for both fields is 89 cm SSD. What is the skin gap?

29. Rotational arc therapy will be used for our prostate cancer boost. The arc will be 270 degrees. Calculated monitor units are 280 MU. What is the monitor unit per degree setting?

30. The starting angle for the above boost is 225 degrees. Rotating clockwise, what is the finishing angle?

URINARY

- Kidney
- Bladder

KIDNEY (RENAL CELL)

General Facts and Epidemiology:

- Median age of onset 55 to 60 years
- Men affected twice as much as women
- Nephroblastomas are kidney cancers seen in children

Etiology

- Direct cause is unknown, but several risk factors have been identified:
  - Smoking
  - Cadmium, lead, asbestos exposure
  - Thorotrast (alpha emitter) exposure
  - Low intake of vitamin A
  - Diabetes
  - Polycystic kidney disease
  - Family history
  - Obesity
  - Hypertension

Clinical Presentation

Signs and Symptoms

- Table 9-13 lists histologic types for the kidney by location
- Hematuria (gross or microscopic)
- Back pain
- Palpable mass in abdomen
- Weight loss
- Fatigue
- Fever

Lymphatic Drainage and Spread Patterns

- Local invasion, regional lymphatics include paraaortic, paracaval, celiac axis, distant metastasis through easily accessible renal artery and vein to lung, liver, bone, brain; adenocarcinomas spread to the fingers, eyelids, and nose

Workup

- CT chest and abdomen
- MRI
- Cystoscopy
- Blood chemistry
- Urine cytology
- IVP
- Ultrasound
- Biopsy (US or CT guided)

TABLE 9-13 Histologic Types for Kidney by Location

Histology—Depends on Location	
Renal Parenchyma	**Renal Pelvis**
Adenocarcinoma	Transitional cell 90%
Clear cell	Squamous cell
Granular cell	Adenocarcinoma
Spindle cell	

Staging and Grading

- TNM staging, grading specified as high or low; Robson staging I-IV expressing confinement to kidney or vein and node involvement and distant metastasis

Treatment

- Radical, simple or partial nephrectomy, and involved veins if positive lymph nodes
- Resectable, early-stage is curable with surgery only
- Solitary metastatic lesions may be resected as well
- Radiation therapy to tumor bed, residual disease optional for T3 or larger to 50 to 55 Gy
- Radiation used most often palliatively
- Chemotherapy is investigational; most renal cell not chemoresponsive
- Interferon or interleukin-2 has low response rate but results outweigh cytotoxic chemotherapy

Radiation Treatment Borders

- Radiation treatment fields to tumor bed AP/PA to include bilateral paraaortic lymph nodes
- Pediatric cases take care to cover the entire vertebral bodies to prevent uneven bone growth along the spine

Treatment Delivery

- AP/PA fields sufficient until cord tolerance
- Beam shaping to spare as much bowel as possible
- Patient supine with arms above head or akimbo for easy triangulation
- Immobilization minimal
- Daily billing simple to intermediate
- Boost fields may add modifiers such as wedges, upgrading daily billing to complex

BLADDER

General Facts and Epidemiology

- High incidence in industrial cities
- Men 2.5 times more likely than women
- Median age 68 years
- Likely occurs in the trigone, posterior/lateral walls or neck of the bladder
- Liver failure and uremia usually cause of death

Etiology

- Dye, rubber, textile, leather, pain working
- Chronic bladder infections
- Smoking
- Previous pelvic irradiation
- Pesticide exposure
- Contaminated water supply

Clinical Presentation

Signs and Symptoms

- Hematuria (most often gross)
- Urinary tract infection
- Urinary frequency, urgency, dysuria

Histology

- Transitional cell
- Squamous cell
- Adenocarcinoma
- Sarcoma
- Lymphoma

Lymphatic Drainage and Spread Patterns

- Direct spread through bladder walls and invade muscle; lymphatics include common, external, internal iliac, and obturator. distant spread first to bone, then liver, lung, and rarely the skin

Workup

- CT of abdomen, pelvis
- Transurethral biopsy of the bladder (TURB)
- Urine cytology
- Urinalysis
- IVP
- Ultrasound
- Chest x-ray for metastasis
- Cystoscopy with brushing

Staging

- TNM and grading specified as high or low

Treatment

- Transurethral resection is sufficient for superficial tumors (T is)
- Segmental or radical cystectomy for low grade
- Instillation/intravesical chemotherapy following surgery lowers recurrence rates
- Radical cystectomy to include removal of the prostate in men, removal of reproductive organs in women; urethra may be partially removed if high risk for local recurrence; will require an ileal diversion
- Radiation used if no surgery or preoperatively for tumors invading the superficial muscle
- Preoperative radiation dose 20 to 45 Gy
- Radiation for palliation/urinary bleeding
- If radiation used definitively, then 60 to 70 Gy total
- Radiation and chemotherapy used together for bladder sparing
- Cisplatin- and methotrexate-based chemotherapy

Radiation Treatment Borders

- Preoperative and postoperative fields are simple AP/PA fields or four field box
- Upper border at S1 and lower border at obturator foramen
- Lateral border to pelvic rim
- Beam shaping to protect bone marrow reserves in iliac crest

Treatment Delivery

- Supine with hands folded on abdomen
- Bladder volume should be consistent so instruct patient to empty bladder before treatment
- Side effects minimal for preoperative and postoperative cases
- Definitive cases may show signs of cystitis, proctitis, diarrhea
- Instruct to drink plenty of fluids, avoid high fiber foods
- Preoperative and postoperative fields likely intermediate to complex due to beam shaping
- Immobilization for the lower extremities with alpha cradle, vac lock, or simple block, and Velcro feet

URINARY SECTION REVIEW EXERCISES

1. Cancers of the kidney usually arise in the:

   a. Cortex
   b. Medulla
   c. Renal pelvis
   d. Adrenal gland

2. Nephroblastomas are also known as:

   a. Wilms' tumor
   b. Ewing sarcoma
   c. Bowen disease
   d. Klinefelter syndrome

3. Common metastatic site(s) for renal cell carcinoma is/are:

   a. Bone
   b. Brain
   c. Lung
   d. All of the above

4. Cancers manifesting in the renal pelvis are most commonly:

   a. Transitional cell
   b. Adenocarcinoma
   c. Clear cell
   d. Squamous cell

5. Cancers manifesting in the renal cortex are most commonly:

   a. Transitional cell
   b. Adenocarcinoma
   c. Clear cell
   d. Squamous cell

6. Which of the following examinations are best used in the detection of bladder cancers?

   1. TURB
   2. Urine cytology
   3. Cystoscopy
   4. DRE
   5. PSA

      a. 1, 2, 3
      b. 1, 4, 5
      c. 2, 3, 4, 5
      d. 3, 4, 5

7. Most bladder tumors arise in the (select three):
   a. Posterior wall
   b. Lateral wall
   c. Trigone
   d. Neck
   e. Urethral opening

8. List three etiologic factors for bladder cancer:

9. List three histologic types for bladder cancer:

10. When treating a patient with bladder carcinoma preoperatively, the treatment portals should be large enough to include the:
    a. Obturator nodes
    b. Obturator, external, hypogastric, and presacral nodes
    c. Hypogastric and presacral nodes
    d. Obturator, paraaortic, and paracaval nodes

11. Briefly define the following:

    Cystectomy

    Intravesical therapy

    TURB

    IVP

12. The ureters attach the ______ surface of the bladder.
    a. Anterior
    b. Posterolateral
    c. Superior
    d. Inferior

13. Renal cell carcinomas have immediate access to the blood route via the:
    a. Portal vein
    b. Superior vena cava
    c. Inferior vena cava and abdominal aorta
    d. Mesenteric and femoral artery

14. The right kidney is slightly lower than the left due to the presence of the:
    a. Diaphragm
    b. Adrenal gland
    c. Liver
    d. Spleen

15. The bladder is ______ to the cervix and ______ to the symphysis pubis.

16. The bladder is ______ to the seminal vesicles and ______ to the ovaries.

17. The most common presenting symptom of bladder cancer is:
    a. Back pain
    b. Hematuria
    c. Abdominal pain
    d. Fever

18. A carcinogen linked to renal cell and bladder carcinomas found in radiation therapy departments is:
    a. Benzene
    b. Asbestos
    c. Cadmium
    d. Leather

19. The ureters enter the kidneys at the:
    a. Renal pelvis
    b. Renal cortex
    c. Adrenal cortex
    d. Medullary zone

20. Urine passes from the bladder to the outside of the body via the:
    a. Ureter
    b. Urethra
    c. Trigone
    d. Calyx

21. Label Figure 9-20 showing the following structures:
    a. Inferior vena cava
    b. Aorta
    c. Kidney
    d. Ureter
    e. Bladder

22. Using Figure 9-21, draw the typical anterior field for preoperative radiation for bladder cancer.

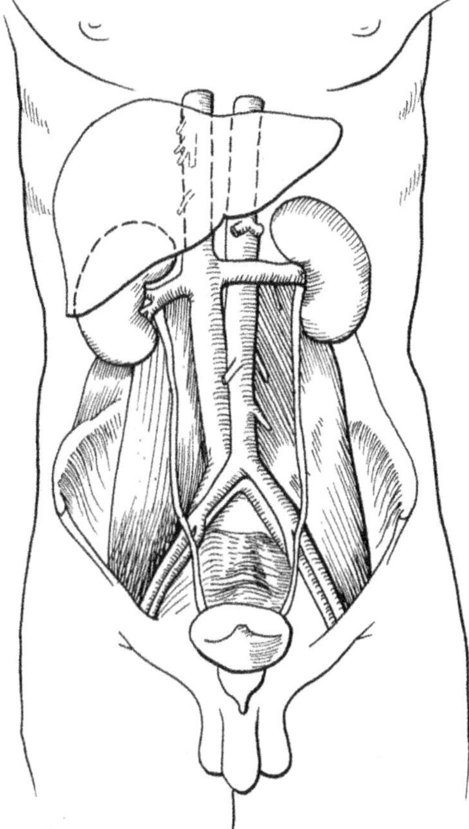

FIGURE 9-21 Anterior abdomen and pelvis.

Think About It

23. The anterior/posterior field for a preoperative bladder cancer patient is 15 × 20. There are two Cerrobend blocks in the upper right and left corners measuring 4 × 5 cm each. Calculate the effective equivalent square.

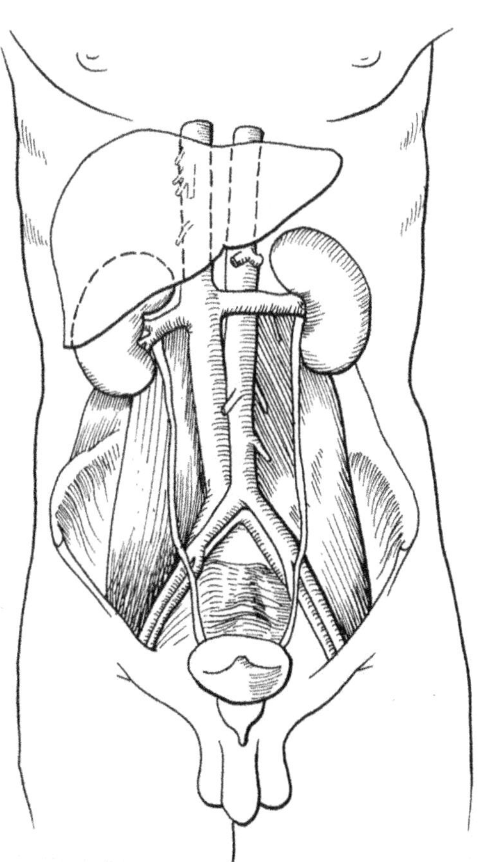

FIGURE 9-20 Anterior abdomen and pelvis.

24. During treatment planning for bladder carcinoma, the patient should be asked to urinate before simulation begins. If any contrast has to be inserted into the bladder, it should not amount to much more than any residual urine left in the bladder after the patient has voided (an additional 25 mL is acceptable). Why is this important?

25. The TD 5/5 of the kidney ranges from 18 to 23 Gy. When treating the pediatric patient, the opposite kidney should be shielded so that dose is limited to less than 15 Gy. Why is the tolerance lower in this case?

CENTRAL NERVOUS SYSTEM: BRAIN, SPINAL CORD, PITUITARY

GENERAL FACTS AND EPIDEMIOLOGY

- CNS malignancies occur at various stages of life.
- Young children have the best prognosis.
- Benign tumors can be life threatening.
- Low-grade, benign tumors may be managed with surgery and radiation.
- High-grade tumors are most threatening but rarely metastasize outside of the central nervous system.
- 80% occur in the brain.
- Most pituitary tumors are benign.
- Pituitary tumors are the most common new growths near the sella turcica.
- Nonfunctioning pituitary adenomas occur at all ages and at equal frequency among men and women.

BRAIN AND SPINAL CORD

Etiology

- Genetics
- History of breast cancer
- Rubber manufacturing and other chemical exposures
- Cystic/polyp conditions of the CNS
- Previous radiation to the head
- Immunosuppression

Clinical Presentation

Signs and Symptoms

- Signs and symptoms depend on the location of the tumor; four functional areas of the cerebrum:
  - Frontal—increased cranial pressure, personality changes, seizures, motor dysfunction, speech impairment, urinary incontinence, cranial nerve VI palsy
  - Parietal—increased cranial pressure, vision loss, seizures, weakness, memory loss, loss of touch
  - Temporal—speech disorders, seizures, loss of smell, weakness of cranial nerve VI, defective hearing, defective memory
  - Occipital—seizures, loss of vision, tingling, weakness, hallucinations
  - Table 9-14 lists the function and location of cranial nerves
- Spinal cord tumors symptoms are a function of local anatomy; within the spinal canal there is a well-defined extradural space containing fat and blood vessels; symptoms reflect involvement of nerves controlling motor and sensory function; some symptoms include the following:
  - Decreased temperature
  - Pain sensation
  - Weakness
  - Reflex changes
  - Paralysis
  - Acute urinary retention

TABLE 9-14 Cranial Nerves

Cranial Nerve	Function	Location
Olfactory I	Conveys impulses related to smell	In the olfactory foramina of the ethmoid
Optic II	Vision	From eye to optic canal
Oculomotor III	Controls eye movement; lens and pupil	In the superior orbital fissure
Trochlear IV	Movement of eye and muscle sense	In superior orbital fissure
Trigeminal V	Chewing movements; touch, pain, temperature sense of head and face	In superior orbital fissure
Abducens VI	Movement of the eye	In superior orbital fissure
Facial VII	Facial expressions; taste	In acoustic canal through to facial canal
Vestibulocochlear VIII	Balance and hearing	Internal acoustic canal
Glossopharyngeal IX	Swallowing and secretion of saliva; aid in blood pressure and respiration	Jugular foramen
Vagus X	Sensations and movement of organs	Jugular foramen
Accessory XI	Shoulder movements; turning of the head; movements of the viscera; voice	Jugular foramen
Hypoglossal XII	Speech and swallowing	Hypoglossal canal

- Incontinence of bowel and bladder
- Impotence
- Radicular pain in the thighs

- 31 pairs of spinal nerves*:
  - 8 cervical nerves
  - 12 thoracic
  - 5 lumbar
  - 5 sacral
  - 1 coccyx

Histology

- Glioma
- Astrocytoma
- Ependymoma (near the cerebellum)
- Meningioma
- Schwannoma
- Medulloblastoma (cerebellum or near the medulla oblongata)
- Neurilemoma
- Craniopharyngioma
- Melanoma (spinal cord)
- Oligodendroglioma
- Hemangioblastoma (spinal cord)
- Pineal gland tumors

Lymphatic Drainage and Spread Patterns

- Astrocytomas, glioblastomas, oligodendroglioma, and meningiomas usually grow locally; some cells may spread to the cerebral spinal fluid (CSF) but do not implant; signs of increased cranial pressure (ICP) must be addressed immediately
- Medulloblastomas, ependymomas, and pineal gland tumors tend to spread throughout the CSF due mainly to close proximity to the lateral and fourth ventricles
- No lymphatic drainage

Workup

- Physical
- Neurologic examination
- MRI
- CT
- CT guided needle biopsy
- Lumbar puncture except for obvious ICP

Staging

- Grade, tumor, metastasis (GTM) system since no lymphatic drainage; World Health Organization (WHO) has recommendations for classifying neoplasms by histology and grade

Treatment

- Stereotactic surgery in order for small tumors like pineal gland growths
- All intracranial tumors should be resected; whenever a complete resection is possible, it should be performed
- Considerations for surgery include neurologic deficits following resection
- Radiation used adjuvant to surgery; conformal techniques desirable to maintain satisfactory sensory and motor function
- Most respond favorably to radiation; resistant tumors may benefit from heavy particle beam therapy
- Small benign tumors, or small recurrent tumors may benefit from single stereotactic radiosurgery using gamma knife or low energy x-rays
- Small malignant tumors benefit from multifraction stereotactic radiation therapy
- Chemotherapy efficacy is limited due to blood-brain barrier
- Chemotherapy drugs need to be lipid soluble if given intravenously
- Chemotherapy may be administered locally directly into the tumor or into the circulating CSF or intraarterially
- Steroids used to help alleviate and control swelling

Radiation Treatment Borders

- Primary tumors with low potential for CSF spread are treated with conformal fields; 2-3-cm margin around the tumor or tumor bed to begin then shrinking to 0.5-cm margin
- Multiple beam arrangements to help spare normal brain tissue, optic chiasm, orbits, and lens
- Primary tumors with high potential for CSF spread require a dose to the entire spinal axis: whole brain helmet technique down to C2 and total spine in single extended field or matched fields

---

*Cervical and thoracic spinal nerves pass out of the spinal canal horizontally; lumbar and sacral descend down before they reach the intervertebral foramina (horse-tail).

Treatment Delivery

- Total dose for primary tumors range from 50 to 70 Gy
- Lower dose for radiation to tumor bed; higher dose for partial resections or no surgery
- Lower dose for those receiving chemoradiation
- Conformal fields may use various portal arrangements; patient may be supine with chin flexed or neutral depending on ports
- Objective is to accurately treat the CTV while consistently sparing normal brain and sensitive tissues such as the lens
- Primary tumors are typically solitary and unilateral; fields will likely be aimed to the affected side only; be mindful of any exit dose to low tolerance tissues; wedged pair is common; multifield IMRT fields also possible
- Reliable immobilization of head imperative since margins are small although movement in the cranium is relatively nonexistent
- When treating entire spinal axis, overlap is eliminated by using half field technique or table kick and collimator angles
- Skin gaps should be carefully measured daily and junction changed every 3 to 5 fractions
- Symptoms of disease may cause patients to be dizzy, weak, confused, or nauseous so be prepared to support during transfer from wheel chair/gurney to PSA or while ambulating; advise patients to always come accompanied to therapy
- Side effects from therapy include skin desquamation and hair loss
- Educate patient on scalp care—no harsh shampoo or razor cutting, no chemical processing, protect from the sun
- Fields will require beam shaping with MLC and use of modifiers; billing charges complex

PITUITARY/HYPOPHYSIS

Etiology

- Heredity as part of endocrine syndromes

Clinical Presentation

Signs and Symptoms

- Symptoms influenced by the portion of gland affected and which hormones are affected
- The anterior portion of the gland produces at least six hormones: prolactin (PRL), adrenocorticotropic hormone (ACTH), follicle-stimulating hormone (FSH), luteinizing hormone (LH), growth hormone (GH), and thyroid stimulating hormone (TSH)
- The posterior portion stores and releases two hormones: vasopressin/anti-diuretic hormone (ADH) and oxytocin
    - Weight changes
    - Excess hormonal levels
    - Uncontrolled diabetes
    - Hyperparathyroidism
    - Multigland hyperplasia
    - Amenorrhea
    - Short stature syndromes
- The presence of a pituitary tumor may also manifest as neuro-ophthalmic disturbances from pressure on nerves and orbit compartment
    1. Headache
    2. Visual disturbances
    3. Cranial nerve III, IV, V, VI palsy
    4. Hydrocephalus
    5. Seizures

Histology

- Traditionally classified pituitary growths by histologic staining and referred to as:
    - Basophil adenoma
    - Eosinophil adenoma
    - Chromophobe adenoma
- Currently classified by hormone function or nonfunctioning such as:
    - GH producing
    - ACTH producing
    - TSH producing

Lymphatic Drainage and Spread Patterns

- No lymphatic drainage
- Regional spread only

Workup

- History and physical
- Thyroid function
- Endocrine profile
- MRI with gadolinium enhancement
- CT

Staging

- Classified by location such as: suprasellar, parasellar, or infrasellar
- Hardy's classification indicates location and tumor size and grade
- Staging not used in radiation oncology practice

Treatment

- Need to treat the hormonal imbalance and reduce the size of the growth
- Dopamine for prolactinomas, GH secreting tumors
- Other pharmacologic therapies as appropriate for hormone manipulation
- Surgery using a transsphenoidal approach for small tumors can be for biopsy or total resection
- Radiation therapy for postoperative treatment after subtotal removal, recurrent disease, or when surgery not possible
- External beam, standard fractionation therapy with low energy x-rays
- Stereotactic radiosurgery with single dose x-rays or gamma knife
- Proton beam and other heavy particles good option due to short range and Bragg's peak in this thin area of the body
- Permanent interstitial implant using Y^{90}; dose range 500 to 1000 Gy rarely used in United States

Radiation Treatment Borders

- No lymphatic drainage and local spread only so small conforming fields needed with tight margins
- Good surface landmarks are just inferior to the glabella at midline; 2.0 cm anterior and 2 cm superior to the external auditory meatus
- Fields are small 6 × 6 cm

Treatment Delivery

- Single fraction dose with SRS need to limit dose to optic chiasm to 8 to 10 Gy to minimize damage to optic pathways
- Reported doses of 12 to 35 Gy using SRS; lower doses for nonfunctioning tumors and higher doses for functioning tumors
- Traditional method with external beam fractionation to 40 to 50 Gy using three field technique (vertex + laterals or anterior + laterals) to spare normal brain tissue, or parallel opposed laterals, or rotational arcs
- Patient may be positioned supine with neutral head position for three field or parallel opposed fields techniques; be mindful of protecting the lens
- Patient may be positioned supine with maximum chin flexion for rotational arcs through the coronal plane or three field vertex and laterals
- Patient may be positioned prone with chin hyperextended for three field technique or rotational arc through the coronal plane
- Reliable immobilization imperative with tight margins
- Arcs may be administered in noncoplanar arrangements requiring couch kicks
- Beam energies may be mixed
- Sophisticated 3-D conformal planning and use of wedges for three field technique and arc techniques, mixed energies, couch kicks incur complex billing charges even though beam shaping is nonexistent or minimal
- Side effects are minimal and may include edema, skin reddening, and hair loss
- Advise patient on scalp care—no razor shaving, no harsh shampoo, protect from the sun

CENTRAL NERVOUS SYSTEM REVIEW EXERCISES

Multiple Choice

1. The lateral ventricles are located within the:

a. Cerebral hemispheres
b. Brainstem
c. Sella turcica
d. Falx cerebri

2. The area of the cerebrum responsible for sensory and association is the:

a. Frontal area
b. Parietal area
c. Temporal area
d. Occipital area

3. The sense of smell is conveyed by the:

a. Olfactory nerve
b. Oculomotor nerve
c. Abducens nerve
d. Facial nerve

4. A glioma spreads by means of:
   a. Local invasion
   b. Cerebrospinal fluid
   c. Lymph nodes
   d. Blood

5. Which of the following brain tumors have the tendency to spread via the CSF?
   a. Glioma
   b. Astrocytoma
   c. Medulloblastoma
   d. Oligodendroglioma

6. Which of the following brain tumors is seen more frequently in the adult?
   a. Medulloblastoma
   b. Ependymoma
   c. Pituitary adenoma
   d. Glioma

7. Single dose stereotactic radiosurgery is most appropriate for:
   a. Multifocal metastatic brain tumors
   b. Recurrent 5-cm brain tumors
   c. Solitary 2-cm primary brain tumors
   d. Solitary 5-cm primary brain tumors

8. Which of the following is *not* a symptom of intracranial tumors?
   a. Headache
   b. ICP
   c. Seizures
   d. Nocturia

9. The primary management modality for primary brain tumors is:
   a. Surgery
   b. Radiation
   c. Chemotherapy
   d. Hormonal therapy

10. Which of the following are symptoms of pituitary adenomas?
   a. Uncontrolled diabetes
   b. Visual disturbances
   c. Sinus pressure
   d. a and b only
   e. All of the above

11. Using Figure 9-22 below, label the following anatomy:
   a. Pineal gland
   b. Pituitary gland
   c. Pons
   d. Medulla
   e. Third ventricle
   f. Fourth ventricle
   g. Sphenoid sinus

12. A primary spinal cord tumor located in the lumbosacral region may demonstrate by:
   a. Tingling sensation in the lower abdomen
   b. Pain radiating along the flank
   c. Incontinence, impotence
   d. Radiating pain down the legs
   e. c and d only

13. Facial pain could be associated with a primary CNS tumor near cranial nerve:
   a. I
   b. III
   c. VII
   d. XI

14. The tolerance dose TD 5/5 for the lens of the eye is:
   a. 5 to 10 Gy
   b. 10 to 20 Gy
   c. 20 to 30 Gy
   d. 30 to 40 Gy

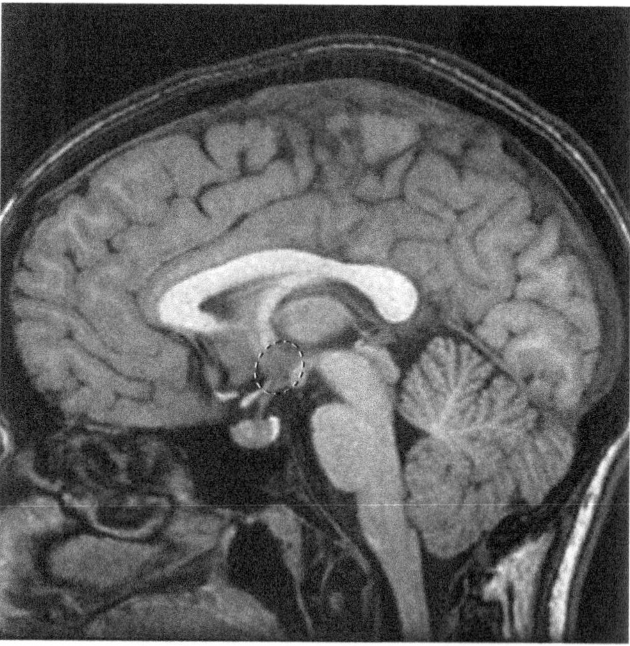

FIGURE 9-22 CT sagittal view brain.

15. The tolerance dose TD 5/5 for the optic nerve or chiasm is:

a. 50 Gy
b. 60 Gy
c. 70 Gy
d. 80 Gy

16. Local hair loss and erythema are the expected side effects from cranial radiation. Patients should be advised to:

a. Use mild shampoo or water only for washing
b. Use a razor to shave the head before the hair begins to thin
c. Apply keratosis cream to scalp daily
d. Apply hot towels daily to restimulate hair growth

17. Symptoms of brain tumors commonly include dizziness, diplopia, and seizures. Patients should be advised to:

a. Come accompanied to each therapy session
b. Take an analgesic before therapy
c. Take an antidiuretic before therapy
d. Apply cold towels to the forehead after each treatment

18. Involvement of cranial nerve ______may manifest as dysphagia.

a. IX
b. VII
c. VI
d. V

19. During primary brain tumor irradiation, dose to normal brain tissue should be kept below:

a. 45 Gy
b. 50 Gy
c. 60 Gy
d. 75 Gy

Think About It

20. Several primary tumors metastasize to the brain. However, primary brain tumors do not spread outside of the central nervous system. Briefly explain.

21. Noncoplanar beam arrangements are useful in treating pituitary adenomas. What is the advantage of this treatment strategy over traditional coplanar field arrangements?

22. Radiation therapy treatment fields often conform to primary brain tumors with about a 2-cm margin. Metastatic brain disease calls for whole brain radiation therapy. Explain.

23. A 270-degree rotational arc will be used to treat a pituitary adenoma through the coronal plane. The starting angle is at the 225-degree gantry position. What is the finishing angle?

24. For the above 270-degree rotation, the calculated monitor units for the arc are 280 MU. What is the calculated MU/degree?

25. If manual calculation was performed, what information would be required for the final monitor unit calculation?

SKIN CANCER

General Facts and Epidemiology

- Skin cancers make up one third of all cancer incidence in men and women in the United States
- There are two main types of primary skin cancers: melanomas and nonmelanomas

- Nonmelanomas are the most common
- Both types are easily visible and extremely curable if detected early
- Many melanomas are not discovered until late so there is greater mortality
- Melanomas are radioresistant
- Nonmelanomas are radiosensitive
- People of Celtic and Irish descent with fair skin are at increased risk

Etiology

- Ultraviolet radiation exposure
- Genetic disorders such as albinism
- Ionizing radiation
- Exposure of skin to chemicals such as arsenic
- Chronic irritation and inflammation

Clinical Presentation

- Symptoms depend on skin cancer type (Table 9-15)

Histology

- Melanomas
  - Lentigo maligna
  - Superficial spreading
  - Nodular
  - Palmar/plantar
  - Acral lentiginous
- Nonmelanomas
  - Basal cell
  - Squamous cell
  - Keratoacanthoma—resembles squamous cell
  - Bowen disease—single plaque with red, scaly border
  - Paget disease—single plaque in nipple, genital area
  - Merkel tumor—asymptomatic nodule
  - Verrucous carcinoma—wartlike, fungating
  - Marjolin ulcer—squamous cell-like with slow growth
  - Kaposi sarcoma—AIDS related
  - Adnexal (sebaceous gland) carcinoma
  - Eccrine (sweat gland) carcinoma

TABLE 9-15 Symptoms of Skin Cancer by Histologic Type

Basal Cell and Squamous Cell	Melanoma
Early signs: small papule with telangiectasia, firm induration of skin, patches of keratosis and scaling	Change in size, thickness, or contour of an existing mole
Late signs: loss of skin markings, change in pigment, hyperkeratosis	Lesions may be tan or black, itching and/or bleeding
Ulcerating lesions show very late	Lentigo maligna: flat, pigmented grow radially, penetrates vertically
As lesion grows, it ulcerates and bleeds and may have a rolled border and look crusty	Superficial spreading: disorderly appearance, extends horizontally and vertically Nodular: grow vertical, uniform blue-black color, sharp delineation

Lymphatic Drainage and Spread Patterns

- Nonmelanomas tend to remain in the dermal layers of the skin
- Melanomas penetrate deep into dermal layers and will metastasize via the blood route easily since blood vessels are in the dermal layers of the skin
- Area lymph nodes are considered when managing melanomas

Workup

- Physical examination: look for asymmetry, borders, color and diameter
- Excisional biopsy both diagnostic and therapeutic in some cases
- Incisional biopsy if lesion is large, expected benign or in a cosmetically compromising location
- Blood markers: keratin, CEA, S-100 protein
- Mohs surgery especially if melanoma suspected

Staging

- TNM system is used for nonmelanomas. Clark and Breslow staging may be used in melanomas.
- Clark method—categorizes lesion according to invasion through the levels of the epidermis and dermis
- Breslow method—categorizes lesion according to vertical thickness between the granular layer of the epidermis and the deepest part of invasion

Treatment

- Surgery for diagnosis and treatment: Mohs technique for recurrent basal cell and squamous cell, questionable borders, or suspicious for melanoma
- Radiation plays definitive role in nonmelanomas, especially if partial excision and/or to preserve cosmesis
- Radiation is adjuvant for nonmelanomas
- Electron or kilovoltage radiation for nonmelanomas
- Topical chemotherapy for nonmelanomas; systemic chemotherapy for melanomas
- Cryotherapy—liquid nitrogen for injury to vasculature for nonmelanomas
- Laser therapy—carbon dioxide laser excises with minimal bleeding in nonmelanomas
- Photodynamic therapy—porphyrin administered to patient then exposure to intense light for nonmelanomas
- Immunotherapy used for melanomas

Radiation Treatment Borders

- Radiation treatment fields for nonmelanomas should be focused with 1- to 2-cm margin around lesion
- Fields for adjuvant radiation in melanoma will have margins of 3 to 4 cm and may include regional lymphatics; deeply invasive, large nonmelanomas may need regional node dose
- Fields should be en face electrons of energies sufficient to cover the depth of lesion and regional lymph nodes if elected or kV photons for improved cosmetic effects
- Need wider margins for Merkel cell; 4 to 5 cm

Treatment Delivery

- Total dose for nonmelanomas range from 45 to 70 Gy depending on location; daily fractionation of 2 GY
- Hypofractionation in single dose of 20 Gy or 32 Gy in four fractions
- Patient surface should be perpendicular to the horizontal axis of the electron beam
- Bolus may be used along with electrons to increase surface dose
- Dose for melanomas is lower since radiation is adjuvant to chemotherapy and depends on patient's life expectancy; 30 Gy in 10 fractions, 36 Gy in 6 fractions, or 50 Gy in 25 fractions for solitary metastatic lesions
- Beam shaping achieved with Cerrobend cutouts or thin-lead cutouts placed on patient's skin surface (use wax or equivalent to absorb scatter radiation on the underside of lead cutout)
- Setups are clinical for nonmelanomas; make sure margin is maintained
- Positioning aids and immobilization typically simple; pillows, sponges, tape
- If larger areas need treatment, adjacent, matched electron fields may be used (overdose areas should be identified using computerized, dosimetric treatment planning and skin gaps may be necessary)
- Anticipate wet desquamation at high dose ranges, especially when electrons are used with bolus
- Patients should be educated on skin care; keep area clean and dry
- Inform patient to protect skin from sun, avoid extreme temperatures and ointments containing perfumes and inorganic additives

SKIN CANCER SECTION REVIEW EXERCISES

For Questions 1-5, indicate whether the statement is true or false

1. Nonmelanomas have higher mortality rates than melanomas. ______
2. The most common cancer type overall in the United States is nonmelanoma skin cancer. ______
3. Melanomas are usually tan or black in color. ______
4. In late stage disease, melanomas tend to ulcerate and have a rolled border on examination. ______
5. Melanomas are not usually treated with radiation because they are radioresistant. ______
6. Control rates for stage I basal cell carcinoma are approximately:
   a. 90%
   b. 70%
   c. 50%
   d. 20%
7. Clark method for classifying melanoma is based on:

a. Width of the growth
b. Depth of invasion
c. Maximum thickness in millimeters
d. Nodal metastasis

8. Write three statements appropriate for increasing public awareness regarding the prevention of skin cancers.

9. The skin serves many functions. List three functions of the skin.

10. The following are etiologic factors for skin cancers except:

a. Ultraviolet radiation exposure
b. Chemical carcinogens
c. Epstein-Barr virus
d. Genetic albinism

11. Melanocytes are found in the ______ layer of the skin.

a. Basal
b. Subcutaneous
c. Corneum
d. Sebaceous

12. Cells most sensitive to radiation are located in which layer of the epidermis?

a. Stratum basale
b. Stratum granulosum
c. Stratum lucidum
d. Stratum corneum

13. Which of the following activities increases risk of developing skin cancer?

a. Working in rubber manufacturing
b. Sweeping and inhaling Cerrobend dust
c. Frequent visits to the tanning salon
d. Swimming in high chlorine pools

14. Nonmelanoma type skin cancers are not usually seen in children. One possible reason is:

a. Children have a strong resistance to damaging UV rays
b. Screening for skin cancer is only recommended for adults
c. Adult skin cells are more mature and are resilient against injury
d. Nonmelanomas are a result of long-term exposure to UV rays

15. Lentigo maligna is a histologic type of melanoma characterized by:

a. Growth in a radial pattern with notches and reddish color
b. Tan or brown flat stainlike patterns on the palms or soles
c. Growth in a radial pattern with tan or black color
d. Raised pattern with black, blue-black color

Think About It

16. What role does immunotherapy play in the management of melanoma?

17. List the expected acute side effects of radiation therapy for nonmelanoma skin cancers (include fractionation schemes and anticipated time of skin reaction)

18. The depth of invasion for a diagnosed squamous cell carcinoma of the skin is 4 cm. The physician will prescribe dose for coverage by the 90% dose line. What electron energy is appropriate for this case?

19. A patient has a nonmelanoma located on the lower eyelid. Briefly discuss positioning and field arrangement strategies.

20. When a lesion on the external surface of the nose is treated, a lead shield should be placed into the nostril. Briefly explain why.

LEUKEMIA

General Facts and Epidemiology

- Heterogenous group of neoplastic diseases of the hemopoietic system
- Heterogenous—not of uniform composition or structure
- Affecting about 44,240 persons per year
- Divided into 2 categories
- Chronic—slower growing with uncontrolled expansion of mature cells
- Acute—progresses quickly and characterized by autonomous proliferation of undifferentiated cells in the bone marrow
- Subtypes (4 main)
  - *Myelogenous* leukemia—arises directly or indirectly from hemopoietic stem cells
    - AML—Acute myelogenous leukemia
    - CML—Chronic myelogenous leukemia
  - *Lymphocytic*—arise from other cells populating in bone marrow
    - ALL—Acute lymphocytic leukemia
    - CLL—Chronic lymphocytic leukemia

History

- 1827—First case documented by Alfred Velpeau, a French surgeon
- 1844—Alfred Donné is credited with the first known observation of leukemic cells and the establishment of the disease as a hematologic condition
- 1845—Rudolph Virchow, German physicist discovered a patient with splenic enlargement and massive accumulation of white blood cells as weisses blut (white blood)
- The advent of the staining technique in microscopy in the late nineteenth century permitted the morphologic subdivision of the myelogenous and lymphocytic

Anatomy

- Leukemia develops during the formation of the constituent elements of the blood and lymphocytes
- Hematopoietic process through which mature erythrocytes, neutrophils, eosinophils, basophils, monocytes, and platelets are formed and lymphopoietic process through which lymphocytes are formed begin at the most primitive level with the pluripotent stem cells
- These cells have a self-renewing capability and generate differentiation cells of multiple lineages
- Myeloid stem cells provide the progenitors for the six types of blood cells, whereas the lymphoid pool provides the progenitors for the classes of lymphocytes
- Cells then become fully mature, functional blood cells and lymphocytes during normal differentiation and maturation
- During leukemic development, the production of the hematopoietic or lymphopoietic progenitors is uncontrolled and greatly accelerated, resulting in incomplete or defective cellular maturation
- Acute leukemia involves the rapid proliferation of primitive, undifferentiated stem cells, whereas cellular differentiation is largely preserved in chronic leukemia
- Symptoms of leukemia result from the leukemic cells' interference with normal processes
- Leukemic cells accumulate in the bone marrow, impairing the body's normal production of adequate supplies of red blood cells, WBCs, and platelets
- Decrease in the number of these necessary blood components results in anemia, thrombocytopenia,

and neutropenia, causing symptoms such as fatigue, pallor, bleeding, and infection

- Normal range of values:
  - WBCs—3.90 to 10.80 thousand/mm^3
  - RBCs—3.90 to 5.40 million/mm^3
  - Platelets—150 to 424 thousand/mm^3
- Acute—the accumulating leukemic cells are immature or have undergone a defect in maturation
  - ALL—characterized by invasion of the bone marrow by leukemic lymphoblasts
  - AML—results from the proliferation of defective or incompletely matured cells derived from the pluripotent hematopoietic stem cell pool
- Chronic—the maturation of the cells is preserved, but unregulated proliferation results in the accumulation of leukemic cells in the bone marrow
  - CLL—disorder of morphologically mature, but immunologically less mature, lymphocytes
  - CML—involves the replacement of marrow cells with mature myeloid cells that are insensitive to the normal proliferation control mechanisms

ACUTE LYMPHOCYTIC LEUKEMIA

Epidemiology

- Acute subtypes account for 50% of all leukemias
- Most common pediatric malignancy—80% of them are *ALL*
- Peak incidence 2 to 3 years of age
- Uncommon after age 15 years of age
- Males predominately
- Hispanic children increased prevalence of ALL compared with African American children and white children
- Disease more common in whites than African Americans
- Higher socioeconomic groups and more developed countries have a higher incidence

Etiology

- Unknown
- Possible association with physical and chemical agents
- Japanese atomic bomb survivors had tenfold to fifteenfold increase in acute leukemia (ALL over AML)
  - Interesting note—no significant increase in leukemia after 1986 Chernobyl, where large amounts of iodine released (but there were significant increase in thyroid cancer)
- Benzene derivatives
- Hydrocarbons
- Alkylating agents—cyclophosphamide increase risk in acute leukemia
- Hereditary—in acute leukemia
- Identical twin risk within 1 year of each other in 20%
- Down syndrome—risk is 10 to 30 times increase change for acute leukemia
- Natural retroviruses and human T-cell, lymphotropic viruses (specific to ALL in adults)

Prognostic Indicators

- 75% of patients with ALL—complete remission (dependent on a number of factors such as age and WBC at time of diagnosis)
- ALL in age 1 or younger, and older than 10 carry a worse prognosis
- ALL in adults over 50 had worse prognosis
- Leukocyte count:
  - Less than 10,000/mm^3 is more favorable
  - 20,000/—49,000/mm^3 is worse
  - More than 50,000/mm^3 is least favorable
- Other features with low prognostic value include: (at time of diagnosis)
  - CNS, mediastinal mass, massive organomegaly and/or adenopathy, biologic qualities of the leukemic cells such as the immunophenotype, cytogenetics, and DNA content
  - Unfavorable prognostic indicators: poor performance status, impaired organ function, low serum albumin levels

Clinical Presentation

Suppressed natural blood components cause:

- Anemia—from fatigue and pallor
- Thrombocytopenia—manifested by:
  - Oozing gums
  - Epistaxis (nose bleeds)
  - Petechiae—tiny red spots on skin from escape of small amounts of blood

- Ecchymoses—discoloration of skin from escape of blood into tissues
- Menorrhagia—excessive menstrual bleeding
- Excessive bleeding after dental procedures

- Neutropenia causes:
  - Increased respiratory problems
  - Dental issues
  - Sinus problems
  - UTI (urinary tract infection)
  - Liver, splenic, and testicular enlargement
  - Mimics rheumatoid arthritis with joint swelling, bone pain, and tenderness (often causes a child to limp or refuse to walk)
  - Symptoms rarely occur 6 weeks before diagnosis
  - Vomiting, headaches, papilledema (swelling of the optic disc), neck stiffness, and cranial nerve palsy are indications of CNS involvement

Detection and Diagnosis

- Blood cell count
- Two thirds of patients have thrombocytopenia and anemia
- Leukocyte counts vary from high to low (abnormal high WBC—poor prognosis)
- Immunophenotyping—morphologic evaluation, special stains, electron microscopic examination and surface marker studies can yield a diagnosis in 90% of patients
- Bone marrow aspiration biopsy for definite diagnosis (amount of leukemic blast cells is the determinant) or 25% of presence of leukoblasts is positive
- Other abnormalities—hyperuricemia, metabolic abnormalities, hyperkalemia, hypomagnesemia, hypercalcemia and hypocalcemia
- Leukemic infiltrates of liver, periosteum, and bone
- A mediastinal mass (seen on chest x-ray)
- Extramedullary leukemia—most common sites in CNS and testes (sanctuary sites, because they are "hidden" from most chemo agents)

Pathology

- Unregulated by proliferation of lymphoblasts
- Disease cells limit the production of other healthy cells by overcrowding and inhibiting cell growth and differentiation

Staging and Classification

- Morphological appearance
- Immunologic classification
- FAB (French-American-British), L1, L2, and L3 are divisions based on cell size, nuclear shape, number, prominence of nuclei, and amount and appearance of cytoplasm
- Most pediatric ALLs are L1
- L3s carry the worst prognosis

Treatment Techniques

Used alone or in combination:

Radiation

- *(TBI)* Total Body Irradiation example—1200 cGy. 3 consecutive days 200 cGy, twice daily*
- Dose rate set for 100 cGy/min at midplane at the central region, the umbilicus. This low dose is necessary to spare late-responding tissues (all visceral organs, most common is lung). Figure 9-23 shows an immobilization device for TBI.
- ***Helmet*** field (Figure 9-24) to encompass the meninges dose example—(1800 cGy; 200 cGy/day × 9 consecutive days). Helmet field covers meninges—encompassing C2 with falloff around the head; special attention to spinal cord in this setup
- *CNS* in combinations with helmet—patient prone in head holder to include total spine and brain field (helmet). Field arrangement is very important. Special techniques such as gapping and feathering help avoid hot spots

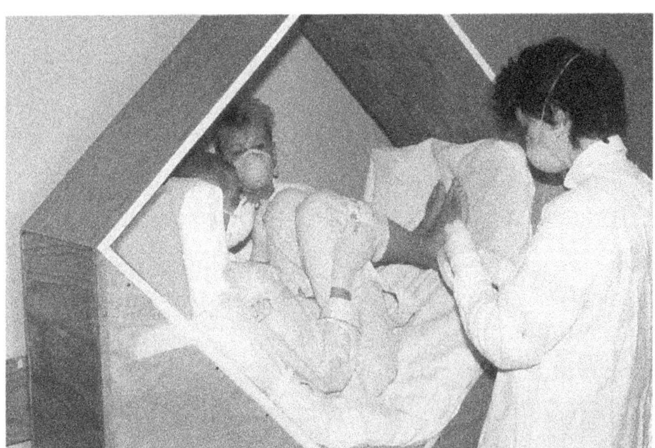

FIGURE 9-23 New England Medical Center's custom-made immobilization device for total-body irradiation.

*Doses may vary from center to center.

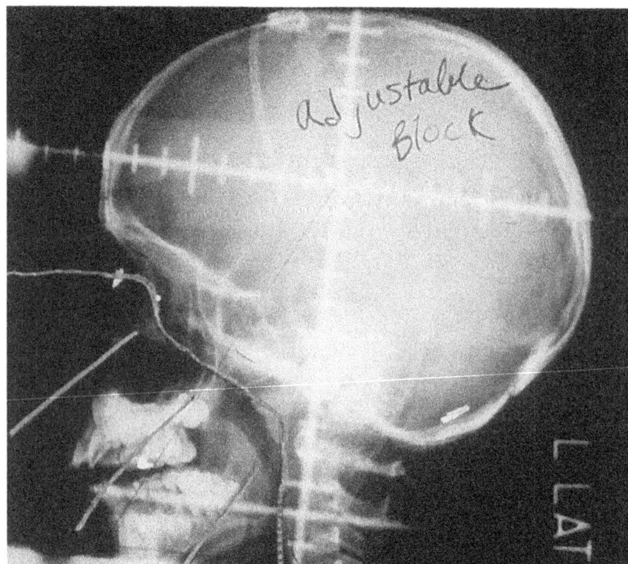

FIGURE 9-24 Simulation film for a helmet field that covers the meninges encompassing C2.

Chemotherapy

***Remission Induction* (given immediately upon diagnosis)**

- Prednisone or dexamethasone
- Vincristine
- L-asparaginase
- High risk patients—also anthracycline, daunorubicin added

***Consolidation* (after remission is achieved)**

- IV methotrexate and L-asparaginase

Maintenance or Continuation Therapy

- IV mercaptopurine (6-MP) and systemic methotrexate

Prophylaxis of Overt CNS

- Methotrexate

Bone Marrow Transplant

- Harvesting of healthy marrow from matched donor
- Diseased marrow has be destroyed or ablated by chemo or TBI
- Harvested marrow injected back into patient
- Transplanted marrow finds its way into bone marrow cavities and begins supplying the patient with normal, healthy hematopoietic cells
- Failures in transplants are recurrent leukemia (primarily in autologous donor) and graft-versus-host disease

Side Effects

Acute

- GI—nausea, vomiting, diarrhea, anorexia, and malaise
- Mucosa of mouth, pharynx, bladder, and rectum
- Normal secretions inhibited impairing their functions
- Integumentary—skin reactions, itching, tingling, bruising and dry and inelastic skin that cracks easily
- Alopecia
- Blanching or erythema of skin and mucous membranes
- Respiratory—intestinal pneumonitis

Chronic

- Permanent sterility
- Cataracts
- Hepatic fibrosis
- Radionecrosis of genital tissue, muscle and kidney

CNS Side Effects

- Skin reactions
- Hair loss
- Decrease in blood counts
- Leukoencephalopathy
- Nausea and vomiting
- Somnolence syndrome
- Serious injury to tissue or blood vessels
- Lhermitte sign
- Neuropsychological deficits, intellectual deficits
- Cataracts
- Growth retardation and hypothalamic-pituitary dysfunction
- Hormonal effects
- Myelopathy

ACUTE MYELOGENOUS LEUKEMIA

Epidemiology

- Incidence—13,290 cases/year
- Median age is 65
- Incidence slightly higher in males and Caucasians
- Represents about 90% of all acute leukemias

Etiology

- Exposure to ionizing radiation
- Increased incidence in military personnel at Nevada bomb test sites
- Patients treated (radiation) for ankylosing spondylitis, menorrhagia, and thymic enlargement

- Thorium dioxide (Thorotrast) an intravenous contrast for angiography test
- (1928-1952)—due to alpha particle emission
- Fanconi anemia and Bloom syndrome (genetic disorder with a chromosome breakage)
- Exposure to benzene and alkylating agents
- Tobacco smoke

Clinical Presentation

- To 6-month prodromal period
- Nonspecific flulike symptoms
- Fatigue, pallor, and dyspnea on exertion
- Anemia
- Petechiae
- Purpura (hemorrhage under skin)
- Epistaxis, gingival bleeding, and GI/GU bleeding (reduced platelet production)
- Neutropenia—susceptibility to infections
- Enlarged spleen

Detection and Diagnosis

- CBC
    - Differential leukocyte and platelet counts and blood smears
    - Chromosomal abnormalities
        - Circulation of Auer rods in leukemic cells, and increase in leukemic blast cells, and a decrease in normal precursors)
        - Biopsy (bone marrow based on percentage of blasts)

Pathology

Unregulated proliferation of early precursor cells that have lost the ability to differentiate in response to hormonal signals and cellular interactions

Staging and Classification

- Morphological evaluation, FAB systems
- Categorization—different saturation states from M0-M7

Treatment Technique and Field Design

Refer to AML above.

Side Effects

- Bone marrow depression
- Nausea, vomiting, esophagitis, stomatitis, diarrhea, and ulceration—(GI effects)
- Renal effects
- Rashes and alopecia
- Reproductive—mutagenic and teratogenic

CHRONIC LYMPHOCYTIC LEUKEMIA

Epidemiology

- 15,110 new cases per year
- 30% of all leukemic cases in United States
- Onset age is 65, most are age 70 (rare under age 40)
- Males over females and less common in Asian population

Etiology

- Heredity (first-degree relatives have a twofold to sevenfold increase in risk)
- Familial clustering—the most notable of all leukemia
- Immunologic factors such as immunodeficiency syndromes and viruses
- Only leukemia *not* associated with radiation exposure

Prognostic Indicators

- Stage at time of diagnosis
- Age
- Doubling time of peripheral blood lymphocyte count
- Pattern of bone marrow involvement
- T-cell variety of CLL—the more aggressive

Clinical Presentation

- Characterized by minimal changes in blood count
- Blood tests at routine doctor visit may indicate lymphocyte counts equal to or higher than 10,000/mm^3
- Asymptomatic
- Fatigue, fever, night sweats, weight loss
- Lymphadenopathy and enlarged spleen
- Chromosomal abnormalities

Pathology

- Bone marrow lymphoid tissue
- Increased proliferation of leukemic cells in bone marrow, blood, lymph nodes, and spleen
- Enlargement of lymph nodes and spleen
- Decreased bone marrow function

Staging and Classification

- Modified *Rai* system (three major prognostic groups)
- Stage 0—low risk
- Stage I and II—intermediate risk
- Stage III and IV—high risk
- Stages based on adenopathy, splenomegaly, anemia, and lymphocytosis
- *Binet* system: three stages based on involvement of five specific anatomic sites: cervical nodes, axillary nodes, inguinal nodes, spleen and liver
- Cytochemistry used to classify CLL into two subtypes: B-cell and T-cell

Treatment Techniques

- Optimal treatment is unknown
- Early stage disease will not benefit from treatment
- Chemotherapy—when progressive anemia and thrombocytopenia—drugs used chlorambucil and alkylating agent and prednisone (chlorambucil prevents the separation of the strands of DNA, which is necessary for cell replication)
- Radiation—used for palliative for localized masses of lymphoid tissue and/or enlarged spleen (AP/PA) total dose of 500 cGy—100 cGy/day × 5; spleen field design would be clinical encompassing a 1-cm margin; simulation of field by palpation of spleen, fluoroscopy, and now CT with contrast
- Surgery—splenectomy (an enlarged spleen causes cytopenia, which is the result of accelerated removal or excessive pooling of platelets or RBCs)

Side Effects

- Chlorambucil causes bone marrow depression
- GI—anorexia, nausea, vomiting
- Dermatitis, urticaria
- Reproductive—mutagenesis, teratogenesis, and sterility
- Prednisone causes GI peptic ulcers and pancreatitis
- Metabolic response—centripetal obesity, hyperlipidemia, hyperosmolar nonketotic coma and immunosuppression
- Neurologic side effect is pseudotumor cerebri
- Glaucoma and cataracts
- Hypertension
- Skin striae
- Amenorrhea
- Impaired wound healing

CHRONIC MYELOGENOUS LEUKEMIA

Epidemiology

- 15% of all adult leukemias
- Peaks at mid-60s
- Slightly more in males

Etiology

- Unknown
- Possible link to radiation and benzene exposure
- Possible link to the Philadelphia chromosome

Prognostic Indicators

- Spleen size, platelet count, hematocrit, gender, and percentage of blood myeloblasts
- Disease typically transforms into acute leukemia after a chronic phase of 3 to 4 years when patient enters a blast crisis
- Survival time approximately 2 years

Clinical Presentation

- Three stages: chronic, accelerated, and acute phase or blast crisis
- Clinical symptoms generally mild—malaise, fatigue, heat intolerance, sweating, and easy bruising
- Symptoms related to splenic enlargement include vague discomfort in the LUQ, early satiety, weight loss, and peripheral leg edema
- 3 to 4 years patient enters blast crisis—fever, bone pain, and pronounced weight loss

Detection and Diagnosis

- Insidious but incidental
- Mild to moderate anemia and leukocytosis

- Myeloblasts, promyelocytes, and nucleated RBCs
- Increased granulocytic and megakaryocytic hyperplasia
- Presence of the Philadelphia chromosome

Pathology

- Abnormal hematopoietic stem cells giving rise to the progeny of the Philadelphia chromosome

Staging and Classification

Three distinct stages:

- Chronic (or stable phase)
- Accelerated phase
- Acute phase (blast crisis)

Treatment Techniques

- Radiation (spleen like CLL, and TBI same as CLL)
- Chemo drugs—Imatinib mesylate (Gleevec), interferon, and hydroxyurea
- Bone marrow transplantation (same as CLL)

Side Effects

- Gleevec—severe skin reactions, fluid retention and edema, GI disturbances, hemorrhage, anemia, neutropenia, thrombocytopenia, liver toxicities, and potential immune suppression
- Interferon—flulike symptoms, fever, chills, malaise, muscle aches, anorexia, and weight loss
- Hydroxyurea—hematopoietic system, bone marrow depression, rapid leucopenia, and erythrocytic abnormalities; GI side effects—anorexia and diarrhea. Facial erythema and maculopapular rash are integumentary reactions; reproductive reaction—teratogenic

Role of Radiation Therapist

- Communication when treating children and with parents
- Sufficient time allotted for explanations
- Eliciting cooperation of younger children
- Scheduling longer times (if treatment may take longer, such as TBI, bone marrow transplants)
- Knowledge of preparation for bone marrow transplantation; BID treatments
- Knowledge of reverse isolation techniques
- Thorough knowledge of treatment techniques

Present Outcomes

- Pediatric leukemia (most common form ALL) with advancement of multidisciplinary therapeutic interventions, the survival rate has gone from 4% in 1962 to current 5-year survival rates of 75 to 85%
- AML—not improved over last 5 years; overall 5-year is 21%
- CLL—due to no definitive therapy for cure—5 year survival rate is 74%
- CML—no treatment cure; survival rate depends on phase of disease

LEUKEMIA REVIEW EXERCISES

Define the following terms:

1. Thrombocytopenia
2. Leukapheresis
3. Splenomegaly
4. Leukopenia
5. Anorexia
6. Teratogenic
7. Neutropenia
8. Toxicity
9. Benzene

10. Bone marrow depression

11. Auer rods

12. Nadir

13. Pruritus

14. Ecchymoses

15. through 19. Complete Table 9-16 to match and define the chemotherapy drug with the correct leukemia.

Drug Type Disease Effect

16. The first documented case of leukemia was by:

a. Alfred Donné
b. Rudolf Virchow
c. Alfred Velpeau
d. Marie Curie

17. When leukemic cells accumulate in the bone marrow, there is an impairment of the body's normal production of adequate supplies of:

a. White blood cells
b. Red blood cells
c. Platelets

18. *Weisses blut* means:

a. White blood
b. Red blood
c. Bone marrow
d. Platelets

TABLE 9-16 Leukemia Review

e.g.	Prednisone	Hormonal Agent	ALL, CLL	GI-Ulcers/ Pancreatitis
15.	Chlorambucil			
16.	Doxorubicin			
17.	Vincristine			
18.	Interferon			
19.	Hydroxyurea			

List the normal values for the following blood values:

19. White blood count ______________________

20. Red blood count ______________________

21. Platelets ______________________

22. Create a diagram of the breakdown of hematopoiesis and lymphopoiesis.

23. List the differential white blood cells:

______________ ______________
______________ ______________
______________ ______________

24. Which of the leukemias is found mostly in children?

a. ALL
b. AML
c. CLL
d. CML

25. Which of the leukemias is not associated with previous radiation exposure?

a. ALL
b. AML
c. CLL
d. CML

26. The most important diagnostic factor for detecting CML is:

a. Nucleated RBCs
b. Philadelphia chromosome
c. Circulation of Auer rods
d. Complete CBC

Explain the following radiation techniques and setup—must define: field size, positioning, immobilization devices, doses, and field arrangements.

27. TBI

28. Helmet

29. CNS

30. Bone marrow transplant

31. Why is a gap calculated when treating total CNS?

32. Define a feathering technique and when it is used in a radiation setup.

33. Factors that lead to failure in bone marrow transplants include:

   1. Recurrent disease
   2. Autologous donors
   3. Graft-versus-host disease

   a. 1, 2
   b. 1, 3
   c. 2, 3
   d. 1, 2, 3

34. Patients treated with methotrexate develop a rapid onset of bone marrow depression, with nadir occurring within a range of:

   a. 3 to 5 days
   b. 5 to 10 days
   c. 10 to 14 days
   d. 15 to 20 days

35. Integumentary system includes which of the following except:

   a. Skin
   b. Nails
   c. Hair
   d. Blood cells

36. Which of the following would be considered integumentary side effects from chemotherapy drugs seen in leukemia patients?

   1. Alopecia
   2. Dermatitis
   3. Hyperpigmentation

   a. 1, 2
   b. 1, 3
   c. 2, 3
   d. 1, 2, 3

37. The field design for treating a spleen clinically, you would need to allow how much margin around the organ:

   a. 1-cm
   b. 2-cm
   c. 3-cm
   d. Margin is not important

38. Patients with ______ always exhibit lymphocytosis:

   a. ALL
   b. AML
   c. CLL
   d. CML

39. Which leukemia has the worst prognosis:

   a. ALL
   b. AML
   c. CLL
   d. CML

40. A patient is treated using two adjacent spinal fields. The collimator setting for field No. 1 is 8 cm width × 10 cm length. The collimator setting for field No. 2 is 8 cm width × 12 cm length. Both fields are treated at 100-cm SSD. Calculate the gap on the skin surface for the fields to abut at 4 cm depth.

41. When treating a TBI, what might be used during the first treatment to check midline doses and are placed at specific areas such as the patient's ankles, knees, and thighs:

    a. TLDs
    b. Film badges
    c. Pocket dosimeter
    d. Ionization chamber

42. In a helmet field treatment, it is very important to cover the meninges and C2. Which of the following is not one of the layers of the meninges?

    a. Dura mater
    b. Pia mater
    c. Subarachnoid mater
    d. Arachnoid mater

43. Which of the leukemias appear to have a hereditary component?

    a. ALL
    b. AML
    c. CLL
    d. CML

44. For a definitive diagnosis for ALL, which of the following is needed?

    a. Biopsy of the spleen
    b. Bone marrow aspiration biopsy
    c. CT with contrast
    d. Definitive white blood count

45. The spleen is located in which quadrant:

    a. LUQ
    b. LLQ
    c. RUQ
    d. RLQ

46. In which of the following phase(s) of the cell cycle may the undifferentiated cells have a decreased proportion of blast cells compared with normal bone marrow blast cells in regards to the pathology of AML?

    1. S
    2. M
    3. G1

    a. 1, 2
    b. 1, 3
    c. 2, 3
    d. 1, 2, 3

LYMPHOMA

GENERAL FACTS

Hematopoietic System

- Blood
- Lymphatic tissue
- Bone Marrow
- Spleen

Three Basic Types of Blood Cells

- Erythrocytes (RBC)—smallest of all blood cells; responsible for transporting oxygen and carbon dioxide throughout the body
- Leukocytes (WBC)—formed in red bone marrow; mainly found in the lymphatic tissue of the spleen and include lymphocytes and monocytes; responsible for the body's defense system
- Thrombocytes (platelets)—necessary for blood clotting and they respond with seconds to initiate the coagulation process

The Lymphatic System

- Subsystem of the circulatory system
- Closely relates to the cardiovascular system
- Composed of specialized connective tissue containing large quantities of lymphocytes
- Consist of lymphatic vessel, organs, nodes, and lymph (white milky substance)
- Occurs throughout the body

Functions

- Vessels drain tissue spaces of interstitial fluid that escapes from blood capillaries and loose connective tissues, filters it, and returns it to the bloodstream. This is important in maintaining the overall fluid levels in the body (most important function).
- The lymphatic system absorbs fats and transports them to the bloodstream.

- The intricate system plays a major role in the body's defense and immunity. Immunity is the ability to fight off infectious organisms, foreign bodies, and diseases. Specifically, lymphocytes and macrophages recognize and respond to the foreign matter.

Lymphatic System

- Lymphatic vessels
  - Contain lymph
  - Start in spaces between cells referred to as lymphatic capillaries
  - Every region of body that has blood supply has these capillaries, (exception—CNS and bone marrow are avascular)
  - Collects cellular debris, sloughed off cells, and foreign substances that occur in the intercellular spaces and transported away for filtration
  - Flow is in one direction only
  - Lymphatic capillaries join to form larger lymphatic vessels
  - Lymphatic vessels resemble veins in structure but have thinner walls and more valves promoting one-way flow
  - These larger vessels follow veins and arteries and eventually empty into one of the two ducts in the upper thoracic—the thoracic duct or the right lymphatic duct, which then flow into subclavian veins
- Lymph
  - Excessive tissue fluid consisting mostly of water and plasma proteins from capillaries; plasma—liquid portion of the blood; 90% water; 10% proteins, nutrients, electrolytes, respiratory gases, etc.
  - Differs from blood by the absence of formed elements in it
- Lymphatic Organs
  - Spleen—largest mass of lymphatic tissue
    - Posterior to and to the left of the stomach in the abdomen
    - It is 12 cm in length
    - Filters blood
    - Removes old red blood cells
    - Manufactures lymphocytes (B) for immunity surveillance
    - Stores blood
    - Has no afferent lymphatic vessels, so does not filter lymph
    - Often removed during laparotomy for biopsy and staging purposes
    - After removal—bone marrow and liver assume the spleen's function
- Thymus
  - Located along trachea superior to heart and posterior to the sternum in upper thorax
  - Larger in children and more active in pediatric immunity
  - Site where T lymphocytes mature
- Tonsils
  - Lymphatic nodules embedded in the mucous membrane
  - Located at junction of oral cavity and pharynx
  - Protect against foreign body infiltration by producing lymphocytes
  - *Pharyngeal tonsils* (adenoids) in nasopharynx
  - *Palatine tonsils* are in posterior lateral wall of oropharynx
  - *Lingual tonsils* are at the base of the tongue in oropharynx
- Thoracic duct
  - Left side of body and larger than right lymphatic duct
  - Serves the lower extremities, abdomen, left arm, and left side of head and neck and drains into the left subclavian vein
  - It is 35 to 45 cm in length and begins in front of the second lumbar vertebra (L2) and is called the *cisterna chyli*
  - Lymph travels through lower extremities to the cisterna chyli, and continues upward to the thoracic duct
- Right lymphatic duct
  - Serves only the right arm and right side of head and neck and drains the right subclavian vein
  - Approximately 1 to 2 cm in length
  - Box 9-3 illustrates an overview of lymphatic flow.
- Lymph Nodes
  - Located along the path of lymph vessels
  - Vary in size from 2 to 30 mm in length and often occur in groups
  - Contain both afferent (one-way valves entering the lymph node at several points) and efferent vessels,

BOX 9-3 Lymphatic Flow Overview

- **Tissue fluid** leaves the cellular interstitial spaces and becomes
- **Lymph**; as it enters a
- **Lymphatic capillary**, it merges with other capillaries to form an
- **Afferent lymphatic vessel**, which enters a
- **Lymph node** where lymph is filtered. It then leaves the node via an
- **Efferent lymphatic vessel**, which travels to other nodes, then merges with other vessels to form a
- **Lymphatic trunk**, which merges with other trunks and joins a
- **Collecting duct**, either the right lymphatic or the thoracic, which empties into a
- **Subclavian vein**, where lymph is returned to the bloodstream.

From Washington CM, Leaver D: *Principles and practice of radiation therapy*, ed 3, St Louis, 2010, Mosby/Elsevier.

smaller in diameter (valves leaving the node, again facilitating one-way flow)

- Slowing of lymph out of node facilitates the effective filtering of the lymph through phagocytosis, the endothelial cells of the node engulfs, devitalize, and remove the contaminants
- If substances are trapped inside the reticular fibers and pathways throughout the node, excessive fluid accumulation occurs producing swelling of node called edema (due to heightened phagocytic activity)
- Swelling goes down as pathogen is devitalized (e.g., if infection-antibiotics may be used)
- Figure 9-25 illustrates lymph node anatomy.

Lymphedema, also known as **lymphatic obstruction,** is a condition of localized fluid retention caused by a compromised lymphatic system. This often becomes a problem in the field of radiation therapy when dealing with patients with breast cancer. When performing surgery to remove and stage breast cancer, surgeons often take out many axillary lymph nodes to see whether the cancer has begun to spread. In doing this, the natural flow of lymph through the arm is disrupted, and without rehabilitation, lymphedema can occur.

In these patients, the arm swells, often reducing circulation, and there is the danger of developing an infection of that limb. Lymphedema can usually be controlled by wearing compression bandages and through therapeutic exercises. Surgeons have also begun using a technique known as the **sentinel node biopsy** in hopes of reducing the risk of lymphedema development by reducing the number of lymph nodes removed during surgery (Washington and Leaver 2010).

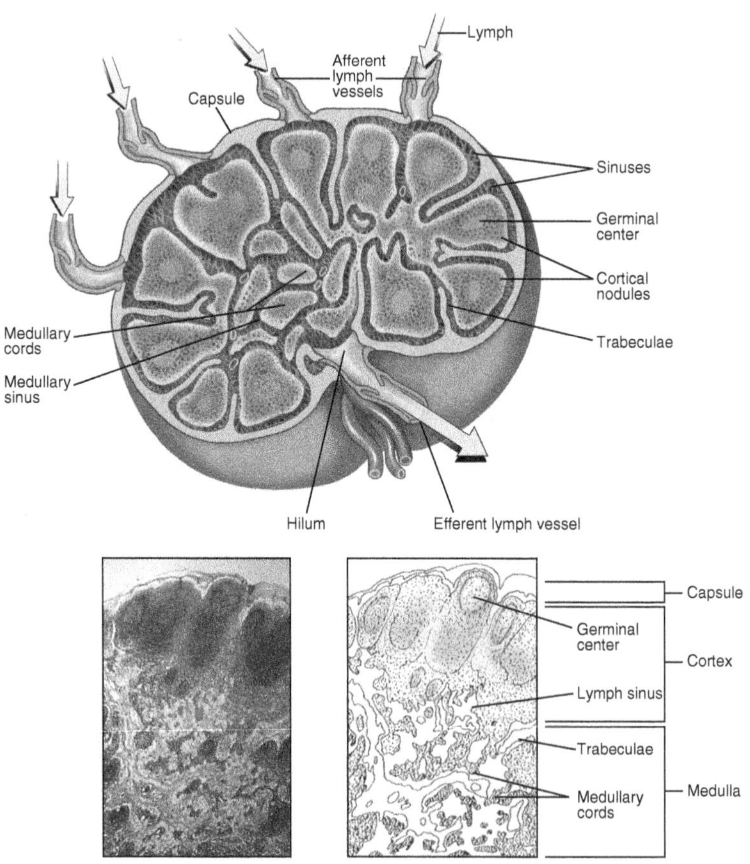

FIGURE 9-25 Lymph node.

Two Main Histologies

Hodgkin Lymphoma (HD)

- Presence of Reed-Sternberg cell
- Spreads contiguous
- Cell contains 1 to 2 large nuclei
- Occurs anywhere that lymph travels

Non-Hodgkin Lymphoma (NHL)

- Spreads randomly
- Lymphoid tissue: primary and peripheral contains B and T precursor cells
- Classified as follicular or diffuse

Epidemiology

Hodgkin

- 2008—8220 new cases; 1350 will die
- Less than 1% of newly diagnosed cancer
- Male over female
- Incidence peak occurs before adolescence in underdeveloped countries but in the mid- to late 20s in industrialized countries
- Occur in younger people (<40); median age 38
- Rare in children under 10

Non-Hodgkin

- Increased incidence of 65%; 2008-66,120 new cases, 19,160 deaths
- Male over female
- White males have higher incidence
- Burkitt lymphoma and AIDS (Africa)
- Median age is 65, peaking 80 to 84
- Third most common childhood malignancy (10% of all childhood cancers)

Etiology

Hodgkin

- Cause unknown
- Viral/contagious
- Epstein-Barr virus (EBV) genome in the DNA cell of the Reed-Sternberg cell
- Defective T-cell function

Non-Hodgkin

- Unknown (genetic alterations of the B or T lymphocytes)
- Identified risk factors*
- Ionizing radiation
- Ankylosing spondylitis

Prognostic Indicators

- Staging has the greatest effect on the prognosis
- Risk of relapse after treatment—greater in later stages due to increased bulky disease
- Prognosis slightly worse in males
- Gender may be a deciding factor in treatment
- Youth—favorable prognosis (teens to twenties)
- Extent of disease, presence of "B" symptoms, sites involved, disease in lower abdomen, spleen involved
- Elevation of serum markers (such as erythrocyte sedimentation rate)

Anatomy and Lymphatics

Major Lymph Nodes (HD/NHL)

- Waldeyer ring (tonsillar lymphatic tissue surrounding the nasopharynx and oropharynx) and cervical, preauricular, and occipital lymph nodes. Tonsils include: (1) nasopharyngeal (2)—tubal (pharyngeal-adenoids), (3)—palatine, (4)—lingual
- Supraclavicular and infraclavicular lymph nodes
- Axillary lymph nodes
- Thorax (hilar and mediastinal nodes)
- Abdominal cavity (paraaortic nodes)
- Pelvic cavity (iliac nodes)
- Inguinal and femoral lymph nodes
- Major lymphatic regions of the body

Clinical Presentation

Hodgkin

- Painless mass in neck and supraclavicular area
- Mediastinal node—chest x-ray
- Most disease above diaphragm

---

*The cause of Hodgkin disease is currently unknown; however, several factors have been identified to be associated with HD. It is important to note that these factors may increase the risk of developing HD, but most people with these conditions still do not develop HD. Infection with the EBV may play a role in the development of certain types. EBV also causes mononucleosis, which is known as mono or kissing disease.

- Systemic symptoms (B symptoms)
- Unexplained fevers (>38 °C)
- Drenching night sweats
- 10% weight loss
- Pruritus
- Alcohol induced pain
- Enlarged lymph nodes
- Neck, clavicular, axilla, groin area node enlargement
- Mediastinal mass if x-ray
- Enlarged spleen or abdomen
- Bony tenderness
- Pleural effusion

Non-Hodgkin
- Similar to HD
- Unlike HD, NHL can arise in lymph nodes, GI tract, Waldeyer ring, CNS (AIDS)
- Similar to Hodgkin
- Shortness of breath—lung involvement
- Abdominal pain or change of bowel habits may indicate pelvic disease
- Headaches, vision, seizures
- GI, CNS, Waldeyer ring

Pathology

Hodgkin
- Reed-Sternberg cell
  - Lymphocyte-rich Hodgkin lymphoma (LRHL)
  - Nodular sclerosing Hodgkin lymphoma (NSHL)—*Most common subtype* in developed countries accounting for 60% to 80%. Mostly in adolescents and young adults. Mediastinum and supradiaphragmatic most often involved sites. Approximately one third of patients have "B" symptoms.
  - Mixed cellularity Hodgkin lymphoma (MCHL) accounts for 15% to 30% of all Hodgkin lymphoma. It occurs at any age, lacking early adult peak of NSHL. Most commonly involved lymph nodes are in the abdomen and spleen.
  - Lymphocyte-depleted Hodgkin lymphoma (LDHL) is the least common subtype in the United States. Occurs in older patients and HIV-infected patients; presents with advanced disease in spleen, liver, and bone marrow and with B symptoms. It carries the worst prognosis.

Non-Hodgkin
- Two types of lymphoid tissues:
- Primary (central lymph tissue)
  - Precursor cells both B and T
  - Occurs in bone marrow and thymus
- Periphery (secondary lymph tissue)
  - Antigen-specific reactions occur
  - Lymph nodes, spleen, and mucosa-associated lymphoid tissue (MALT) found in epithelium of nasopharynx and oropharynx (Waldeyer ring), GI tract, distal ileum (Payer patches), colon, and rectum

NHL Histologic Classification
- Follicular (nodular)—40%
  - B-cell origin
  - It runs an indolent course with prolonged survival (5 to 7 Years)
  - Usually appear below diaphragm and involve mesenteric lymph nodes
  - Usually not found in children; do not commonly involve the Waldeyer ring
- Diffuse—60%
  - B- or T-cell origin
  - It runs a more aggressive course spreading quickly to other nodes and extranodal sites
  - Increased involvement in bone marrow and Waldeyer ring

Lymphatic Drainage and Spread Patterns

Hodgkin
- Predictable pattern of spread: referred to as *contiguous*
- Spread is predictable to adjacent lymph node or region (viscera spread)
- Rapidity of the growth is not predictable
- Late stages and spread may include spleen, liver, and/or bone marrow
- Very late stage—lungs, skeletal

Non-Hodgkin
- Nonpredictable, noncontiguous
- Spread randomly
- May involve upper digestive tract, CNS, skin, GI tract, Waldeyer ring, or Peyer patches

Workup

Hodgkin

- Complete history and physical
- Lab studies (CBC/platelet)
- Liver/renal function
- Blood chemistry, thyroid function
- Chest, CT, MRI, PET/CT with FDG
- Gallium, bone scan
- Bone marrow biopsy
- "B" symptoms

Non-Hodgkin

- Complete history and physical
- Cytologic evaluations
- HIV test
- Blood chemistry
- Urinalysis
- LDH
- Liver function
- Serum alkaline phosphate
- Same x-ray with GI and SB
- Bond marrow biopsy
- CT, MRI, PET

Staging

Hodgkin

- Stages—I thru IV
- Subdivided into A or B groups
- Fever, night sweats, weight loss will be indicated as B symptoms (e.g., IIB)
- B symptoms indicate worse prognosis
- Ann Arbor Staging Method

Non-Hodgkin

- Patients usually have more advanced disease
- Diaphragm has less significant role than in HD
- NHL is usually more bulky disease
- Staging—Ann Arbor is used mostly, but not significant with NHL

Treatment

- Chemotherapy is primary for both HD and NHL.
- Combination chemotherapy is used carefully to limit the risk of known latent effects, such as the development of leukemia (i.e. AML) and infertility.
- HD sample combinations—MOPP (Nitrogen Mustard, Oncovin [vincristine], procarbazine, and prednisone); COPP (cyclophosphamide, Oncovin, procarbazine, prednisone); ABVD (Adriamycin, bleomycin, vinblastine, dacarbazine) and other derivatives of these combinations; etoposide has been increasingly incorporated into treatment regimens to reduce gonadal toxicity.
- NHL sample combinations—CHOP (cyclophosphamide, doxorubicin, vincristine, prednisone; MACOP-B (methotrexate, doxorubicin, cyclophosphamide, vincristine, bleomycin, prednisone)

Radiation Treatment Borders

Hodgkin

- Traditional total-nodal irradiation (stage I and II)—the contiguous lymphatic chains irradiated, which included the supradiaphragmatic lymph nodes to the anterior and posterior fields called the *mantle field*; mantle includes the following lymph nodes: submandibular, occipital, cervical, supraclavicular, infraclavicular, axillary, hilar and mediastinal areas; borders include:
- Anterior—superior border is at the inferior portion of mandible
  - Inferior—is at the level of insertion of diaphragm (T10)
  - Posterior—the superior border includes the occipital nodes and the inferior border is the same as it is anteriorly (T10)
  - Laterally—axilla nodes are included
  - Blocking is extremely important—
    - Lungs (AP/PA), but inclusive of adequate margin
    - Humeral heads blocked
    - Larynx block anteriorly unless bulky disease adjacent
    - Cord block posteriorly, dependant on total dose
    - Heart—cardiac silhouette treated to 15 Gy; block to apex of heart thereafter; at 30 to 35 Gy add a subcarinal block (5 cm inferior to the carina)
- Mantle field (Figure 9-26)—patient is supine with arms akimbo (elbows bent) and hands on the hips or above head; chin must be extended as much as possible to prevent exposure to mouth from exit dose of posterior field; treatment in posterior field forces the

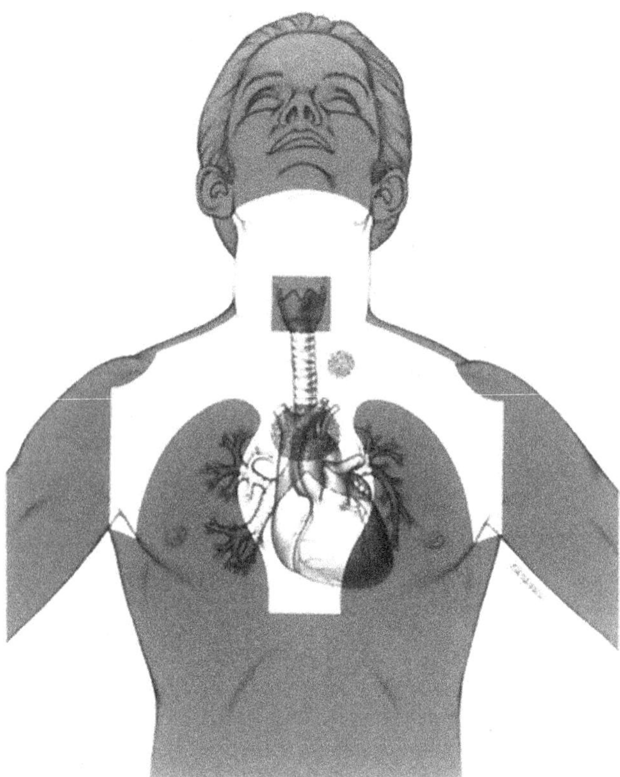

FIGURE 9-26 Mantle field for treatment of Hodgkin disease.

chin superiorly and eliminates the exit dose to the oral cavity; body molds are helpful for these treatments.

- Followed by the AP/PA subdiaphragmatic lymph nodes including the paraaortic nodes and the spleen (or splenic pedicle if spleen was removed); the combination of the mantle and *paraaortic fields* are referred to as extended field irradiation (Figure 9-27).
- Total nodal irradiation would refer to treatment of the pelvic, retroperitoneal, and inguinal nodes in addition to supradiaphragmatic and subdiaphragmatic nodes.
- Today, standard treatment for Hodgkin is the ABVD regimen alone or in combination with radiation (30 to 36 Gy) to just the involved lymph node region (Figure 9-28).

Radiation Treatment

Non-Hodgkin

- Non-Hodgkin lymphomas vary in comparison to that of Hodgkin
- Very sensitive to radiation
- Are much more lethal

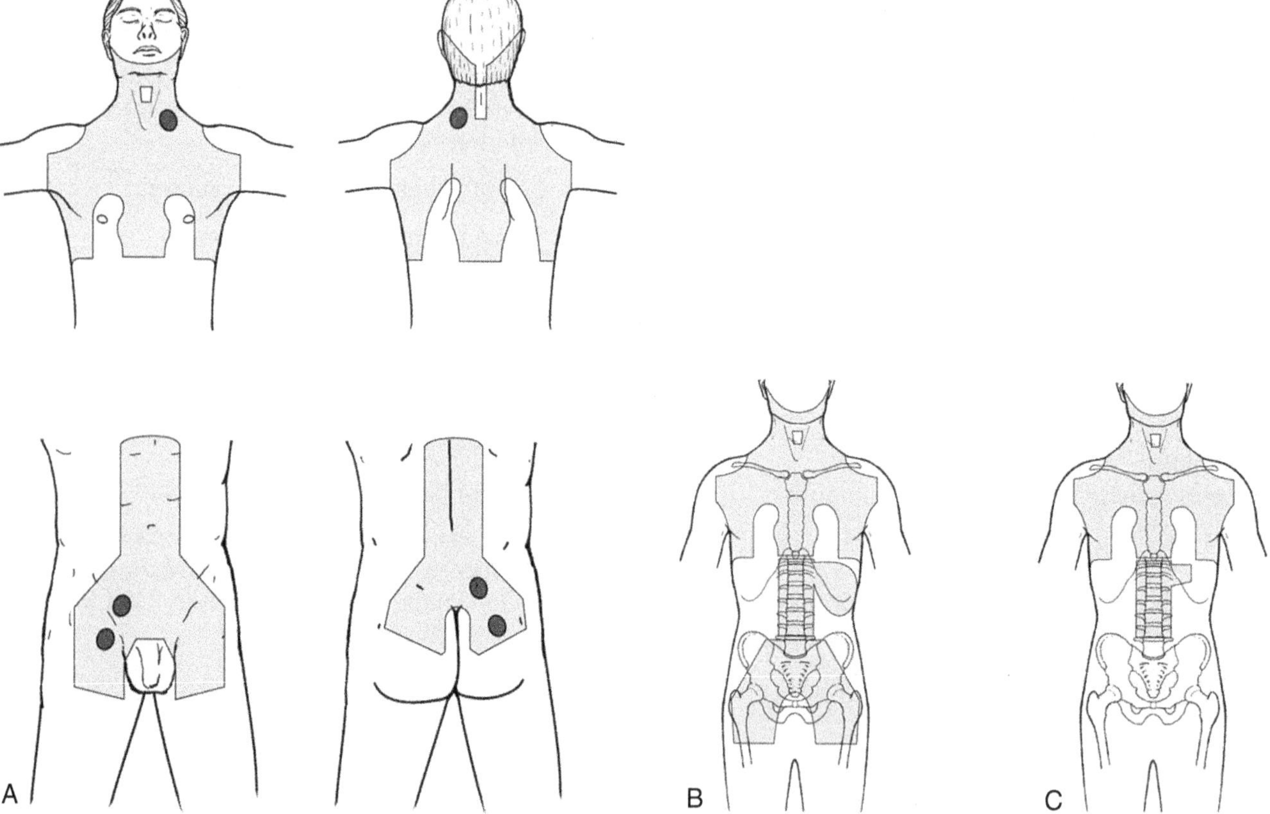

FIGURE 9-27 Extended field irradiation.

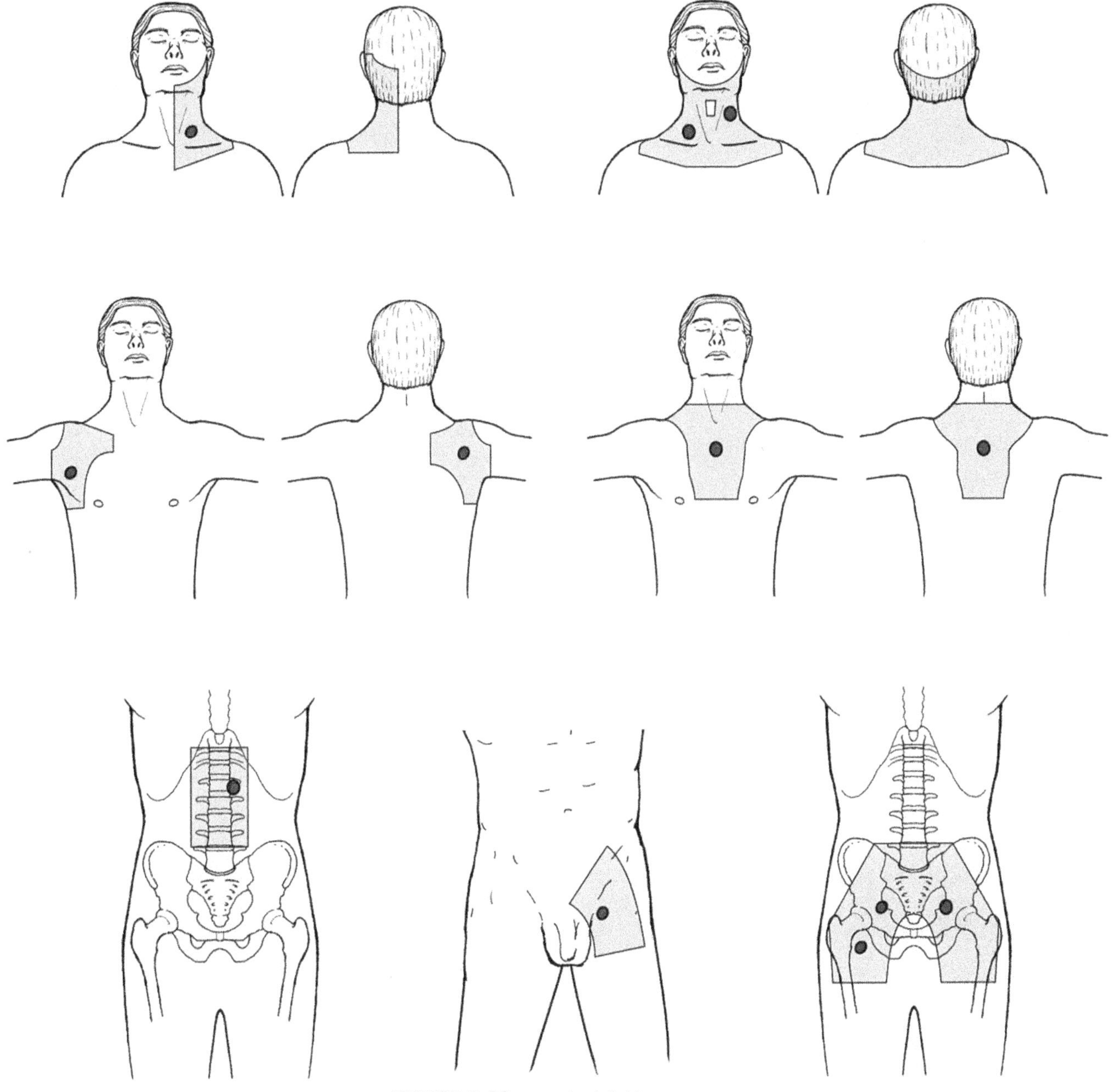

FIGURE 9-28 Involved field treatment.

- Treated with both radiation to involved site (and draining nodal groups on the same side of the diaphragm) and chemotherapy for systemic treatment
- 35 to 45 Gy suggested for local control
- Radiation and chemotherapy will vary due to staging of disease
- CNS and gastric lymphomas in NHL is about 60 times more common in patients with AIDS than general population
- GI tract lymphomas are the most common of the extranodal lymphomas

Treatment Delivery and Side Effect Management

Hodgkin. Acute side effects dependent upon field size and area treated:

- Fatigue
- Occipital hair loss (may be permanent)
- Skin erythema
- Sore throat (esophagitis)
- Altered taste (with preauricle nodes)

- Transient dysphagia from radiation-induced esophagitis
- Dry cough
- Nausea
- Occasional vomiting
- Diarrhea (rare)

Side effects are managed by advising:

- Antiemetics
- Nongreasy skin creams
- Protection from sunlight
- Rest
- Altered diet (soft bland foods, no alcohol)
- Throat lozenges
- Diarrhea medication or low residue diet

Non-Hodgkin

- **Side effects dependent on area treated**
  - If mouth and neck treated—
    - Dry mouth
    - Difficulty swallowing
    - Loss of appetite
    - Mucositis
    - Mouth sores
    - A *Candida* infection
    - Altered taste
    - Redness of skin
    - Sore throat
    - Hair loss
    - Transient dysphagia from esophagitis
    - Dry cough
  - If abdomen treated—
    - Nausea and vomiting
    - Fatigue

When Delivering Therapy:

- Pay attention to abutting fields and the importance of blocking critical structures, such as the liver, spine, and kidneys
- Abutting fields will likely call for periodic feathering of field junctions
- Closely monitor blood counts especially when large amounts of bone marrow are irradiated
- Communication is most critical in helping your patient maintain good nutrition and electrolyte balance when large amounts of GI are involved in the radiation field
- Pediatric patients will need special considerations; take time getting acquainted; allow parents to participate, encourage and observe; encourage young patients to be creative about dealing with changes in physical appearance and any interruptions to their normal routine

LYMPHOMA REVIEW EXERCISES

1. List the components and major functions of the lymphatic system.

2. List the three basic types of blood cells and their functions.

3. What are the two types of lymphocytes that participate in adaptive immune responses?

4. What are the smallest vessels of the lymphatic system, which are located in the spaces between ells?

5. Explain the flow of the lymph.

6. Which lymphatic vessels empty into the cisterna chyli, and which duct receives lymph from the cisterna chyli?

7. What happens to foreign substances in lymph that enter a lymph node?

8. Lymph flows through a node in one direction entering ______ lymphatic vessels and flowing out by way of ______ lymphatic vessel.

9. What is the purpose of the spleen?

10. If a spleen is removed, which other organs take over some of the functions of the spleen?

11. How do lymphatic vessels differ in structure from veins?

12. What is the role of the thymus in immunity?

13. The largest single mass of lymphatic tissue in the body is:

a. Liver
b. Spleen
c. Bone marrow
d. Thymus

14. Which of the following is not considered a tonsil?

a. Pharyngeal
b. Palatine
c. Lingual
d. Vallecula

15. Which of the following organs atrophies after puberty?

a. Thymus
b. Thyroid
c. Spleen
d. Liver

16. B cells mature in which of the following?

a. Thymus
b. Bone marrow
c. Spleen
d. Liver

17. The lymphatic system consists of:

1. Fluid
2. Vessels
3. Arteries
4. Organs
5. Nodes

a. 1, 2, 3
b. 2, 3, 4. 5
c. 1, 2, 4, 5
d. 1, 2, 3, 4, 5

18. Lymph nodes are what length?

a. 4 to 6 cm
b. 10 to 15 cm
c. 1 to 25 mm
d. 2 to 4 in

19. The thymus gland functions in immunity by producing:

a. Blood
b. T cells
c. B cells
d. C cells

20. Which of the following might describe non-Hodgkin lymphoma?

1. Originates in lymph nodes or in extranodal tissue
2. Most likely to spread randomly
3. Commonly arising in GI tract

a. 1, 2
b. 2, 3
c. 1, 3
d. 1, 2, 3

21. The thoracic duct is the main collecting duct of the lymphatic system and begins in the:

a. Suprasternal notch
b. Cisterna chyli
c. Inguinal areas
d. T-12

22. Seventy-five percent of all Hodgkin disease will have:

a. Lymphocytic predominance
b. Lymphocytic depletion
c. Nodular sclerosis
d. Mixed cellularity

23. The most common presenting symptom for Hodgkin disease is:

a. Abdominal mass
b. Painless axillary node enlargement
c. Painless cervical node enlargement
d. Painless inguinal node enlargement
e. Mediastinal mass

24. A large binucleate or polynucleate cell present for a diagnosis of Hodgkin is referred to as:

a. Ann Arbor cell
b. Reed-Sternberg cell
c. Thomas Hodgkin cell
d. Epstein-Barr cell

25. Classification for staging of lymphomas is traditionally:

a. TNM
b. Ann Arbor
c. Duke classification
d. AJC

Staging of lymphomas may also include the following letters denoting organ. (MATCH)

26. S ____	A. marrow
27. H ____	B. lung
28. L ____	C. liver
29. M ____	D. spleen
30. P ____	E. osseous
31. O ____	F. skin
32. D ____	G. pleura

33. T or F
Irradiation is the primary treatment modality for the majority of patients with early stages of Hodgkin disease.

34. A 23-year-old male patient has an enlarged cervical lymph node. Diagnostic workup reveals positive mediastinal and axillary nodes as well.
Based on this information, the patient would be Stage:

a. I
b. I E
c. II
d. II E

35. Staging for Hodgkin disease also includes an A-B grouping. Which symptom is not one of the classical B symptoms?

a. Profuse night sweats
b. Weight loss greater than 10% of body weight
c. Unexplained fever above 38° C
d. Unexplained pruritus

36. In Hodgkin disease, involvement of several nodal regions of both sides of the diaphragm accompanied by localized involvement of an extralymphatic site is stage:

a. II
b. II E
c. III
d. III E

37. In the treatment fields of Waldeyer ring for non-Hodgkin lymphoma, the fields' delineation closely resembles that of carcinoma of the:

a. Supraclavicular fossa nodes
b. Orbit
c. Pelvis
d. Nasopharynx

38. Which lymph node groups are treated in a mantle field?

a. Mediastinal
b. Axillary
c. Both a and b
d. Neither a nor b

39. Which of the following are common side effects of radiation therapy to the abdomen?

1. Nausea
2. Vomiting
3. Fatigue

a. 1 only
b. 2 only

c. 3 only
d. 1, 2, and 3

40. T or F
Non-Hodgkin lymphoma (NHL) differ in a couple of ways from Hodgkin (HD), one is that it occurs primarily in older persons.

41. T or F
NHL is most likely to spread randomly, rather than orderly as HD does.

42. A young woman has swelling in her lower neck for suspected HD. A chest x-ray also revealed mediastinal adenopathy. She had not experienced any fever, night sweats, or weight loss. Staging would likely be:

a. I A
b. II A
c. II B
d. III A

43. The most favorable of the four subtypes of Hodgkin disease is:

a. Lymphocytic predominance
b. Nodular sclerosis
c. Mixed cellularity
d. Lymphocyte depletion

44. NHL may arise in:

1. Lymph nodes
2. Gastrointestinal tract
3. Waldeyer ring

a. 1 only
b. 1, 2
c. 1, 3
d. 1, 2, 3

45. In NHL, lymphocytes pathologically arrange themselves in pattern(s) called:

a. Follicular
b. Nodular
c. Both a and b
d. Neither a nor b

46. The optimal dose to the mantle field:

a. 2000-3500 cGy
b. 3000 cGy
c. 3500-4400 cGy
d. 5000-6500 cGy

47. Which nodes are included in the inverted Y field?

1. Retroperitoneal
2. Common iliac
3. Inguinal
4. Popliteal

a. 1, 2
b. 2, 3, 4
c. 1, 2, 3
d. 1,2, 3, 4

48. Radiation carditis is a chronic side effect after irradiation to the mantle field; this is inflammation of the:

a. Pharynx
b. Heart
c. Lung
d. Axilla

49. Transient dysphagia is an acute side affect after irradiation for Hodgkin. Dysphagia is:

a. Difficulty breathing
b. Difficulty swallowing
c. Discomfort to stomach
d. Difficulty urinating

50. When extremely large fields are treated (as is mantle and paraaortics) above and below the diaphragm, an appropriate separation must be left between the fields:

a. Shrinking field
b. Gap
c. Algebraic formula
d. Geometric formula

PEDIATRICS

GENERAL FACTS AND EPIDEMIOLOGY

- Males have higher incidence
- Treatment varies by site but requires multidisciplinary approach because of late effects
- Multidisciplinary approach is appropriate since long-term, disease-free survival is intended; single

management modalities would be so intense that the late effects (Table 9-17) would outweigh the benefit of cure

- Surgeries are typically conservative to preserve limbs and function
- Cancer is the No. 2 killer of children; accidents are No. 1
- Since children have not had time to accumulate adverse affects of poor diets, chemical exposures and other carcinogenic situations, the study of pediatric cancers has given the opportunity to explore certain genetic/chromosomal abnormalities
- Approximately 66% of children survive their cancer
- Young children will require sedation and elaborate immobilization
- Older children through young adults need special age-appropriate considerations; Table 9-18 lists some age-appropriate considerations for pediatric patients

Neuroblastomas

- Originates in the neural crest cells of the sympathetic nervous system
- Most common in infants, most younger than 5 years old
- Younger than 2 years old tend to have localized disease
- May be linked to abnormal maturation of fetal neural crest cells
- A unique characteristic is that it has been known to spontaneously regress

Clinical Presentation

- Symptoms and signs depend on location (Table 9-19)
- Can show up anywhere along the sympathetic nerve chain

TABLE 9-17 Long-Term Side Effects of Radiation and Chemotherapy

Radiation	Chemotherapy
Cataracts, impaired growth, impaired cognition, abnormal dentition, hypoplasia of bone, hypothyroidism, lung fibrosis, pericardial thickening, secondary cancers, hypoplasia of abdominal and pelvic organs	Myocardial damage, lung fibrosis, infertility, sterility, leukemia, hearing impairment, liver and/or kidney dysfunction, impaired cognition, peripheral neuropathy

TABLE 9-18 Age Appropriate Considerations for Pediatric Patients

Age Group	Care Considerations
Toddlers	Very attached to their parents but beginning to assert some independence; can communicate in 2- to 3-word sentences; use familiar names; talk in calming tones; allow parents to come along
Preschoolers 3-5 yr	Conversational and have increased independence; can cooperate but may be fearful, so ask them to participate; be honest, use terms they understand and analogies; do not punish them for crying or wanting to retreat
School age 6-12 yr	Can think logically about concrete things; be specific and honest; use demonstration to explain procedures
Adolescent 13-18 yr	Greater emotional needs; modesty and privacy important; show empathy, keep in mind they fear threats to their physical appearance; establish rapport by having general conversations about what they like or do in their free time

TABLE 9-19 Neuroblastoma Symptoms

Localized	Disseminated
Chest: cough, dyspnea	Fever, weight loss, malaise, fatigue
Neck: Swelling	Bluish skin nodules
Pelvis: bowel or bladder changes	Rapid liver enlargement
Brain: Uncontrolled eye movements, mental retardation	Lytic bone lesions with pain

Lymphatic Drainage and Spread Patterns

- Metastasis may be to the skin, liver, and bone marrow

Workup

- Physical examination
- Chest x-ray
- Urine sampling
- CT abdomen, chest, and pelvis
- MRI
- X-rays of bone
- Bone marrow biopsy for suspected metastasis

Staging

- Evan and D'Angio stage I-IV
- Pediatric oncology group stage A-D
- International system stage 1-4

Treatment

- Very sensitive to radiation and chemotherapy
- Local disease is usually managed with surgery alone
- Complete or partial resections are followed by multiagent chemotherapy (cyclophosphamide, doxorubicin, etoposide, cisplatin)
- Radiation often given in late stage disease; 1000 cGy for palliation, 2000 to 3000 cGy to region of residual disease following surgery
- Survival favorable with intensive management, such as multi-agent chemotherapy and/or bone marrow transplants
- Radioimmunotherapy being investigated with I^{131}

Radiation Treatment Borders

- Total body radiation (TBI) therapy in the setting of bone marrow transplant preparation
- For hepatomegaly or primary mass palliation, fields are limited to the mass or liver with margin

Treatment Delivery

- TBI requires complex dosimetric calculations
- Patient may be positioned standing or semirecumbent with knees bent up toward chest or lying supine at an extended treatment distance
- This age group suitable for supine position at extended distance
- Even dose distribution is of great concern so tissue compensators made with rice bags or gelatin may be placed at thinner areas such as the lower extremities and neck
- Arms bent along chest could compensate for low density lung tissue from the lateral aspect
- Care to keep doses low to lens using lens shields and lungs, using specially fabricated blocks
- Local, palliative fields are likely arrangements for reduced dose to neighboring tissues and beam shaping
- TBI would incur complex treatment charges
- Local fields would incur various levels of charges depending on field arrangement and beam modification

NEPHROBLASTOMA (WILMS' TUMOR)

- Occurs mostly between 2 to 5 years old; median age 3
- Genetics is a risk factor, so may manifest sporadically
- Multiple genitourinary abnormalities increase risk
- Treatment very successful, overall cure rate is more than 80%
- Arises in embryonal kidney cells
- Can contain renal tubular, glomerular, and connective tissue elements
- Highly anaplastic, clear cell sarcomas and rhabdoid tumors are unfavorable histologies

Clinical Presentation

- Abdominal mass
- Hypertension
- Hematuria (microscopic most frequent)
- Recurrent urinary tract infections

Lymphatic Drainage and Spread Patterns

Usually infiltrate the kidney capsule to adjacent structures then through the blood; renal hilar, paraaortic nodes are commonly positive at diagnosis; distant metastasis to lung, brain, or bone

Workup

- Physical examination
- Abdominal ultrasound
- CBC, urinalysis
- IVP
  - CT
  - Liver/kidney function
  - Chest x-ray for suspected metastasis
  - Blood serum to check for elevated lactate dehydrogenase (LDH)

Staging

- National Wilms' Tumor Study (NWTS) uses stages I-V; stage V indicates bilateral kidney involvement.

Treatment

- Surgery is nearly always the first step with careful exploration of the opposite kidney and lymph nodes.
- Chemotherapy and radiation can be used to debulk the tumor before surgery.
- Radiation can be used adjuvantly to prevent local recurrence to tumor bed and associated areas of residual disease; dose ranges from 10 to 40 Gy.
- Chemotherapy includes actinomycin-D and vincristine.

Radiation Treatment Borders

- Irradiation to the tumor bed defined by presurgery imaging or surgical placement of radiopaque markers
- The whole abdomen is treated in those with peritoneal seeding or tumor rupture before or during surgery; dose 10 to 12 Gy.
- Paraaortic nodes should be included with the entire width of the spine to avoid scoliosis.
- Boosts may be used for residual disease.

Treatment Delivery

- Need beam shaping to protect bowel and normal kidney
- Patient positioned supine using immobilization appropriate for age; arms up for easy triangulation
- Parallel opposed fields to avoid opposite kidney
- Sedated children will be accompanied by parents, nursing, and/or respiratory care staff, respiratory staff; be prepared to educate parents and accompanying staff
- Low dose so likely skin reactions minimal

RHABDOMYOSARCOMA

- Arises from embryonal mesenchyme, with potential for differentiating into skeletal muscle
- Most common pediatric soft tissue tumor
- Can arise almost anywhere in the body where striated muscle or mesenchymal tissue is located
- Can invade and spread quickly
- Age group 5 to 14 years
- About 40% are younger than 5 years old
- Incidence in U.S. Caucasian:African American is 4.4:1.3
- Histologic subtypes embryonal, alveolar, pleomorphic

Clinical Presentation

- Painful mass
- Swelling
- Limitation of function
- Obstruction
- Discomfort

Lymphatic Drainage and Spread Patterns

- Spread varies with histologic type but usually local (from muscle insertion to insertion) then through blood or regional lymphatics

Workup

- X-rays
- CT
- MRI
- Myelogram to check for CNS involvement
- CBC
- Liver function
- Bone marrow biopsy

Staging

- International Rhabdomyosarcoma Studies (IRS) system used "grouping" based on extent of disease at time of treatment; stages I-IV; later a TNM system based on International Union Against Cancer was developed to reflect disease characteristics including grade

Treatment

- Surgery is always in order.
- Complete resection versus gross resection is influenced by the site, cosmetic effect, and function (i.e., orbit RT to tumor and margin and surgery avoided).
- Those staged at II or above may require radiation in the range of 40 to 50 Gy, conventional or hyperfractionation protocols—60 Gy
- Multiagent chemotherapy is always in order as well (vincristine, actinomycin D, cyclophosphamide, etoposide, ifosfamide, doxorubicin, melphalan).

Radiation Treatment Borders

- Concentrate on sparing lymphatic vessels (preserve a strip of soft tissue) and ends of bones to retain relative bone growth to extremities; RT to tumor and margin
- Complex planning required to ensure that extensively infiltrating tumors have sufficient margins while growth plates are spared
- Total dose ranges influenced by patient age and size of tumor
- Most desirable to include the entire muscle compartments in extremities with several shrinking fields
- Abdominal tumors also require multiple shrinking fields

Treatment Delivery

- Hyperfractionation protocols incur complex charges; keep an eye on time intervals between doses
- Immobilization critical

- Positioning influenced by location
- For head and neck area, all positive lymph nodes should be irradiated
- CNS tumors only need 2 cm margin
- In pelvis, take care to shield femoral epiphyseal plates and proximal femur
- Extremities—regional lymph nodes only treated if they were found positive
- Low-dose lung radiation for pulmonary metastasis
- Patients receiving high dose need skin care education

EWING SARCOMA

- Arises in nonosseous portion (medullary canal) of the bone and occasionally in soft tissues
- If it arises in the canal, it may break through the cortex/periosteum forming a soft tissue mass
- The periosteum is a natural barrier for spread
- Has an onion skin appearance on x-ray
- Age range 5 months to 60 years with peak incidence between 11 and 17
- Most common bone tumor in children younger than 10 years old
- Tumor is rare in children younger than 5 years old
- Primarily occurs in large, long bones and bones in the pelvis

Clinical Presentation

- Bone pain
- Tenderness, swelling
- Neurologic abnormalities if spine/nerves are compressed
- Weight loss, fatigue
- Fever

Lymphatic Drainage and Spread Patterns

- May spread through the blood to the lung, bone, lymph nodes, and CNS

Workup

- MRI
- CT
- Chest x-ray
- Bone marrow biopsy
- Lumbar puncture
- CBC
- Kidney and liver function
- LDH serum

Staging

- No accepted system has been adopted; tumors are classified as localized or disseminated

Treatment

- Surgery for biopsy
- Surgery for tumor resection is determined by location, extent, cosmesis, and function
- Ewing very chemosensitive (vincristine, cyclophosphamide, doxorubicin, ifosfamide)
- Chemotherapy is likely the induction then followed by radiation/surgery
- Radiation for local control of primary or sites of metastasis
- If tumor extends or is near the meninges, prophylactic radiation to CNS is good

Radiation Treatment Borders

- Keep a margin of soft tissue for lymphatic drainage preservation
- Entire bone with shrinking fields to decrease chances of bone growth retardation
- Need many field reductions; total 55 to 60 Gy
- Controversy on sparing one end of the bone when lesion is centrally located in bone

Treatment Delivery

- Position depends on location
- Extremities need to be positioned away from opposite limb and body
- Reliable immobilization is critical
- Keep an eye on multiple cone down doses
- Parallel opposed fields with beam shaping and modifiers such as bolus to increase dose to surgical scar
- Dry and wet desquamation expected at doses at high range
- Educate patient and parents on skin care

MEDULLOBLASTOMA

- One of the most common pediatric CNS primaries; close to low grade astrocytomas
- Peak age 5 to 8 years old; another peak 20 to 30 years old

- Male:female ratio is 2:1
- Comes from primitive neuroepithelial cells of the cerebellum
- Usually detected in the fourth ventricle and expands causing obstruction of cerebral spinal fluid (CSF) circulation
- CSF obstruction causes hydrocephalus
- High potential for CNS spread

Clinical Presentation

- Specific symptoms depend on location of tumor
- Hydrocephalus may occur with nausea, vomiting, changes in level of consciousness

Lymphatic Drainage and Spread Patterns

- No lymphatics in the CNS but spread likely throughout the CNS in circulating spinal fluid

Workup

- CT
- MRI
- Neurologic assessment
- Biopsy
- Lumbar puncture (avoid puncture if intracranial pressure increased)

Staging

- TGM for tumor, grade, and metastasis through the CNS

Treatment

- Surgical resection, even if not total, could restore CSF flow.
- For children younger than 2, radiation is avoided and intense chemotherapy is given (cisplatin, vincristine).
- Chemotherapy is last resort or used for those with unfavorable prognostic factors; blood-brain barrier presents an obstacle.
- Have to use lipophilic agents, local therapy (directly into the tumor or intrathecal)
- Lipophilic agents are the nitrosoureas.
- New drugs have recently been developed with promise of crossing the blood-brain barrier.
- Certain drugs may render the brain and tumor capillaries more porous and penetrable.
- Radiation is the most important postsurgical treatment.
- Radiation doses to total 54 Gy to posterior fossa/tumor bed

Radiation Treatment Borders

- Whole brain with lower border at C2 for margin on the fourth ventricle; total dose 35 Gy
- Entire spinal compartment from C2 to S2 to cover all circulating spinal fluid; total dose 24 Gy
- Boost posterior fossa with opposed lateral fields with an extra 10 to 20 Gy

Treatment Delivery

- Treatment of entire spinal axis requires careful field matching/skin gaping.
- Beam geometry will require use of collimation, couch rotation to prevent overlap.
- Match points should be moved during treatment course; every 3 to 5 days the match point should be moved (feathered).
- Patients positioned prone with arms at sides in immobilization at least covering head to pelvis
- Treatment charges will be complex.
- Be prepared to counsel patient and family on skin care as hair loss, dry desquamation likely

RETINOBLASTOMA

- Most common intraocular tumor in children but occurs rarely
- Small blue cell of neuroectodermal origin
- Occurs in children 6 months to 4 years
- Hereditary pattern has been observed
- 65% are unilateral

Clinical Presentation

- Abnormal retinal light reflex (white rather than red)
- Visual abnormalities

Lymphatic Drainage and Spread Patterns

- Lymphatics not typically involved, local extension into sinus or brain

Workup

- No biopsy; risk of severe bleeding is too great
- CT

- Bone marrow biopsy
- Lumbar puncture

Treatment

- Good response to chemotherapy
- Radiation has been the classic way to manage
- Cryotherapy may provide local control
- Total enucleation leads to almost certain cure while sacrificing the globe
- Radioactive plaques of cobalt of iodine possible; can deliver 40 to 60 Gy in a week
- Cure rates with plaques is greater than 80% with visual preservation

Radiation Treatment Borders

- Real challenge to treat retina and spare the cornea and lens
- AP and lateral field with hanging lens block; 3-D conformal therapy ideal, no lymphatics included

Treatment Delivery

- Dose 180 to 300 cGy per fraction to total 4000 cGy
- May hypofractionate; must consider under growth of facial bones
- Fields are small, need reliable head immobilization
- Watch margin on opposite orbit and lens
- 90-degree pair likely will need wedges with minimal field shaping
- Use of wedges incur complex treatment charges

PEDIATRIC REVIEW EXERCISES

1. When treating the tumor bed for Wilms tumor, care should be taken to include the entire width of the spine to prevent:

   a. Scoliosis
   b. Bowel obstruction
   c. Pericardial thickening
   d. Lung fibrosis

2. Which of the following is *not* an associated risk factor for pediatric solid tumors?

   a. Parasites
   b. Environment
   c. Ionizing radiation
   d. Prenatal factors

3. The most common symptom of Wilms' tumor is:

   a. Hematuria
   b. Pain
   c. Abdominal mass
   d. Nocturia

4. Nephroblastomas metastasize most commonly to the:

   a. Bone
   b. Lung
   c. Liver
   d. Brain

5. Neuroblastomas originate in the:

   a. Neural crest tissue
   b. Kidney
   c. Ventricles
   d. Bone

6. Which of the following primary brain tumors typically spreads to the cerebrospinal fluid (CSF)?

   a. Medulloblastoma
   b. Craniopharyngioma
   c. Teratoma
   d. Astrocytoma

7. The most common symptom of Ewing sarcoma is:

   a. Weight loss
   b. Neurologic abnormalities
   c. Pain
   d. Fever

8. The most frequent orbital malignancy in children is:

   a. Retinoblastoma
   b. Lymphoma
   c. Rhabdomyosarcoma
   d. Osteoblastoma

9. Wilms' tumors originate from what cell type?

   a. Neuroblasts
   b. Nephroblasts
   c. Nephroclasts
   d. None of the above

10. Which type of childhood cancer is mostly associated with *prophylactic* irradiation of the CNS?

    a. Ewing sarcoma
    b. Wilms' tumor

c. Retinoblastoma
d. Acute lymphocytic leukemia

11. Stem cell transplantation is successful in treating childhood cancers such as ALL. Transplanted blood cells may come from a compatible donor, the patient, or an identical twin. Match the following:

____ **Allogeneic donor**	A. self
____ **Autologous donor**	B. compatible match
____ **Syngeneic donor**	C. Identical twin

12. The most important latent side effects from radiation therapy to the pediatric patient include (select two):

a. Impaired bone growth
b. Radiation-induced puberty
c. Secondary cancers
d. Epilation

13. An aggressive management for retinoblastoma is an enucleation. An enucleation is:

a. Surgical replacement of the orbit
b. Surgical placement of orbital prosthesis
c. Surgical removal of the orbit
d. Surgical removal of cataracts

14. When caring for preschool aged children, it is important to:

a. Be authoritative and firm
b. Make sure that they do not cry
c. Keep communications simple and honest
d. Allow them to have lots of choices

15. When caring for an adolescent, it is important to:

a. Be authoritative and firm
b. Make sure that they do not cry
c. Give them extra time for dressing and undressing
d. Acknowledge that modesty and privacy are paramount

16. Your 17-year-old Hodgkin disease patient is worried about not having her hair back in time for the prom. An acceptable response may be:

a. Do not worry about it, no one will be looking at your head
b. Beauty is in the eye of the beholder; forget what others say
c. I know someone you can speak with about some creative alternatives
d. Your hair should be back within 2 weeks following chemotherapy

Think About It

17. The entire spinal axis will be treated using whole brain fields with a field size 15 × 20 and spine field with field size 8 × 30 in your pediatric patient using a SAD technique, 6 MV beam. To avoid overlap at the field junction, table kicks will be used during treatment of the lateral brain fields. The SSD for both lateral fields is 93-cm SSD. Calculate the table kick.

18. Calculate the monitor units required for the lateral brain fields in the above case using the additional information below.

Prescription: 36 Gy in 24 fractions
Output/reference dose rate = 0.996 cGy/MU
Field shaping using MLC

Field size	Output factor for TAR
12^2	1.008
13^2	1.013
15^2	1.021
16^2	1.024
17^2	1.028

TAR table for 6 MV
Field size→

Depth ↓	12^2	13^2	15^2	16^2	17^2
3 cm	0.951	0.952	0.954	0.957	0.959
5 cm	0.890	0.892	0.894	0.896	0.897
7 cm	0.786	0.789	0.790	0.792	0.794
9 cm	0.773	0.775	0.776	0.779	0.810
11 cm	0.752	0.753	0.756	0.757	0.758

19. A similar case was planned during the previous week. The child was a tall, 12-year-old and his spine field was treated with a field area 8 × 48 cm at the skin. The limits of the collimator, on the 100-cm isocentric linear accelerator, is 40 × 40 cm. The minimum extended treatment distance for this case is:

a. 100 cm
b. 120 cm
c. 140 cm
d. 148 cm

20. The actual collimator setting for the above case would be:

a. 8.0 × 40
b. 5.0 × 40
c. 6.7 × 40
d. 6.7 × 35

SARCOMAS: PRIMARY BONE AND SOFT TISSUE

PRIMARY BONE

General Facts and Epidemiology

- Increased incidence in adolescent years and at around 60 years old
- Osseous and nonosseous cell types
- Most bone malignancies are metastatic (60% to 65%)
- Various types have different epidemiology
- Table 9-20 lists primary bone histologies and epidemiology

Etiology

- Radiation exposure
- Genetic disorders
- Viruses
- Development abnormalities

Clinical Presentation

Symptoms

- Pain
- Mass
- Swelling

TABLE 9-20 Primary Bone Histologies and Epidemiology

Histology	Epidemiology
Osteosarcoma	Adolescents and young adults
Chondrosarcoma	Over 50 years old; incidence increases with age
Fibrosarcoma/Malignant fibrous histiocytoma	Very rare; 6-81 years old; most older than 40
Round cell/Ewing sarcoma	Ewing occurs in childhood; age range 10-30 years old
Giant cell	Usually benign; shows up in the metaphysis or epiphysis of long bones in young adults
Multiple myeloma	Actually a blood malignancy originating in the bone marrow; elderly affected the most; solitary multiple myeloma known as plasmacytoma

- Fracture
- Compressed nerves
- Weight loss, fever associated with hypercalcemia (rare, except for Ewing)

Histology

- Fibrosarcoma
- Osteosarcoma
- Chondrosarcoma
- Ewing sarcoma
- Hemangiosarcoma
- Chordoma

Lymphatic Drainage and Spread Patterns

- Periosteum keeps primary bone tumors contained
- Lymphatics are not usually invaded
- Blood vessels are throughout the layers of the bone so spread is to distant sites via the blood route to the lung
- Any nodes found positive automatically puts the patient at stage III at the least
- Primary will spread along the bone

Workup

- X-ray
- CT
- MRI
- Nuclear bone scan

- White blood cell count
- Alkaline phosphatase
- Calcium levels
- Biopsy

Staging

- TNM staging; grading is included. Musculoskeletal Tumor Society (MSTS) has a recommended staging system that focuses on compartmental localization—bone, joints, skin, and subcutaneous tissues

Treatment

- Benign tumors are excised whenever possible.
- Bone grafts can fill spaces.
- Protective internal fixation may be necessary to maintain skeletal support.
- Conservation surgery option for all to avoid amputation; contraindicated if there is invasion of regional nerves, blood vessels, and/or pathologic fracture
- Surgery with an intralesional margin cuts into the primary and leaves some behind but is at least necessary for biopsy
- Surgical margins may be modest to wide (entire bone is taken with wide margin and prosthesis may follow).
- Surgery not recommended for plasmacytoma
- Radiation possible for benign lesions and those that cannot be resected or preserved for limb salvage; keep in mind radiation carcinogenesis possible for those young patients
- Chemotherapy for multiple myeloma, Ewing sarcoma, osteosarcoma, and histiocytic types

Radiation Treatment Borders

- Traditional radiation fields would begin large enough to cover the entire bone
- Due to normal tissue toxicity, wide margins such as 5 cm on either side of the primary is accepted (growth plates on one end may be spared to preserve growth in young patients)
- Only need margin on the bone
- If entire limb radiated, then fields will shrink after 20 Gy in the young
- If wide margins only include a portion of the bone, may shrink after 40 Gy in the adult
- Final boost field will conform to primary tumor

Treatment Delivery

- Total dose for primary tumors range from 50 to 70 Gy
- "Shrinking fields" watch out for field reductions
- Spare soft tissue and lymphatics to avoid chronic lymphedema
- Parallel opposed commonly used with as much soft tissue spared as possible
- Parallel-opposed with minimal field shaping may incur simple charges, although planning is complex with multiple field size changes
- Side effect expected is skin desquamation; be prepared to educate patient on skin care—avoid sun exposure, wash with water, no scratching or scrubbing

SOFT TISSUE SARCOMA

Etiology

- Direct cause is unknown
- Genetic and environmental factors such as previous radiation, herbicide exposure
- People with Von Recklinghausen disease, Li-Fraumeni syndrome at increased risk

Clinical Presentation

Symptoms

- Mass (usually painless)
- Joint pain
- Obstruction of blood flow (phlebitis)
- Weight loss

Histology. There are several histologic subtypes (Table 9-21):

- Liposarcomas
- Leiomyosarcomas
- Fibrosarcomas
- Synovial
- Malignant fibroblastic and histiocytic
- Rhabdomyosarcoma
- Neurofibrosarcoma

Lymphatic Drainage and Spread Patterns

- Spreads mainly by local invasion in a longitudinal direction within the muscle group where they originate

TABLE 9-21 Soft Tissue Sarcoma Histologies and Epidemiology

Histology	Epidemiology
Liposarcomas	Average age is 40-60 years; Seen mostly in lower extremities
Leiomyosarcomas	Commonly found in the GI, GU, along smooth muscles and vascular systems;
Fibrosarcomas	Seen mostly in ages 20-50 years old; special subtype known as Desmoid tumor
Synovial	Young adults; occur mostly in articular areas and tendon sheaths
Rhabdomyosarcoma	Seen in children 5-20 years old; occurs anywhere there is striated muscle; mostly in extremities
Kaposi sarcoma	Most common neoplasm occurring in people with AIDS; age group >50 years; of vascular origin but manifests as purplish lesions on the skin or mucosal surfaces; typically multifocal

- Usually no spread to lymph nodes except for synovial sarcoma
- Distant spread through blood to lung, bone, brain, liver

Workup

- CT
- MRI
- Soft tissue x-ray
- Bone scan
- CT guided core-needle biopsy

Staging

- AJCC and UICC has TNM system
- Grading is important
- If there are positive nodes, this is considered equivalent to a metastasis and takes precedence over the anatomic stage
- Initial invasion along local, anatomically defined planes

Treatment

- Surgery for biopsy at least; compartmentectomy takes the entire muscle compartment
- Total excision desired but consider cosmetic result and limb/organ function following surgery
- Goal is to preserve the muscle or limb so debulking may be the extent of surgery
- Chemotherapy may be used but still controversial
- Radiation helpful postoperatively; may also be beneficial preoperatively if tumor larger than 5 cm
- Radiation most appropriate for chest, limbs, and pelvis; harder to use for abdomen because of low tolerance tissue in the abdomen
- Brachytherapy would involve placement of catheters in the long axis of the extremity administering 45 Gy; if used as boost dose ranges from 16 to 30 Gy
- No accepted chemotherapy regimen; intraarterial chemotherapy being explored and isolated limb perfusion with chemotherapy also under investigation
- Radiation for pain relief, bleeding, or edema in Kaposi sarcoma; dose 30 Gy in 10 fractions or one single fraction of 8 Gy

Radiation Treatment Borders

- GTV plus 4-cm margin in the longitudinal aspect to 50 Gy; shrink to GTV plus 2-cm margin to final dose for preoperative radiation
- For postoperative, radiation then irradiate the limits of the excision including surface scar and drainage sites plus 4-cm margin to 50 Gy; shrink to final dose with 1-cm margin
- Lateral margins may vary by practice; range from 2 to 3 cm
- Fields should be shaped to preserve normal soft tissue and lymphatic vessels
- Brachytherapy remains within the limits of the surgical bed plus 2-cm margin
- In the abdominal area, margins are tighter; IMRT to restrict dose to low tolerance organs (kidneys, bowel)
- Palliative Kaposi fields very localized; electron therapy may be appropriate depending on location of lesions

Treatment Delivery

- Total doses may range from 50 Gy (abdomen and microscopic disease) to 80 Gy for extremities
- Total doses lower for abdominal tumors; 45 to 50 Gy
- High doses require elaborate treatment planning and will likely involve multiple ports at oblique angles, use of IMRT to spare normal soft tissues and bone marrow in adjacent bone
- Shrinking fields to spare normal tissue
- Expect skin desquamation at higher doses

- Charges incurred will likely be complex
- Patient position will need to be appropriate for site treated (Figures 9-29 and 9-30); objective is to isolate the soft tissue mass/tumor bed from adjacent tissues and achieve reproducibility; immobilization critical with alpha cradle, vac lock systems
- Lower extremities may need to be positioned reversed on PSA; table kicks may be necessary to execute treatment plan
- Extremities need to be positioned so that the beam's horizontal axis is parallel to the limb to maintain dose uniformity

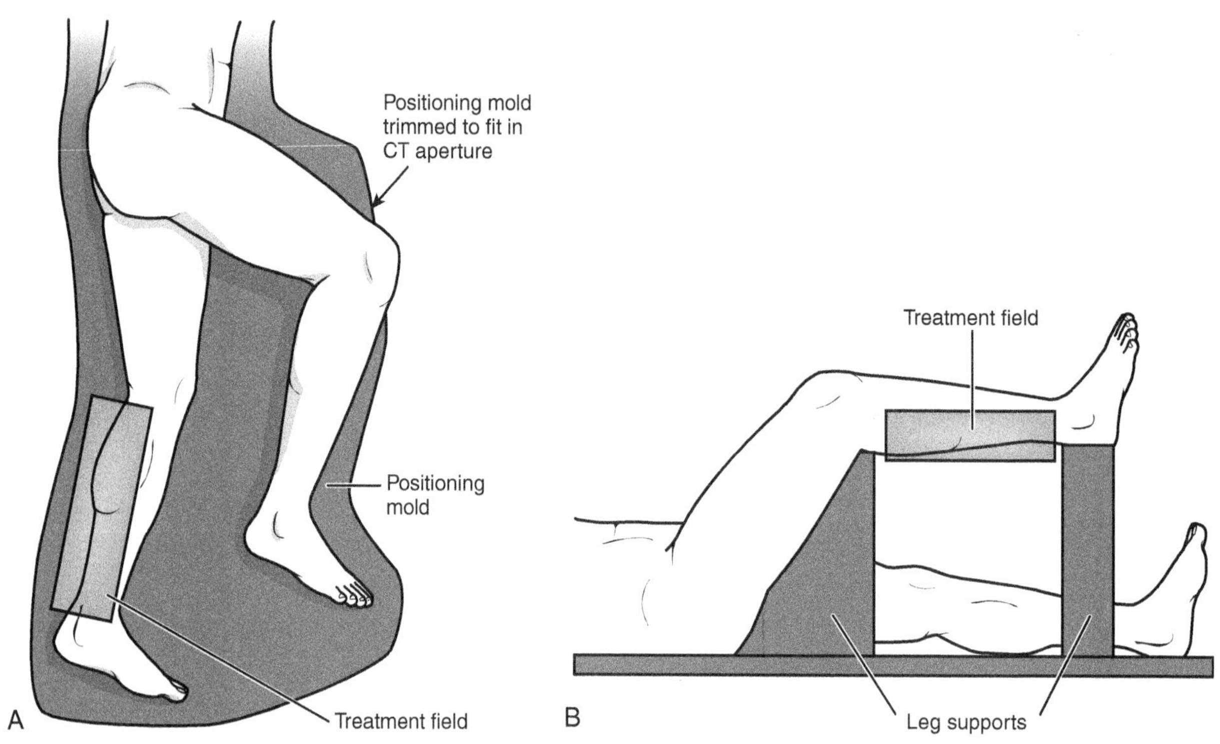

FIGURE 9-29 Potential positions for a tumor in the lower leg.

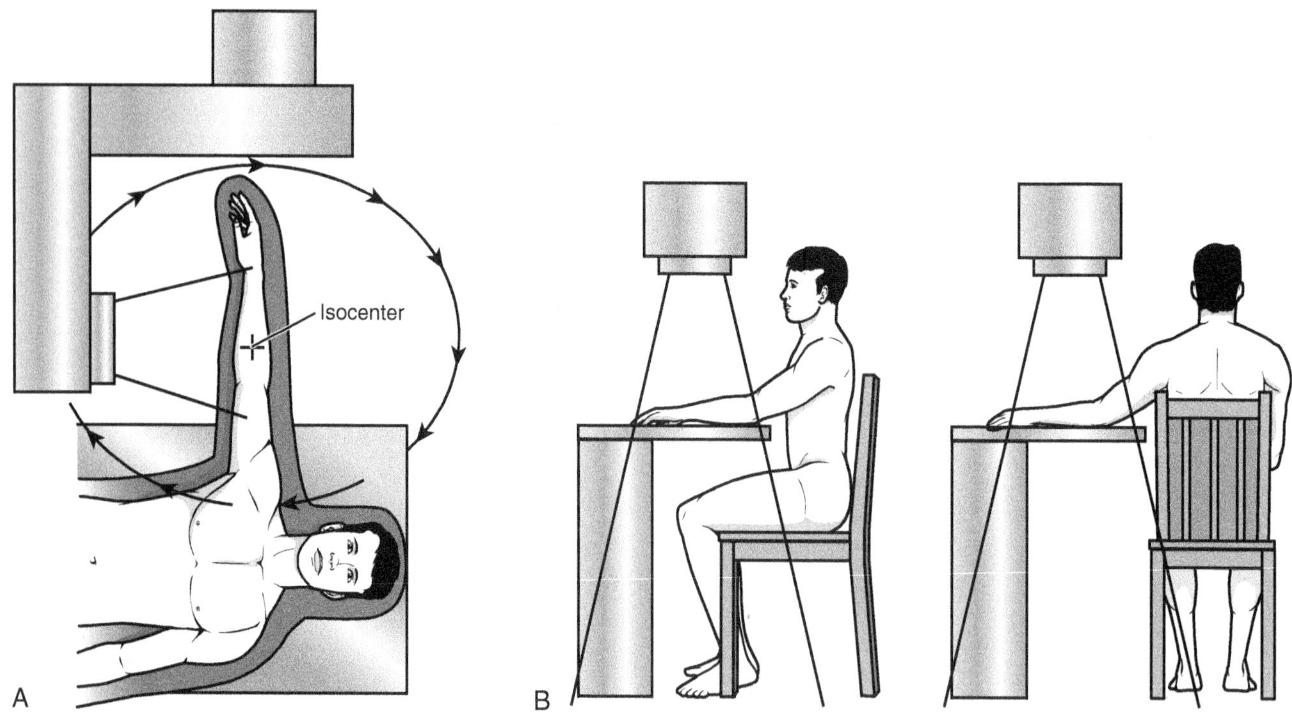

FIGURE 9-30 Potential positions for tumors in the forearm.

- Advise patient to protect skin from sun, no harsh soaps, decrease friction in the area, if wet desquamation keep clean and dry and open to the air whenever possible

SARCOMAS: PRIMARY BONE AND SOFT TISSUE REVIEW EXERCISES

Multiple Choice

1. Soft tissue sarcomas usually spread:

   a. Through several muscle compartments
   b. Locally, along the longitudinal muscle plane
   c. Locally, along the vascular supply in the muscle
   d. Toward the distal joint

2. When extremities are treated with radiation, it is important to spare:

   a. A strip of soft tissue to prevent obstruction of blood flow
   b. A strip of bone to prevent obstruction of lymph flow
   c. A strip of soft tissue to prevent obstruction of lymph flow
   d. A muscle compartment to prevent obstruction of blood flow

3. When treating a lower extremity, it is almost always necessary to position the patient:

   a. Reversed on the PSA with feet in toward the gantry
   b. Prone with arms above the head
   c. In the lateral position with both legs flat on the PSA
   d. In the supine position with both legs flat on the PSA

4. Sarcomas originate in the _______ tissue layer.

   a. Endoderm
   b. Mesoderm
   c. Ectoderm
   d. DuoDerm

5. A rhabdomyosarcoma is a malignant tumor arising from:

   a. Smooth muscle
   b. Glandular epithelium
   c. Striated muscle
   d. Mammary tissue

6. Liposarcomas originate in:

   a. Muscles
   b. Articular joints
   c. Tendons
   d. Fat

7. Primary osseous tumors metastasize to the lung via:

   a. Local invasion
   b. Seeding
   c. Lymphatics
   d. Blood

8. Limb salvaging surgery would include:

   a. Intralesional incision
   b. Wide margin excision with bone grafting
   c. Marginal margin excision with internal fixation
   d. All of the above

9. What feature would be present on an x-ray image of a lytic primary bone tumor?

   a. Increased density in the region of the tumor
   b. Decreased density in the region of the tumor
   c. Expansion of the boney compartment
   d. Expansion of the adjacent muscle

10. What is the likely explanation for weight loss and fever in the patient suspected to have primary bone cancer?

    a. Presence of the tumor causes infection and loss of appetite
    b. Presence of the tumor causes physiologic cachexia
    c. Presence of the tumor causes hypercalcemia
    d. Presence of the tumor causes hyperthyroidism

11. Radiation to the abdomen for soft tissue sarcomas in the peritoneum is limited by low tolerance organs such as the kidneys. The TD 5/5 for the whole kidney is:

    a. 45 Gy
    b. 37 Gy
    c. 23 Gy
    d. 10 Gy

12. A natural barrier for regional spread of primary bone tumors is the:

    a. Periosteum
    b. Articular cartilage

c. Endosteum
d. Medullary canal

13. Compact bone is arranged in concentric circle patterns known as:

a. Volkmann canals
b. Lacunae
c. Haversian systems
d. Lamellae

14. The area of spongy bone is found in the:

a. Diaphysis
b. Epiphysis
c. Medullary canal
d. Canaliculi

15. A solitary multiple myeloma tumor is known as a:

a. Plasmacytoma
b. Histiocytoma
c. Osteogenic sarcoma
d. Desmoid tumor

16. Which of the following has an onion skin appearance on x-ray?

a. Giant cell sarcoma
b. Ewing sarcoma
c. Histiocytic sarcoma
d. Chondrosarcoma

17. A common symptom for soft tissue tumors is:

a. Hemorrhage
b. Fracture
c. Painless mass
d. Palpable lymph nodes

18. The most common childhood bone cancer is:

a. Chondrosarcoma
b. Fibrosarcoma
c. Osteosarcoma
d. Ewing sarcoma

19. The most common primary bone cancer overall is:

a. Chondrosarcoma
b. Fibrosarcoma
c. Osteosarcoma
d. Ewing sarcoma

20. Kaposi sarcoma is the most common neoplasm in those diagnosed with:

a. Li Fraumeni syndrome
b. Von Recklinghausen disease
c. Epstein-Barr virus
d. AIDS

21. The primary treatment of choice for local control of soft tissue sarcomas located in the extremities is:

a. Surgery
b. Radiation therapy
c. Chemotherapy
d. Immunotherapy

22. The variables that are used for staging soft tissue sarcomas are:

1. Histologic grade
2. Tumor size
3. Regional lymph node involvement
4. Presence of distant metastases

a. 1, 4
b. 2, 3
c. 2, 3, 4
d. 1, 2, 3, 4

True/False

Place a T for true and F for false in the space provided, then correct false statements so that they are true without changing the intent of the original statement.

23. _______ Soft tissue sarcomas are relatively rare.

24. _______ Rhabdomyosarcoma is the most common primary orbital malignancy of childhood.

25. _______ Regional lymph nodes must be included in treatment ports for primary bone tumors.

Think About It

26. What possible positioning strategy could you use for a patient with a soft tissue sarcoma in the calf of the leg?

27. What possible positioning strategy could you use for a patient with a soft tissue sarcoma on the right flank?

28. How does Ewing sarcoma differ from osteosarcoma?

29. How do the total radiation doses differ for metastatic bone disease versus primary bone malignancy?

30. How do the field arrangements differ for metastatic bone disease versus primary bone malignancy?

PALLIATIVE CARE

GENERAL FACTS

- Plan of care should be individualized
- Patient's performance status should be considered (Karnofsky, level of function I-IV, ECOG status)
- Extent of disease must be established quickly; palliative care or emergent care is not always given during late-stage disease, exclusively
- Life expectancy will influence plan of care
- Previous treatments will influence plan of care
- Patient convenience and expense must be considered
- Short courses of radiation have demonstrated similar results as longer courses
- Duration of response, acute side effects, chronic complications, re-treatment rates and results must be considered

BRAIN METASTASIS

General Facts and Epidemiology

- Most common anatomic primary sites are breast and lung
- Metastasis from gastrointestinal or gynecologic regions are rare
- Melanoma has highest percentage of brain metastasis than any other primary cancer
- 40% of CNS tumors are metastatic
- Median survival is 3 months
- Favorable factors: Karnofsky greater than 70, absent or controlled primary, age less than 60 years, metastasis limited to brain

Clinical Presentation

- Headache
- Impaired cognition
- MRI can detect multiple lesions and meningeal involvement
- CT helpful also
- Lesions are usually multifocal
- Depending on location of tumor, can also see nausea, vomiting, somnolence, loss of speech, memory impairments, disturbed vision, disturbed hearing, motor impairment, personality changes

Workup

- CT
- MRI
- Neurologic assessment
- Cognitive and motor assessments

Treatment

- Surgery for single, isolated lesions
- Surgery if metastasis is to the cerebellum, causing severe ataxia
- Large cavitating lesions in the cerebrum are best removed

- Radiation may be combined with surgery and potentially doubles survival; see 70% to 90% symptom relief for those treated with radiation
- 20 Gy in 5 fractions yield similar results as 40 Gy in 20 fractions
- Whole brain radiation is intended to limit tumor progression and to limit the prolonged use of steroids
- Small, recurrent, single focus lesions may benefit from stereotactic radiosurgery with linac or gamma knife; no larger than 3 to 4 cm in size
- Single dose SRS can be 20 to 30 Gy
- Steroids can relieve symptoms alone within 48 hours
- Steroids improve neurologic function, but do not affect the length of response
- Anticonvulsants may also be beneficial

Radiation Treatment Borders

- Radiation treatment fields are typically opposed laterals
- Fields should cover the entire cranium
- Inferior border at the supraorbital ridge, through the external auditory meatus, and at the mastoid process
- If lesion is at the inferior portion of the temporal lobe, inferior border may be lowered with care to protect the lens of the eye

Treatment Delivery

- Physically support patients who have impaired ambulation to prevent falls
- Advise patients to refrain from driving and come accompanied to treatments
- Remind patients to use mild soap for hair washing or warm water only, protect head from the sun, take all medications as instructed; no razor shaving of the head
- Be prepared to handle seizures, syncope, dizziness
- Parallel opposed fields will likely call for simple positioning aids such as a neutral head rest and tape, or immobilizing masks are appropriate for patients with cognitive deficits or lowered levels of consciousness
- No field shaping and simple positioning aids incur billing charges
- Use of immobilizing masks and MLC to protect the orbits, lens, and sinuses advances to complex billing charges

INCREASED INTRACRANIAL PRESSURE (ICP)

General Facts and Epidemiology

- May be caused by primary tumors or metastatic tumors of the central nervous system
- Identified by expanding lesions in the brain causing pressure in the cranial compartment
- CNS hypoxia is the danger
- Brain shifts may lead to tentorial herniation and brain stem injury

Clinical Presentation

- Headache, nausea, and vomiting
- Blurred vision, diplopia impaired motor function
- Altered mental function
- Seizures, paralysis
- Difficulty speaking, writing

Workup

- CT, MRI
- Stereotactic biopsy
- Lumbar puncture should be avoided if disease is intracranial because a sudden shift in brain tissue can be fatal

Treatment

- Steroids initially for reduction of edema
- Anticonvulsants if seizures present
- Radiation for those with confirmed brain metastasis 30 Gy in 10 fractions
- Radiosurgery if solitary lesion
- Surgical resection if primary brain tumor suspected

Radiation Treatment Borders

- Standard whole brain
- Inferior border at the supraorbital ridge, through the EAM, and just below the mastoid process

Treatment Delivery

- Supine on neutral headrest or chin slightly flexed
- Immobilize with tape or mask depending on patient ability to cooperate

- Field size typically 21 × 18 for the adult; treated with lateral fields to midline
- Field is simple with no beam shaping; collimation to avoid lens, sinuses, and oral cavity incurs simple billing charges
- Be prepared to assist patients with motor difficulties
- Be prepared to handle seizure episodes
- Patients should always be accompanied
- Although short course, scalp alopecia and moderate dry desquamation expected
- No harsh shampoo, protect scalp from sunlight, no razor shaving to the scalp, no chemical processing of the hair

SPINAL CORD COMPRESSION

General Facts and Epidemiology

- Of 100 spinal cord compressions, only 60 will finish radiation; 20 will have disease progression; 20 will not be referred because of paraplegia or early death
- Tumors arising in or metastasizing to the bone may cause spinal cord compression
- Most commonly secondary to involvement of spinal column and anterior to spinal cord
- Less frequently posterior to cord and occasionally in epidural space
- Lung, breast, unknown primaries, lymphomas, myeloma, sarcoma, prostate, and kidney primaries are the frequent culprits
- Those ambulatory after treatment have median survival of 8 to 9 months; nonambulatory less than 1 month
- Less than 20% with paraplegia will ambulate again
- Compressions caused by lymphomas or myelomas have better prognosis

Clinical Presentation

- Specific symptoms depend on location
- Long-standing back pain
- Radiating pain from middle back to flank or from lower back to pelvis/lower extremities
- Weakness, sensory deficits, incontinence, urgency
- Paralysis
- Common site is the thoracic region

Workup

- MRI most informative; shows good contrast between bone and soft tissue
- Conventional x-ray can show blastic or lytic bone lesions, compression in the spinal cord space
- Neurologic assessment
- Look for elevated alkaline phosphatase

Treatment

- Emergency decompressive, stabilizing surgery especially for fracture dislocation of the spine, acute paraplegia, RT resistant tumors, or no steroid response
- Surgery may include laminectomy and placement of stabilizing rods
- Radiation at 30 Gy in 10 fractions *or* an initial 12 to 15 Gy in 3 fractions followed by 18 to 30 Gy in 6 to 15 fractions for a total of 45 Gy show similar results
- Steroids may relieve pain and improve symptoms
- Analgesics/narcotics until pain is under control
- Chemotherapy may help if the primary is chemosensitive

Radiation Treatment Borders

- Should include the entire vertebral body, spinous processes and cord, with at least one vertebral body above and below the compression
- Location of compression determines the field arrangement; cervical may be delivered posterior only or opposing laterals; thoracic typically posterior only; lumbar may be posterior or AP/PA for deeper section of lumbar spine

Treatment Delivery

- Give adequate support to regions of compression
- Patients may come with spine braces; if braces must be removed, do so with extreme care
- Slightest jerking or twisting may worsen compression and possibly lead to paralysis; avoid using shoulder retractors for cervical spine fields
- Prone position with head in neutral and arms at sides accommodates lateral cervical spine fields, thoracic and lumbar spine
- Avoid having the patient ambulate or transfer themselves from gurney to PSA

- Use assisted sheet lift methods or low impact sliding board methods
- Give skin care instructions as usual
- Regular pain assessment advised
- Pain should be adequately managed; if not, consult with attending physician or oncology nurse
- Treatment fields rarely need field shaping and incur simple charges

BONE METASTASIS

General Facts and Epidemiology

- 50% to 80% breast and prostate primary spread to bone
- 40% to 60% lung and Hodgkin lymphoma spread to bone
- 40% to 50% thyroid carcinomas spread to bone
- 30% to 50% renal cell carcinomas spread to bone
- Thoracic and lumbar spine most common location
- Pelvis is the second most common location
- Bone mets may also be seen in the skull, ribs, cervical spine, humerus, and femur
- Bone metastasis is the second most common cause of pathologic fracture after osteoporosis
- Life expectancy varies widely:

  Lung primary—3 months
  Breast primary—22 months
  Prostate primary—29 months

Clinical Presentation:

- Pain and impaired mobility
- Fracture
- Lytic or blastic lesions
- Neurologic symptoms from spinal cord compression

Workup

- MRI
- Conventional x-ray
- Nuclear bone scan
- PET scanning
- Serum calcium levels
- Tumor markers associated with suspected primary, such as PSA

Treatment

- Prophylactic internal fixation for impending fracture
- Surgical fixation for lytic lesions in high-stress areas
- Radiation can foster healing and reossification in 65% to 85% of patients with lytic lesions
- Radiation brings pain relief to 80% to 90% of patients
- Local radiation with 30 Gy in 10 fractions or single dose of 6 to 8 Gy
- Hemibody radiation appropriate for wide spread metastasis with 6 to 7 Gy total; lungs must be protected and falloff beyond the skin is important to manage
- Radionuclide therapy with rhenium-186, phosphorus-32, strontium-89, or samarium-153
- Analgesics for pain control
- Hormones as appropriate to control primary breast or prostate carcinomas

Radiation Treatment Borders

- Localized fields to include area of metastasis and generous margins especially in extremities
- Spine fields should include entire vertebral body, transverse and spinous processes; include affected vertebrae and at least one vertebral body above and below
- Allow a length of 1.5 cm for each cervical spine, 2.5 cm for each thoracic spine, and 3.0 cm for each lumbar spine to be included in treatment field
- Field widths will likely range from 6 to 8 cm to cover the transverse processes depending on region of spine
- Bone metastasis at L5 or sacrum should be wide enough to include the entire sacrum out to sacroiliac joints
- Spare soft tissues in extremities when possible

Treatment Delivery

- Take care to avoid unnecessary pressure to metastatic sites
- Extremities should be positioned parallel to the horizontal axis of the beam for even dose distribution
- If patient positioned prone for radiation to the spinal column, take advantage of the opportunity to palpate spinous process to verify daily alignment
- Cervical spine should be treated with patient on neutral head rest to avoid stress-increasing pain or the potential for collapse and subsequent cord compression

- As in compressions, cervical spine may be treated using posterior only or opposing laterals to midline; dorsal spine typically treated using posterior only to depth corresponding to region of spine; lumbar may be treated with single posterior or AP/PA fields to midline
- Bone metastasis is painful so make patient comfortable, make sure pain is assessed regularly and properly managed
- Fields usually require very little field shaping, simple positioning aids, no complex immobilization, and incur simple charges

AIRWAY OBSTRUCTIONS

General Facts and Epidemiology

- Lung, trachea, esophagus tumors may compress the trachea, mainstem bronchi, or carina
- Long-term survival is rare

Clinical Presentation

- Dyspnea
- Hemoptysis
- Stridor
- Cough
- Chest pain
- Anorexia

Workup

- Conventional x-ray
- CT

Treatment

- Expandable metallic stents can help maintain the airway
- Oxygen therapy
- External beam radiation for compression due to extrinsic masses with 200 cGy; each fraction to 40 to 50 Gy
- Two 8.5 Gy fractions 1 week apart or a single fraction of 10 Gy, palliates 50% of symptoms; similar results are seen with 10 fractions
- If total atelectasis, begin within 2 weeks of collapse and there is a higher possibility of reexpansion of the lung
- HDR intraluminal radiation with 15 to 20 Gy at 1 cm from the source is as effective as high dose external beam
- Steroids may be used to reduce inflammation

Radiation Treatment Borders

- Local, conforming fields if immediate symptom relief is desired
- If complete workup shows primary lung or esophageal carcinoma, then fields will include the compressive tumor, margin, and regional lymphatics

Treatment Delivery

- As patients are experiencing dyspnea, use positioning strategies to ease oxygen exchange, such as supine position with upper torso slightly elevated or patient positioned sitting
- Arms above the head expands the chest and may help with more effective oxygen exchange
- If patient on oxygen therapy, follow the prescribed liter flow
- Be prepared to help assist with portable oxygen taking care to support the entire tank when transferring
- Watch out for episodes of syncope and dizziness assist as needed
- Localized emergent fields will likely have no field shaping and simple positioning aids incur simple charges
- Fields designed to treat primary disease with curative intent will likely begin with simple arrangements and advance to complex arrangements with field shaping and beam modifiers and required complex immobilization devices

SUPERIOR VENA CAVA (SVC) SYNDROME

General Facts and Epidemiology

- Often this emergency is the first diagnosis and does not mean end-stage disease
- Most are from lung cancer but can also be from lymphoma and germ cell tumors, and sometimes benign conditions such as goiter or aortic aneurysm
- Thrombosis of the superior vena cava is common but death is unusual unless there is a complication, such as brain metastasis or tracheal obstruction
- Must verify histology so we know how to proceed following the relief of symptoms

- Overall survival is poor as most patients have lung cancer; more than 80% with lymphoma can have complete response

Clinical Presentation

- Dyspnea
- Facial edema
- Orthopnea
- Engorged conjunctiva
- Headache, dizziness
- Venous distention
- Cyanosis
- Tachypnea
- Upper extremity edema

Workup

- CT
- Conventional x-ray
- Sputum cytology
- Bronchoscopy
- CT guided biopsy

Treatment

- Radiation in large doses initially such as 3 to 4 Gy in 3 fractions, then tapering to standard fractionation as diagnosis is confirmed
- Adding chemotherapy does not improve symptoms but may be appropriate as management for the primary
- Diuretics, steroids, anticoagulants may be helpful
- Expandable stents if previous radiation therapy
- Usually a good, prompt response to radiation is seen within 3 to 4 days

Radiation Treatment Borders

- Localized fields for the initial high doses for symptom relief
- Once diagnosis is confirmed, fields will include tumor, margin, and regional lymphatics
- Since tumors are often located at the apex of the lung, slight neck extension is required for margin on the lung apex

Treatment Delivery

- Patient should be positioned to ease breathing and oxygen exchange
- Initial emergent fields will be small, simple with no field shaping; patient may lay supine on slight incline with arms at sides and AP/PA arrangement; simple charge
- Following workup, strategy may include off-cord fields, and reduced fields with total doses approaching 60 Gy; immobilization devices, beam modifiers, and beam shaping with MLC advances to complex daily charges
- Be prepared to assist with changes in the level of consciousness, syncope, dizziness, and potentially advancing respiratory distress

LIVER METASTASIS

General Facts and Epidemiology

- Since the liver filters blood from the remainder of the intraabdominal gastrointestinal tract, those originating there have a high tendency to metastasize to liver; such as primaries of the stomach, colon, rectum, esophagus, pancreas
- Other primaries metastasizing to the liver include breast, lung, melanoma, lymphoma, ovarian, bladder
- Common finding in patients with end-stage cancers; liver mets present in 50% to 70% of cancer patients on autopsy
- Mean survival is 75 days if untreated; following treatment, then 9 months with substantial response

Clinical Presentation

- Abdominal pain
- Nausea, vomiting, anorexia
- Jaundice
- Ascites
- Fever

Workup

- Liver function
- Prothrombin time
- Physical examination of abdomen
- CT

- MRI
- Ultrasound
- CT-guided biopsy

Treatment

- Partial hepatectomy if solitary lesion
- Chemotherapy with 5-FU base is shown to get 20% to 30% response
- Intrahepatic arterial chemotherapy infusion
- Radiation doses of 28 to 30 Gy in 14 to 15 fractions to the whole liver known to give significant pain relief, reduce the size, and improve function in 55% to 75% of patients
- Whole liver radiation can lead to radiation-induced liver disease

Radiation Treatment Borders

- Whole liver should be included if possible
- Partial liver can be dosed using intensity modulation or HDR liver implants or selective hepatic artery with radioisotopes
- Medial border across midline, lower border at the level of L2 with right lateral flash
- Beam shaping to protect the kidneys as much as possible, small bowel and colon
- AP/PA fields most appropriate

Treatment Delivery

- Patient should be supine with arms akimbo or above the head for triangulation
- Regularly assess pain and make sure appropriate referrals made for optimal pain management
- If patient is nauseous or vomiting, advise bland diet and plenty of fluids; clear liquids if solid foods are not well tolerated

GYNECOLOGIC/URINARY HEMORRHAGE

General Facts and Epidemiology

- Bleeding may come from late stage, ulcerating tumors in the endometrium, cervix or bladder; bleeding may also be caused by fistulas
- Pain not necessarily an accompanying symptom

Clinical Presentation

- Excessive bleeding from the vagina or urethra
- Catheterized patients with bladder cancers may show bright red blood in catheter bag

Workup

- Suspected primary need confirmed pathology
- Cervical or endometrial biopsy
- Cystoscopy with biopsy
- CT of pelvis

Treatment

- Ferric sulfate to the site stops the bleeding while awaiting complete workup and planning therapy
- Radiation to the local site can stop the bleeding by activating coagulating cells
- Initial large doses such as 3 to 4 Gy per fraction for 3 to 5 days may be applied, followed by tapered doses as primary diagnosis and disease staging dictates

Radiation Treatment Borders

- In either situation, a large pelvic field is used to include the bleeding tumor, and generous margin
- To relieve symptoms right away, a standard stop-sign shaped pelvic field from the top of the sacrum to the obturator foramen and wide enough to include the true pelvis; bone marrow in the iliac crests, head of femurs should be shielded
- Borders may change as histology and stage of disease is confirmed

Treatment Delivery

- Patient may be positioned supine with arms on abdomen for initial emergent doses; simple immobilization of lower extremities
- Use additional barriers on PSA for bleeding
- Dispose of stained coverings using biohazard bags
- If treatment goal changes to more definitive or curative nature, more may be done to spare small bowel, protect normal colon and bladder
- Initial fields with minimal beam shaping are likely AP/PA and incur intermediate charges
- Follow-up fields may include 4 to 6 fields, using complex beam shaping, intensity modulation, alternative positioning to spare small bowel, complex pelvic immobilization, and will incur complex charges

PALLIATIVE CARE REVIEW EXERCISES

1. What area of the brain would you expect to find involved if a patient had vision problems?
   a. Parietal
   b. Frontal
   c. Temporal
   d. None of the above

2. What is the average survival for patients with brain metastasis?
   a. 10 years
   b. 5 years
   c. 3 months
   d. 1 month

3. Distinguish between osteolytic and osteoblastic lesions as they may appear on a conventional x-ray.

4. Compare/contrast palliative doses of radiation for brain metastasis to curative doses for primary brain malignancy.

5. Define the following:

   Superior vena cava syndrome

   Laminectomy

   Partial hepatectomy

6. Steroids are used to:
   a. Stop hemorrhage
   b. Decrease nausea
   c. Restore hydration
   d. Decrease inflammation

7. A patient with brain metastasis may report:
   a. A loss of memory
   b. A change in gait
   c. Nausea
   d. Any of the above

8. Compression of the cauda equina will likely manifest as:
   a. Numbness in the arm
   b. Central back pain
   c. Incontinence
   d. Pain in the right flank

9. Which of the following radionuclides may be used in treating metastatic bone disease?
   a. Technetium-99
   b. Iodine-131
   c. Strontium-89
   d. Iodine-125

10. In spinal cord compression and superior vena cava syndrome, high doses of radiation are given in the first few treatments. The following doses are typical:
    a. 300 to 400 cGy per fraction
    b. 180 to 200 cGy per fraction
    c. 500 to 700 cGy per fraction
    d. 700 to 800 cGy per fraction

11. Which one of the following oncologic emergencies is not typically managed by radiation therapy?
    a. Spinal cord compression
    b. Superior vena cava syndrome
    c. Painful pathologic fracture
    d. Radiation pneumonitis

12. Which one of the following sites is the least likely site of bony metastasis?
    a. Humerus
    b. Femur
    c. Thoracic spine
    d. Lumbar spine

13. Metastatic brain disease differs from primary brain malignancy in that:

a. Metastasis is usually multifocal and primaries are solitary at the time of diagnosis
b. Primary brain tumors are usually multifocal and metastatic lesions are solitary
c. Metastatic brain lesions are associated with longer overall survival than primary malignancy
d. Metastatic brain disease shows symptoms specific to vision impairments whereas primary malignancy may show various symptoms depending on location

14. When treating a patient who has spinal cord compression in the cervical spine, the best position among the following would be:

a. Supine with the chin hyperflexed using shoulder retractors
b. Supine with the chin hyperextended using shoulder retractors
c. Prone with the chin tucked in a total body alpha cradle
d. Prone with the chin and forehead in a horizontal plane and arms at sides

15. A typical field size for the treatment of thoracic vertebrae 5 to 10 would be:

a. 15 × 20 cm
b. 8 × 36 cm
c. 36 × 8 cm
d. 8 × 15 cm

16. A T-shaped radiation treatment field would likely be seen in the treatment of:

a. Spinal cord compression in the upper thoracic region
b. Spinal cord compression in the lower lumbar or sacral region
c. Spinal cord compression in the lower cervical region
d. Spinal cord compression in the upper lumbar region

17. Single posterior fields are not usually adequate for lower lumbar or sacral bone metastasis because:

a. This region of the spine has lordotic curvature
b. This region of the spine has kyphotic curvature
c. This region of the spine has scoliotic curvature
d. This region of the spine is not as dense as the rest of the spine

18. A patient with brain metastasis begins to have a tonic-clonic seizure right before his treatment. The therapist should:

a. Immediately place a hard, sugary candy on his tongue
b. Place a tongue depressor between his teeth
c. Call for assistance and begin CPR
d. Assist the patient to a safe position for the prevention of injury

19. A patient with SVC syndrome appears to have fainted during administration of therapy. The therapist should:

a. Stop treatment and call a Code Blue
b. Stop the treatment, assess vital signs, and call physician or nurse
c. Continue treatment as long as the patient does not roll
d. Complete treatment and place patient in holding area until conscious

20. A common symptom of liver metastasis is:

a. Jaundice
b. Numbness in the upper extremities
c. Venous distention
d. Cyanosis

21. Using the diagram below, draw typical radiation treatment field(s) for confirmed boney metastasis to T6.

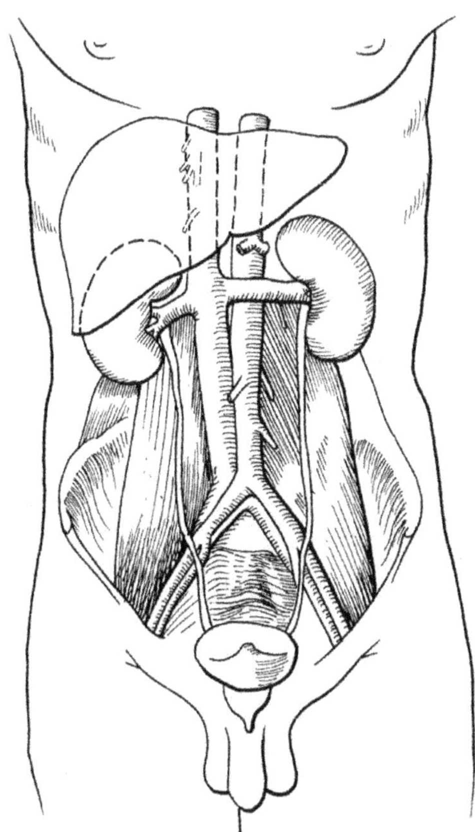

22. Using Figure 9-31, draw the typical whole brain radiation treatment field(s).

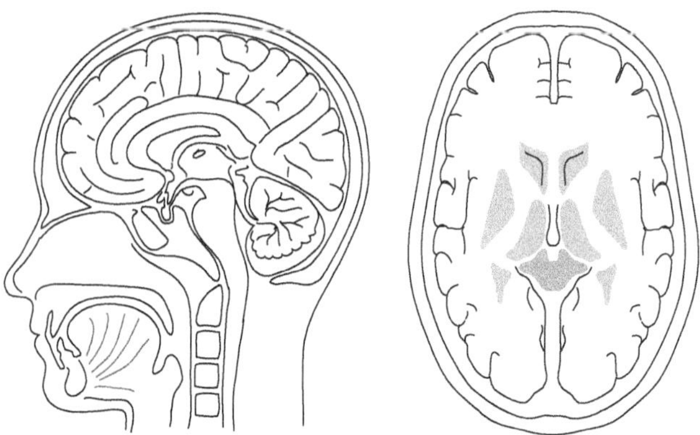

FIGURE 9-31 Sagittal and axial sections brain.

23. Using Figure 9-32, identify whether the treatment portals drawn are likely for:

a. Primary adenocarcinoma of the middle lobe
b. Superior vena cava syndrome initial field
c. Primary mesothelioma of the upper lobe
d. Chronic obstructive pulmonary disease

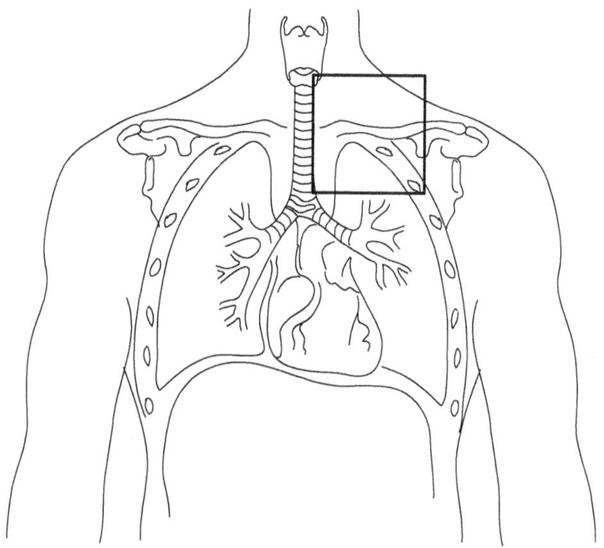

FIGURE 9-32 Anterior chest.

24. Regional lymphatics are not usually included in radiation fields for palliation because:

a. Disease spread is assumed to have already taken place
b. Lymph nodes are less responsive after metastasis
c. Long-term side effects are too great
d. The prognosis is better without treating regional lymphatics

25. Daily treatment charges for a single field spine with no field shaping or beam modifiers would be:

a. Simple
b. Intermediate
c. Complex

26. Collimator rotation for the left lateral whole brain field is 30 degrees (neutral collimator angle is 0 degrees). The collimator angle for the right lateral field should be:

a. 60 degrees
b. 330 degrees
c. 300 degrees
d. 240 degrees

27. The total separation of my patient's skull at the approximate location of isocenter is 15 cm. Opposing, midline treatment ports will require monitor unit calculations for a depth of:

a. 7.5 cm
b. 15 cm
c. 7.0 cm
d. 9.0 cm

BIBLIOGRAPHY

Portal Design in Radiation Therapy; 2nd edition; Van, Dasher, Chestnut, Wiggers.

Bontrager K, Lampignano J: *Textbook of radiographic positioning and related anatomy*, ed 7, St Louis, 2010, Mosby.

Deangelis R: *The integrated radiography workbook*, ed 4, Rutland, 2006, Health & Allied Science Publishers.

Gunderson LL, Tepper JE: *Clinical radiation oncology*, ed 2, Philadelphia, 2007, Churchill Livingstone.

Lenhard RE, Osteen RT, Gansler T: *Clinical oncology*, ed 1, Atlanta, 2001, American Cancer Society.

Rubin P, Williams JP: *Clinical oncology*, ed 8, Philadelphia, 2001, Saunders.

Tortora GJ, Derrickson BH: *Principles of anatomy and physiology*, ed 12, 2008, Wiley-Blackwell.

Washington CM, Leaver D: *Principles and practice of radiation therapy*, ed 3, St Louis, 2010, Mosby.

INTERNET RESOURCES

www.rt-review.com.

CHAPTER 1

Developing Good Habits in the Health Professions

1. Before going to class, activities that will aid focus and identify the most important ideas to note are:
   - Read or preview the topic to be covered
   - Review previous notes
   - Write down any questions you may have
   - Come prepared by having read and completed assignments
2. Studying can be more productive when you set a specific objective for your studying time. The four elements to establish an effective purpose are:
   Goal—Make it specific
   Obstacles—Identify potential problems
   Action—Apply effective methods
   Learned—Confirm what you learned
3. Distractions and interruptions interfere with deep learning and result in the need to repeat and review more often. Put phones on vibrate or have voice mail pick up calls. Place your phone where it is not easily available while you are studying. Establish a reputation with others that your designated time is not to be disrupted.
4. When the answers are narrowed down, consider the following to set priorities and select an answer among the remaining items.
   - The underlying principle or theory that is involved in the overall question
   - Any indications or contraindications for a procedure
   - The steps or priorities within a process or procedure, and their purpose
   - Where the test item lies within a process, and the next step to be executed
   - The type of equipment and instrumentation required and how it works
5. **b.** Mnemonics is a memory device, usually verbal, that makes an association between words or letters and information to be remembered. The first letter of each word of this phrase aids in how to spell a word.
6. **b and d.** Goals should be SMART which includes Specific and Timely.
7. **a and d.** Proper diet and sleep are important to effective learning and memory.
8.

	Note Taking	Reading
Before	Read or preview topic Review notes List your questions Complete assignments	Establish a reading plan Survey or skim Notice headings, titles and terms List your questions
After	Review notes Rewrite notes where needed Compare notes with others Reflect Identify your remaining questions	Review "Talk to the author" Answer end of chapter questions and exercises Find answers to your questions

9. Any suggestions similar to the following would help Michael.
   - Work on his paper before other assignments.
   - Break the job into smaller parts and attempt to do only one part.
   - Work for just a short time.
   - Schedule it in his calendar.
   - Promise to reward himself when it is completed.
   - Think of the consequences.
10. Active/Sensory/Verbal/Sequential
    - Suggestions might include:
    - Active—Study in a group; Walk and talk; Teach it
    - Sensory—Apply concepts in practice; Make connections; Look for specific examples
    - Verbal—Talk about what you learn; Work in a study group; Read your book aloud
    - Sequential—Rewrite notes in a logical pattern; Outline material; Write out steps for procedures
11. Time management tools can help Jose accomplish all his important tasks and attend important events.
    - Calendar or planner
    - Create daily schedules
    - To-do Lists
    - Scheduling study time
    - Break large projects, like the presentation, into smaller steps
    - Use small periods of time for review

12. Techniques:

Candles
Dance
Deep breathing
Eat right
Exercise
Find cheerleaders
Humor
Imagery
Jog
Meditation
Networks
Plan ahead
Play
Read
Set priorities
Sing
Smile
Swim
Walk
Yoga

N	O	P	L	E	N	T	S	A	A	M	U	S	R	E	F
A	D	E	E	A	T	R	I	G	H	T	H	M	E	D	I
N	I	K	X	T	N	D	F	Y	D	H	K	I	P	T	E
B	D	F	E	S	A	E	O	B	O	L	V	L	C	A	H
W	E	P	R	N	L	D	U	E	N	G	A	E	A	L	T
N	E	H	C	L	K	Q	O	G	O	Y	A	X	N	P	E
E	P	E	I	K	F	P	K	G	M	E	D	T	D	N	R
T	B	V	S	W	I	M	I	W	F	L	G	N	L	I	B
W	R	S	E	T	P	R	I	O	R	I	T	I	E	S	D
O	E	H	X	W	L	Z	S	R	E	A	D	J	S	H	K
R	A	D	N	J	A	G	X	I	A	Y	B	Z	H	U	G
K	T	L	S	I	N	L	P	K	N	F	P	R	D	M	E
S	H	D	E	D	A	H	K	E	O	G	E	A	J	O	G
F	I	N	D	C	H	E	E	R	L	E	A	D	E	R	S
J	N	E	H	O	E	N	H	G	R	E	X	E	I	W	U
A	G	F	I	M	A	G	E	R	Y	A	L	V	N	F	Q
P	N	K	M	E	D	I	T	A	T	I	O	N	I	I	Y

CHAPTER 2

An Overview of Cancer and Management Modalities

1.

Benign tumors	Malignant tumors
Encapsulated	Unencapsulated
Rarely fatal	Potentially fatal
Little effect on the host	Substantial effect on the host
Differentiated	Differentiated–undifferentiated
Slow growth	Rapid growth
Low mitotic activity	High mitotic activity
Little tissue destruction	Potentially metastatic
Abnormal proliferation of cells	Invasive and destructive to tissue
	abnormal proliferation of cells

2.

Men:

a. Colonoscopy beginning at age 50, annual or longer interval if low risk
b. Fecal Occult Blood test at 50; annual or longer interval if low risk
c. Manual testicular exam beginning at late adolescence, annual
d. Digital Rectal examination beginning at age 45, annual
e. PSA beginning at age 50, annual; earlier if family history

Women:

a. Manual breast examination beginning at late adolescence, monthly; or each gynecological visit
b. Pelvic exam and pap smear beginning at the time of sexual activity, yearly
c. Mammogram, baseline at age 40 or earlier if family history; annually thereafter
d. Colonoscopy beginning at age 50; annual or longer intervals if low risk
e. Fecal Occult Blood test at 50; annual or longer intervals if low risk

3.

1. Curettage or exfoliation—**scraping of cells**
2. Excisional biopsy—**complete removal of suspicious tissue and margin**
3. Incisional biopsy—**cutting into and taking a portion of suspicious tissue**
4. Fine needle aspiration (FNA)—**use of needle and syringe to draw out fluid from suspicious tissue**
5. Core biopsy—**use of large bore needle to withdraw a section of tissue**
6. Sputum cytology—**sampling of sputum**
7. Washing or irrigation—**introduction of saline into a cavity and analysis of returned solution containing cells**
8. Open biopsy—**surgical procedure exposing area of suspicious tissue for the visual investigation of local area**

4.

Group 1: Glioma. Glioma is a malignancy originating in glial tissue, all others originate in epithelial.

Group 2: Antiemetics. Antiemetics are for management of nausea, vomiting, all others are used to manage cancer

Group 3: Tamoxifen. Tamoxifen is a hormonal agent, all others are cytotoxics; could also discuss Purinethol as not belonging as the others are often used in combination for the management of breast carcinoma

5. Prophylactic management is used to prevent the future manifestation of cancer in a location with no declared disease but possibly microscopic disease not yet detectable. It sterilizes the potential area of metastatic disease.

6.

Adenocarcinoma___E_____	A. malignant tumor occurring in striated muscle
Myeloma___D________	B. malignant tumor occurring in bone
Leukemia___F________	C. malignant tumor originating in the central nervous system
Osteosarcoma___B________	D. abnormal proliferation occurring in the bone marrow
Rhabdomyosarcoma___A__	E. malignant tumor of glandular epithelium
Glioma________C_________	F. abnormal proliferation occurring in the bone marrow, especially the white blood cells

7.

ONCOGENE
CARCINOGENESIS
BIOPSY
TUMOR
DIFFERENTIATION
METASTASIS

8.

Phase specific cytotoxic drugs	Phase non-specific cytotoxic drugs
Effective on dividing cells	Effective on non-dividing cells
One such class would be- Antimetabolites	One class would be alkylating agents
Examples: 5-FU, cytarabine, floxuridine, 6-mercaptopurine	Examples: Nitrogen mustard, cisplatin, cyclophosphamide
Toxicities include: myelosuppression, anorexia, nausea	Toxicities include: myelosuppression, kidney toxicity, nausea, anorexia, neurotoxicity

Refer to chemotherapeutic drug class and side effects table for other possible answers

9.

- Hyperplasia is an increase in the number of cells and is associated with both malignant and benign tumors; typically a response to an acute injury
- Metaplasia is the replacement of a cell type that usually is not present and is commonly associated with malignant conditions
- Anaplasia is the loss of differentiation and is also associated with both malignant and benign conditions
- All three conditions may correct themselves without intervention.

10. c. Mortality rates are based on the number of persons per 100,000 people in a population.

11. b. A substance that can potentially initiate cancer is known as a carcinogen.

12. c. Pain is not a common sign of cancer. Any masses or physiological changes present without pain in the early stages of disease. Refer to the American Cancer Society's 7 warning signs acronym CAUTION.

13. d. The TNM system evaluates the extent of disease by evaluation of the tumor, any positive nodes and distant metastases. Grading evaluates the degree of malignancy or the status of the abnormal cells.

14. c. Malignant conditions that originate in the lymphatic tissues are known as lymphomas.

15. a. Concurrent means simultaneously or at the same time. Multiple modalities are often use as management but not necessarily at the same time.

16. a. Alkylating agents can be toxic to the skin. Special care is required when drugs in this class need to be handled manually.

17. d. Tumors located in the large bowel or rectum may cause a change in bowel habits such as diarrhea, constipation, or change in the caliber of stools

18. c. Adriamycin, also known as Doxorubicin, is known to cause cardiac toxicity.

19. c. The generic TNM classification system with a designated tumor as level 3 typically classifies the tumor as Stage III. At the same time, lymph nodes are likely positive at this time. Without distant metastases, a large tumor with positive nodes is typically less than Stage IV.

20. a. The term carcinoma indicates tissues of epithelial origin.

21. c. All screening listed are helpful in diagnosing malignancy. However, the histopathological study is what confirms that any abnormal growths are malignant.

22. b. Adeno- is the prefix for gland. Carcinoma is the base word for epithelial tissue. So, any malignant tissue of glandular epithelium would be referred to as an adenocarcinoma

23. d. Rhabdo- is the prefix for striated, myo- is the base term for muscle, sarcoma the base term for connective tissue. As muscle is a connective tissue, a malignancy of striated muscle would be known as a rhabdomyosarcoma.

24. b. A laparoscopy is a surgical procedure in which incision is made in the abdomen to explore the anatomy within.

25. **prostate, breast.** Refer to the recent American Cancer Society statistics on cancer incidence in adults.

26. **carcinogenesis.** Carcinogenesis describes the process from health y state to cancerous

27. **myelosuppression.** As cytotoxic drugs affect both normal and abnormal cells, highly proliferating blood cells are most often affected causing a decrease in blood components.

28. **sporadic.** The majority of cancers are caused by repeated mutating events rather than pre-existing genetic predisposition.
29. **curettage.** Scraping away cells is known as curettage.
30. **grade.** Grading a tumor establishes the degree of malignancy by measuring levels of differentiation of cells.
31. c. Bergonie and Tribondeau established that the most sensitive cells are those that rapidly divide, divide often and will continue dividing for a long time.
32. a. DNA synthesis occurs during the 'S' phase of cellular division
33. Mr. Jones' T2 tumor is likely smaller in size and is less invasive to neighboring tissues than Mr. Smith's T4 tumor
34. b. To palliate means to relieve symptoms
35. F. Depending on location, benign tumors may be fatal
36. F. Radiation effects are local so only effects would be to the abdominal organs such as nausea, vomiting if irradiating over the stomach or diarrhea if irradiating the colon
37. T
38. F. Anti-oncogenes are known as tumor-suppressor genes
39. F. Older persons have the highest incidence of cancer
40. F. Surgery is sometimes used prophylactically; an example would be a prophylactic mastectomy for a patient with a strong family history and no definite diagnosis of cancer at the time of surgery
41. e. Cytotoxic drugs may cause many different side effects. Nausea, cardiac toxicity, myelosuppression and alopecia are possible side effects and vary across drugs.
42. d. Before the medical oncologist prescribes a certain drug or combination he refers to the cancer type, whether the tumor would be accessible to a systemic drug, how quickly the drug will be absorbed and if there has been any evidence of resistance to the drug(s) as well as the patient's health status.
43. c. Surgery is the first documented approach to managing cancerous growths.
44. c. Malignant tumors tend to divide often and invade neighboring tissues and distant organs by blood invasion or direct extension. Benign lesions may have abnormal growth patterns but tend to stay local and have a unique 'encapsulation' feature.
45. b. Only a small sub-set of cytotoxic drugs can cross the blood brain barrier. Substitute ureas can cross this barrier.
46. c. The most common symptom of breast cancer is a painless lump.
47. d. When looking at the incidence of cancer in a certain population, we may categories frequencies by race, sex, environment, culture, socioeconomic status, religion and other factors
48. b. Lung cancers are easily detected with routine radiography.
49. d. Beta HCG and AFP are tumor markers frequently associated with tumors of germ cell origin.
50. c. Beginning at age 45 men and women should have at minimum a baseline colonoscopy to check for colon polyps or malignancy.
51. No other factors considered, Mrs. Anthony is at greater risk at this point in time. She has been exposed to a carcinogenic factor over a longer period than Mr. Anthony. The longer the exposure period, the greater the potential for cellular and molecular damage that may ultimately lead to an irreversible injury manifesting as a cancer.
52. No other factors considered, ten years later, Mr. Anthony has had a repeated exposure for 15 years. Although this exposure is shorter than Mrs. Anthony's 25 years of repeated exposure, after such a long period of exposure, quitting will not lessen Mr. Anthony's risk by a remarkable amount.

For discussion: We encourage smoking cessation even after such a long period of direct exposure to cigarette smoke because chronic smoking leads to and compounds other chronic conditions like heart failure, COPD/emphysema and the development of blood clots. We've also become more aware of the carcinogenic effect of second-hand smoke for nonsmokers

53.

Prostatectomy—**the removal of the prostate gland**

Radical mastectomy—**removal of the breast and underlying muscle**

Modified radical mastectomy—**removal of the breast while sparing underlying muscle**

Exenteration— **total removal of multiple organs in a body cavity; i.e. orbital exenteration removes the entire globe of the orbit, pelvic exenteration removes all pelvic organs like the bladder, uterus and rectum**

54. d. Prophylactic therapy is meant to prevent the future manifestation of disease.
55. c. Curative therapy is intended to put the patient in remission.
56. Both clinical and laboratory testing have led to optimal chemotherapy administration delivery methods. Some methods require successive doses with static breaks. Dosages have been refined to allow normal tissue repair. Each successive dose of drug cause a fraction of cell kill, time between doses gives normal tissue time to repair. Normal cells can more readily repair injury than abnormal cells. Cell survival curves are similar in chemotherapy to cell survival curves in radiation therapy.
57. Good vasculature is necessary for the distribution of chemotherapy drug to the tumor and throughout

the tumor's lattice or cells. The effect of radiation is enhanced with the presence of oxygen. Vasculature assures sufficient delivery of oxygen to the tumor.

58. When considering the right management modality for patients, we must consider the main objectives: eradicate disease and maintain a quality life. A quality life could include normal function of organs after therapy. Radiation for the above cancer types would leave the patient with a preserved cervix or uterus (sacrifice of which may lead to emotional trauma for female patients), a preserved voice without the use of a mechanical voice box and preserved cosmesis without excessive scarring or noticeable skin defects.

59. Survival for breast cancer survival is usually at 10 to 20 year increments. Such tremendous progress in managing breast cancers has led to patients living longer without a recurrence of disease.

60. Treatments may fail due to:
  1. Noncompliance of patients to prescribed regimens
  2. Overdosing or underdosing (chemotherapy and radiation)
  3. Geometric miss of the tumor from technical errors
  4. Unexplained resistance of cancer to chemotherapy and/or radiation
  5. Late diagnosis
  6. Misdiagnosis

61. Local chemotherapy is currently used for central nervous system malignancies and other resistant malignancies like primary liver cancers. Local chemotherapy is accomplished by direct injection of the cytotoxic into the tissue or body cavity with or without the implementation of embolization techniques. *Note that lipid soluble drugs may cross the blood brain barrier with the help of a carrier molecule; a select group of drugs may be used in the management of central nervous system malignancies.*

62. a. Fractionation or giving small amounts of dose over time allows the normal tissue time to repair from cellular damage

63. c. Chemotherapy is most often given systemically. Therefore, chemotherapy is appropriate for systemic disease

64. d. Hippocrates, a Greek physician, is credited for identifying cancer

65. c. The youngest and ever-evolving cancer treatment modality among the listed is chemotherapy. Chemotherapy had its beginnings during World War II (1940s)

66. e. Effective cancer management involves every member of the cancer management team from surgical oncology, medical oncology and radiation oncology

67. d. An excisional biopsy takes all of the tumor plus margin and can be the cure for early localized disease and also provide cell sample for histology.

68. e. Cytotoxic drugs may be administered in various routs including IV, topical, enteral or surface applications.

69. b. Actinomycin D belongs to the anti-tumor antibiotic class of chemotherapy drugs.

70. a. Grading establishes the degree of differentiation of cells.

71. d. A tumor that is confined and small, with no associated positive lymphatics and no distant metastasis is likely classified as Stage I.

72. d. Excessive exposure to ionizing radiation, asbestos, and UV light are associated with the development of certain cancers.

73. a. Response to radiation is local. One irradiated to the brain will likely experience localized effects like hair loss, skin erythema and some neurological signs like dizziness and imbalance although it is difficult to associate these symptoms with radiation dose or the presence of CNS disease.

74. d. Common Signs of testicular cancer include a painless lump or swelling in the scrotal area.

75. b. The most widely used and universal staging system is the TNM system which evaluates the tumor, regional lymphatics and distant metastasis.

CHAPTER 3

Radiation Therapy Physics

1. b. 1 mCi is equivalent to 3.7×10^7 dps. Conversion of dps to dpm means multiplying by 60 seconds. Then converting mCi to Ci requires multiplying by 1000 or 10^3

2. d. Given by the formula $\lambda = \ln 2/T\ ½$

3. Electrons are light, negatively charged particles; they can collide and interact with other particles. Protons are heavy, positively charged particles; only interact with electrons.

4. b. Types of nuclear decay include alpha, beta negative and positive, electron capture, internal conversion, fission and fusion aftermaths

5. d. During ionization characteristic x-rays may be produced. If the electron comes close to the nucleus, bremsstrahlung radiation may result. Auger electrons may be emitted as a result of another electron filling an empty space left by the ejected electron.

6. a. In the basic x-ray tube, the anode receives the streaming electrons and is known as the positive side of the tube

7. c. Use the activity formula. $A = Ao\ e^{-\lambda t}$

8. d. Use the formula Average life = 1.44(T ½)

9. c. As the maximum energy increases, more of the converted energy becomes photons

10. b. The decay constant expresses how many atoms are lost over time

11. a. In elastic collisions the incoming electrons gives up all of its energy. On the other hand, inelastic collisions may allow bounce back where the incoming electron shares its energy

12. d. The electromagnetic spectrum shows wavelengths shortening as energy increases.

13. a. The outgoing photoelectron has an energy that is the difference between the incoming electron and the binding energy of the electron collided

14. a. The electromagnetic spectrum shows that the frequency increases as the energy of radiation increases

15.

Photon interactions	Electron interactions
Photodisintegration	Bremsstrahlung
Coherent scattering	Characteristic
Photoelectric effect (Rayleigh)	
Compton effect	
Pair production	

16. b. As radioactive Cobalt transforms, gamma rays and beta negative particles are emitted

17. **protons.** Radionuclides with the same number of protons but different number of neutrons are known as *isotopes*

18.

	Mass (kilograms)	Rest energy	Charge
Electrons	9.11×10^{-31}	.511 MeV	−1
Positrons	9.11×10^{-31}	.511 MeV	+1
Protons	1.67×10^{-27}	938.2 MeV	+1
Neutrons	1.68×10^{-27}	939.5 MeV	0
Alpha particles	6.65×10^{-27}	3729 MeV	+2

19.

Isotopes__B_____	A. Ir^{192} Ir^{192m}
Isobars___C_____	B. $_{27}Fe^{59}$ $_{27}Fe^{58}$
Isotones___D____	C. $_{28}Ni^{60}$ $_{31}Ga^{60}$
Isomers___A____	D. $_{11}Na^{22}$ $_{10}Ne^{21}$

20. 0.496 KeV

Use the formula showing the relationship between wavelength and kinetic energy.

Answer:

$E = 12.4/\lambda$

$E = 12.4/25$ A

$E = .496$ KeV

21. 0.0154 sec

Use the formula showing the relationship between decay constant and half-life.

Answer:

T ½ = $.693/\lambda$

T ½ = .693/ 45 sec^{-1}

T ½ = .0154 sec

22. 7.59 years

Use the formula showing the relationship between half-life and average life.

Answer:

Ta = T ½ /.693

Ta = 5.26 /.693

Ta = 7.59 years

23. 0.1036 or 10.36%

Use the formula below.

$F = 3.5 \times 10^{-4}$ (74) (4 MeV)

F= 0.1036

24. b. The electromagnetic spectrum shows UV light with higher energy and frequency than the other photons mentioned

25. **decreases, increases.** The probability of photoelectric interactions decreases as enery increases. The probability of photoelectric interactions increases as the atomic number of the medium increases.

26. b. Bohr's model shows the massive part of the atom being the nucleus where protons and neutrons reside

27. d. Loss of an electron leaves an imbalance to the atom. Positive charge would then be greater than negative charges

28. c. An alpha particle is composed of 2 neutrons and 2 protons. Loss of these particles would be a loss of 4 atomic mass units

29. b. The emitted photon has an energy that is the difference between the binding energies of transitioning electrons

30. **a. alpha decay b. beta positive**

31. a. Electrons have negative charge, protons positive charge. When equal, they neutralize the atom

32. d. During pair production, two particles of equal energies –.511 MeV are emitted. The incoming photon has to have at least that combined energy.

33. Use the formula showing the relationship between decay constant and activity.

Answer:

$A = Ao\ e^{-\lambda t}$

$5\ mCi = 18\ mCi\ e^{-\lambda(50)}$

$5/18 = e^{-\lambda(50)}$

$\ln 5/18 = \ln (e^{-\lambda(50)})$

$-1.28 = -\lambda\ (50)$

$\lambda = .0256^{-1}$ hours

34. Use the formula showing the relationship between original activity and half-life.

Answer:

$\lambda = .693/8hrs$, $\lambda = .087^{-1}$ hours

$10\ mCi - Ao\ e^{-.087(22)}$

$10\ mCi = Ao\ e^{-1.91}$

10 mCi = Ao (0.148)

67.57 mCi = Ao

35. a. Activity is expressed in units of Curie or Becquerel. The Becquerel is the SI unit

36. b. Photoelectric effect occurs when a photon interacts with a tightly bound electron. Its energy has to be equal to or greater than the binding energy

37. a. Characteristic radiation is emitting when electrons switch places in the shells of the atom
38. c. The farther away from the nucleus, the lower the binding energy
39. a. Isomers are the same element but in an excited state.
40. b. Electromagnetic radiations have the potential to travel at the same speed, they have virtually no mass and carry no charge
41. c. Use the formula Average life = 1.44 (T ½)
42. c. Isobars have the same mass.
43. a. 1 Ci = 3.7×10^{10} dps. Convert to minutes by multiplying by 60.
44. d. The number of electrons per gram has been computed using Helium as a reference. For Helium 3×10^{23} is the number of electrons per gram. Tissue in the question has not been specified as soft tissue or bone, both having a different atomic weight than helium
45. b. 24 days have elapsed. This would be 3 half-life periods for this isotope. 3 half lives would leave about 12.5% of the initial activity. 80 mCi (12.5%) = 10 mCi. The activity formula could also be used
46. d. The half-life of Cobalt is 5.26 years. 10 years is approximately 2 half lives, leaving about 25% of the original atoms.
47. d. The Angstrom is the unit of measure for the wavelength
48. c. C in Einstein's equation is the speed or velocity of light. Option D has incorrect time units
49. c. Photoelectric effect often occurs with an electron tightly bound and in the inner shells of the atom.
50. c. All radiations in the electromagnetic spectrum have the same speed/velocity regardless of wavelength or frequency
51. a. Use the formula $C = \lambda \upsilon$
52. d. Use the formula T ½ = $.693/\lambda$
53. a. Bragg peak shows maximum ionization at the end of the range for heavy, high LET particles
54. b. Isotopes have the same number of protons and different neutrons. The number of protons and electrons are equal in a neutral atom
55. e. The time elapsed has been 4 half-lives. The activity may be found by multiplying the initial activity by 0.5^4. Or the formula $A = Ao\ e^{-\lambda t}$ may also be used.
56. c. The average life is given by the formula: Ta = 1.44 (T ½). So, the half-life is less than the average life. The average life comes close to what may be thought of as the life span for a radioactive nuclide.
57. b. The symbol in the activity formula is the decay constant and expresses the constant fraction of atoms decaying in a certain amount of time
58. b. Secular equilibrium occurs when the parent nuclide has a longer half-life than a daughter product
59. a. Ultrasound is not electromagnetic radiation.
60. d. The electron's mass is low compared to its kinetic energy so it must be traveling at about light speed. The alpha particle has the greatest total energy.
61. d. Protons, neutrons and nucleons have a mass about 1800 times that of an electron
62. c. When an atom is ionized, an electron is ejected from the atom.
63. a. The number in the upper right indicates the atomic mass.
64. c. Unstable radioactive nuclides has excess energy in its nucleus. The nucleus achieves stability by redistributing energy between the nucleons.
65. b. The total attenuation coefficient represents the sum of all possible interactions.
66. b. Energy loss is proportional to the square of particle charge and inversely proportional to the square of its velocity
67. c. This maximum energy loss is known as Bragg peak.
68. c. Electrons have low mass and therefore deposit energy as it moves quickly through the medium.
69. c. The energy transferred is not enough to eject the electron. The incoming electron does not have an energy higher than the binding energy of the orbiting electron.
70. b. The strong electromagnetic field of the nucleus decelerates the electron as it approaches. In the deceleration, some of the energy is lost in the form of an x-ray photon called bremsstrahlung.
71. A. The mass of an alpha particle is three to four times heavier than neutrons and protons
72. A. Alpha particles have the highest LET of about 166 KeV/micrometer
73. N. Neutrons have a neutral charge
74. A. Alpha particles and positrons (+ Beta) do not exist naturally in the atom and occur during radioactive decay
75. B. Beta particles can carry positive or negative charge
76. A. The Helium nucleus has a mass of 4 and consists of 2 protons and 2 neutrons. Combined making the alpha particle
77. P. The Hydrogen nucleus has 1 proton in its nucleus
78. A. Alpha particles have the heaviest mass and carry charges that could cause the most biological damage.
79. N. Since neutrons have no charge they are not directly ionizing. The interaction with atoms is attributed to recoiling and redirection of energy
80. B. A beta particle is an electron if negatively charged, and called a positron if positively charged.
81. Q. Increasing the time of exposure increases the amount of radiation
82. Q. Changing the incoming current changes the quantity of radiation.
83. H. The type of target affects the quality of radiation
84. Q / B. Distance will affect the quantity of radiation by divergence and the intensity of radiation by the inverse square rule. Intensity may be used synonymously with quality.

85. H / B. Filtration in the low energy tube hardens the beam and improves the quality. At the same time, this phenomenon is influenced by the beam energy and type of material. In reference to photon fluence, some energy is absorbed and scattered in the filter so some original energy is lost.
86. H. Changing the tube potential changes the beam quality
87. B. The generator controls the tube voltage, tube current and exposure time
88. d. The electromagnetic spectrum shows x-rays having energy of at least 124 eV
89. a. Alpha particles have a positive charge
90. a. Radiation is energy in motion
91. d. The formulas show the element Iodine which has the same chemical properties. The mass number is different, and the z number is the same at 53 protons so the number of neutrons are different.
92. b. Inverse square law says the intensity of radiation is inversely proportional to distance by a square of distance change
93. Use the formula showing relationship between HVL, photon fluence and transmission.
    Answer:
    $N = N_0\, e^{-\mu\, t}$
    $N = 10^{6}\, e^{(-0.63\ (1.5))}$
    $N = 389{,}000 \quad 3.89 \times 10^5$
94. Use the formula showing the relationship between photon fluence, transmission, and linear attenuation coefficient.
    Answer:
    $N = 10^{8}\, e^{(-11.55(0.2))}$
    $N = 9{,}900{,}000 \quad 9.9 \times 10^{6}$
95. Use the formula showing the relationship between HVL and linear attenuation coefficient.

    Answer:

$$\mu = \frac{0.693}{\text{HVL}}$$

$$11.55\ \text{m}^{-1} = \frac{0.693}{\text{x}}$$

$$\text{HVL} = 0.06 \text{ meters of water}$$

CHAPTER 4

Radiation Biology

1. c. TD 5/5 indicate 5% chance of injury within 5 years following exposure
2. a. LD 50/30 is the lethal dose to 50% of the population in 30 days following exposure
3. c. The TD 5/5 for the whole kidney is about 23 Gy. Lower volumes of the kidney would increase the tolerance dose up to 50 Gy.
4. c. TD 5/5 for the whole brain is 45 Gy. Lower the volume of brain would increase the tolerance up to 60 Gy.
5. b. Organogenesis, or the formation of organs, occurs during the second through the eight weeks of fetal development.
6. a. Oxygen enhances the sensitivity to radiation by increasing the possibility of free radical production.
7. b. The "S" phase is most resistant to radiation. The "S" phase is the stage of DNA synthesis.
8. d. The prodromal syndrome occurs immediately after a large acute radiation exposure. Nausea, vomiting, diarrhea and anorexia are the symptoms of the prodromal stage of radiation sickness.
9. e. Cells that are highly mitotic, undifferentiated and have a long dividing life are most responsive to radiation according to Bergonie and Tribondeau.
10. **stochastic.** Stochastic effects occur long after radiation exposure; typically years following exposure.
11. **prodomal.** Symptoms of the prodromal syndrome include nausea, vomiting, diarrhea, and anorexia.
12. **randomly.** The effects of radiation in tissue are a consequence of random interactions.
13. **OER.** OER is the acronym for oxygen enhancement ratio. This ratio compares the effects of radiation in oxygenated tissue to hypoxic tissues.
14. **M.** The phase of mitosis is the most sensitive phase of cell division.
15. **growth.** During division, a portion of the cells are dividing causing growth of the tumor and another portion is dormant. The portion of cells dividing is known as the growth fraction.
16. **protraction.** Protraction is the time over which radiation is delivered. Protraction is tracked by documenting elapsed days during the therapy regimen.
17.

Type of Chromosomal damage	Consequences to chromosomes	Consequences to the cell
Single break, single chromosome	Restitution; inversion	No damage; change in gene sequence
Single break, two chromosomes	Acentric and dicentric chromosomes; translocation	Loss of genetic information; eventual loss of major parts of the chromosome
Double break, one chromosome	Deletions; inversion	Change in gene sequence; possible dysfunction
Double break, two chromosomes	Inversion; acentric fragments; ring formation	Loss of genetic information; change in gene sequence; severe damage i.e. death

18.

Mitotic rate	Differentiation	Sensitivity	Examples
High	Undifferentiated	High	Blood cells, germ cells
Moderate	Moderate differentiation	Intermediate	Intestinal cells, myelocytes, skin
Low	Moderate differentiation	Low	Liver, mature bone, muscle
Low to none	Well differentiated	Low	Nerves, adult brain

19.

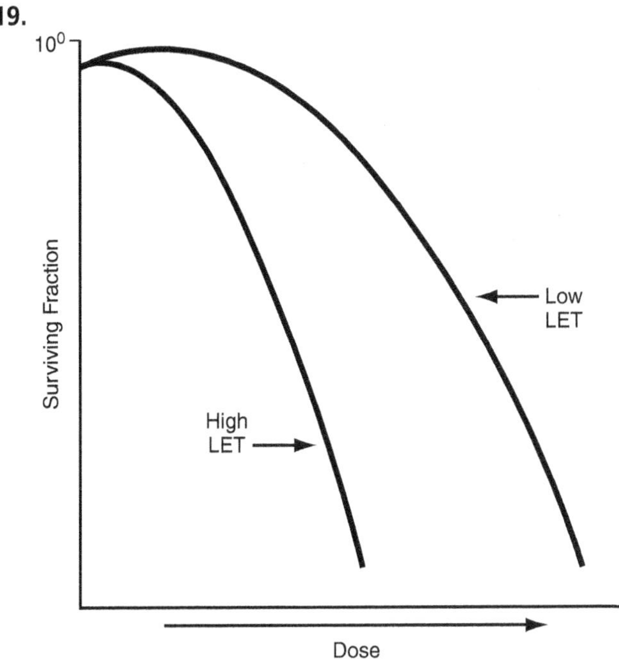

20. a. Erythema, or skin redness, is a result of vascular dilation.

21. c. Epilation, or hair loss, is typically observed after 15 Gy during standard fractionation (i.e. 2 Gy/day, 5 days/week)

22. a. Free radicals are a result of the breaking of the chemical bond between hydrogen and oxygen molecules in water

23. b. Protracted or fractionated doses allow for the repair of normal tissue

24. a. Cross-linking of broken segments of chromosomes are a consequence of DNA injury caused by radiation

25. b. The cumulative effect of radiation dose is the decreased ability for tissue to recover. This is desirable in the cancerous tissue and is demonstrated by increased severity of normal tissue injury as doses accumulate. Although normal tissue can recover more readily than cancerous tissue, more dose means longer delay in recovery.

26. b. Threshold dose-response curves indicate that there is no overt response by exposed tissue below certain doses

27. b. Hematopoietic syndrome is caused by reduced blood cells. Leukocytes are most sensitive of blood cells are the first to show decrease leaving victims feeling fatigued and vulnerable to deadly infections

28. a. LET or linear energy transfer is the energy deposited in an absorber as radiation passes through

29. b. Compared to the others, the epithelial cells in the alimentary tract have a longer mitotic future and divide more often that mature central nervous and connective tissues found in muscle and cardiovascular systems

30. b. The four Rs include reoxygenation, repopulation, redistribution and repair

31. c. At this dose range, a decrease in peripheral blood cells and depression of the bone marrow is likely to occur.

32. d. The development of radiation induced lung cancer would occur 10-20 years following exposure. A stochastic effect is one that occurs much later after initial exposure.

33. a. The Do value on the cell survival curve most accurately represents the sensitivity of certain cells to radiation. The smaller the Do, the more radiosensitive

34. a. RBE value compares a test radiation to 250 keV x-rays

35. b. The single whole body dose of 5000 cGy or greater, would likely cause the exposed to suffer from the CNS syndrome

36. a. Single whole body dose of about 10 Gy, or 1000 cGy would cause bone marrow suppression. Blood transfusion may rescue, but without this intervention death would likely occur within 10 days

37. d. Normal tissue may recover from radiation exposure by regeneration of cells or repair of cellular damage

38. d. High doses above 40 Gy may lead to permanent reduction in saliva.

39. c. Beyond the tolerance of the spinal cord, there would likely be swelling and cell death.

40. a. The more volume exposed the greater the injury. A smaller proportion of cells are left to repair and repopulate damaged cells when a greater volume is exposed.

41. lower. TD 5/5 is the dose for 5% incidence for injury in 5 years. TD 50/5 is the dose for 50% incidence of injury in 5 years. The larger dose would cause more of the exposed population to experience the selected effect.

42. lower. Tolerance for immature cells that are highly mitotic is lower than for mature cells with little mitotic activity.

43. lower. Giving radiation in single doses lowers the tolerance of tissue because there is no time for cellular repair and repopulation

44. **fistula.** Fistula is a possible endpoint for the colon exposed to fractionated doses of radiation up to 55 Gy.

45. **lower.** Germ cells in the ovary are highly mitotic making these cells more sensitive to radiation and manifesting a response sooner than lung tissue having lower mitotic activity and sensitivity to radiation

46. d. Non-stochastic is deterministic and manifest early in the individual exposed. The effects increase in severity as dose increases

47. c. The lens of the eye shows an adverse late effect at doses as low as 500 cGy.

48. b. The cell has an outer membrane and central nucleus. The section between the two is the cytoplasm.

49. d. The effect of radiation depends on the type of radiation, the fractionation and protraction, how much tissue is irradiated and the total dose.

50. d. The nucleus contains the DNA and RNA

51.
R E P A I R
1 (R), 2 (R)

52.
E R Y T H E M A
3 (E), 4 (E), 5 (A)

53.
D E S Q U A M A T I O N
6 (D), 7 (A), 8 (I)

54.
F R A C T I O N A T I O N
9 (F), 10 (R)

55.
L E T
11 (L)

56.
FREE RADICAL

57. a. The lens is more sensitive to radiation than the skin. Early effects will be seen at lower doses

58. d. Radiation protection standards are in place to prevent radiation-induced responses, both acute and latent.

59. d. According to RTOG morbidity scoring, a grade 1 side effect for the colon is a mild change in bowel habits

60. a. According to RTOG morbidity scoring, a grade 3 skin reaction would mean confluent moist desquamation

61. d. The onset dose for wet desquamation using standard fractionation is 40 Gy.

62. a. Somatic effects are limited to the individual exposed and may be acute or latent.

63. c. Ellis formula includes the total dose, nominal standard dose in RETS, the elapsed time and number of fractions.

64. a. Ellis' formula was based on connective type tissue response and was not designed to adjust for variable tissue sensitivities and biological end points

65. c. Fractionation came about during experiments to sterilize rams and spare the skin of the testicles from acute side effects

66. Head and neck cancers originating in the mucosa have a high mitotic activity and short intervals between mitotic events. Hyperfractionation attempts to delay mitotic activity and synchronize cells to most sensitive phases of division to increase cell kill. The spleen stores blood cells that are very radiosensitive. Hypofractionation provides the opportunity to cause cell death in any malignant cells infiltrating the organ and at the same time providing time for the sensitive normal cells to repair.

67. The physician and physicist/dosimetrist should be informed immediately. This is an ideal situation for use of the BED formula to determine what dose and fractionation scheme would lead to the same biological effect as the intended fractionation scheme.

68. This is not a feasible plan. Radioprotectors should be given prior to radiation within an hour or two.

69. This is not a feasible plan. Multiple fractions need to have an interval of 6 hours to allow for normal cellular repair. The interval should consider the understood growth and dividing behavior of the cells to be irradiated.

70. The 3-week break gives the normal and abnormal cells adequate time to repopulate. An adjustment to his total dose and fraction size may need to be made using the BED formula due to his prolonged absence. The original 6 weeks may need to be altered.

71. d. There are 4 signs of injuring including redness, swelling, heat and pain

72. b. The more tissue irradiated the lower the tolerance.

73. a. Ellis' formula used the reference dose of 1800 rets.

74. b. Lethal damage leads to cell death and cannot be repaired.

75. d. 60 Gy and above may cause latent stricture in the esophagus during standard fractionation schemes

76. d. Chemical bonds can be disrupted by ionizing radiations.

77. a. Adenine, thymine, guanine, and cytosine are the nitrogenous bases found in DNA.

78. c. DNA looks like a double helix or twisted ladder.

79. b. Mitosis is the term for cellular division in somatic cells.

80. a. DNA synthesis takes place between G1 and G2.

81. d. Cellular division begins in the M phase, then through G1, S, G2 and M again.

82. a. The cell survival curve for human cells usually has a shoulder region and a straight-line portion.

83. c. Higher LET radiations have mass and charge and therefore cause greater radiobiological effects.

84. d. A linear curve will show the changes in factors proportional.

85. c. Fractionating dose of radiation lessens the biological effects due to repair periods.
86. b. Proliferation describes growth and development as cells multiply.
87. d. The principle target in the human cell is DNA.
88. b. The greatest amount of the cell is about 85% water.
89. c. The extrapolation number is denoted by the 'n' or the measure of the shoulder on a cell survival curve.
90. b. Increasing the protraction, or period over which radiation is given, decreases the effects on the cell.

CHAPTER 5

Radiation Protection and Safety

1. d. According to the current dose limits, the hands of the pregnant therapist has the highest annual dose limit
2. b. Cumulative exposure is given by 10 mSv × age in years
3. b. One disadvantage to film badge monitoring is that there's time required for badge to be sent to an agency for reading.
4. b. For the entire gestation period, exposure should not exceed 0.5 rem or 5 mSv.
5. c. The cutie pie is not normally used to monitor personnel. Rather this ionization chamber is appropriately used for area surveys.
6. b. The Roentgen measures exposure or ionization events in the air.
7. d. Excessive heat, submersion in fluids or damage to the light-tight wrapper can cause damage to the film or unnecessary fogging, affecting accurate reading of the badge.
8. a. The quality factor, also known as radiation weighting factor, parallels the linear energy transfer of the radiation type. Radiations with high LET have higher quality factors or radiation weighting factors.
9. c. Wrappings and storage containers for radioactive materials should bear the sign Caution Radioactive material.
10. **NRC.** Nuclear Regulatory Commission (NRC). The NRC recommends radiation dose limits.
11. **150 mSv or 15 rem.** According to most recent NRC recommendations as of this writing.
12. **500 mSv.** According to most recent NRC recommendations as of this writing.
13. **use factor.** The use factor is the fraction of time the beam is aimed at a particular wall or ceiling.
14. **200 mrem/year.** Radon contributes about 200 mrem/year to internal radiation exposure

15a. Answer: 30 mR
Step 1: 6 minutes = 0.1 hours
Step 2: 0.1 hr (300 mR/hour) = 30 mR

15b. Answer: 67.5 mR
Step 1: Apply the inverse square law
Step 2: 30 mR $(3/2)^2$ = 67.5 mR

16. Answer: 5.7 TVLs
Step 1: 8 hrs/day × 5 days/week = 40 hrs/week = 2400 minutes/week
Step 2: Dose at office; Inverse square law = 0.5 rem/min $(40/20)^2$ = 2 rem/min or 2000 mrem/min
Step 3: 2000 mrem/min × 2400 minutes/week = 4,800,000 mrem/week
Step 4: 10 mrem/ 4,800,000 mrem = 0.0002 % or 0.000002;
Step 5: $0.1^x = 0.000002$
Step 6: $\text{Log}(0.1^x) = \text{Log}(0.000002)$
Step 7: $-1x = -5.6989$
$x = 5.6989$

17a. Answer: 31,500 cGy/week or 315 Gy/week
Step 1: Apply workload formula
Step 2: 35 pts/day × 5 days/wk × 4 flds/pt × 45 cGy/field = 31,500 cGy/week or 315 Gy/week

17b. Answer: 0.0000126
Step 1: Apply the barrier transmission factor formula
Step 2: 1 Gy = 1 Sv (gamma and x-rays), 1 mGy = 1 mSv

$$\text{Step 3: } B = \frac{1 \text{ mGy/week } (1\text{meter})^2}{315{,}000 \text{ mGy } (1/4)(1)} = .0000126$$

18. Answer: 6.25 %
Step 1: Ask how many half value layers of material is 4.4
Step 2: 4.4/1.1 = 4 HVLs
Step 3: 4 HVLs = 0.5^4 = 0.0625 or 6.25 %

19. Crystals in the emulsion on the film badge are transformed, film is processed, and density is read by a densitometer to determine dose. Lithium fluoride crystals trap electrons when exposed in the TLD. When the TLD is heated, trapped electrons are released in the form of light. Light photons are proportional to absorbed dose.
20. Ion chambers measure ionization of air, or migration of charges between charged plates by the liberation of electrons. The Fricke dosimeter relies on a chemical reaction. Ferrous sulfate, Fe^{2+} is oxidized when exposed to radiation and becomes Fe^{3+} ions.
21. c. Dose equivalent is measured in the traditional unit-rem or system international unit-Sievert.
22. F Exposure rate from a patient following insertion should be measured with an ion chamber.
23. T Two HVLs reduces transmission to 25%. 0.05^2 = 0.25
24. T Barrier protection is reduced when there is a beam stopper on the unit as found in Cobalt rotational units.
25. d. The Food and Drug Administration regulates the use of radiation producing machines.

26. d. Although there is a latent period for the development of cataracts, the latent period is far shorter than the typical period of 5-20 years for stochastic effects.
27. b. The GM counter measures the presence of radiation and would be useful in locating a misplaced radioactive source.
28. b. Radon contributes about 2/3 of total background radiation exposure.
29. a. Skin erythema dose was the first unit used to measure radiation response and set the standard for setting dose limits to personnel.
30. d. The Gray is the system international unit for absorbed dose.
31. C. Cosmic radiation is a result of interactions in upper atmosphere.
32. T. Terrestrial is defined as pertaining to the earth.
33. C. Higher altitudes bring exposure to interactions in the upper atmosphere closer.
34. I. Potassium, Carbon, Hydrogen, and Strontium are some contributors to internal radiation.
35. I. There is no shielding for internal sources of radiation.
36. T. Some geographic locations have greater concentrations of natural radioactive materials in the soil and rock.
37. b. The main types of background radiation are cosmic, terrestrial, and internal.
38. c. Higher altitudes bring you closer to irradiative events occurring in the upper atmosphere.
39. d. Terrestrial radiation comes from the soil and rock and can vary based on geographic location.
40. b. The TLD has properties most like living tissue and measures absorbed dose.
41. d. Following brachytherapy procedures, the room should be surveyed after the patient leaves to ensure that no radioactive material is left behind.
42. d. Transfer, burning, or burial are all appropriate for the disposing of depleted radioactive sources
43. c. The use of long forceps allows the handler to take advantage of the inverse square principle. Increasing the distance decreases the dose.
44. a. Hot labs containing solid radioactive sources should have a sign that reads Caution Radioactive Material
45. a. The workload is an expression of beam-on time
46. a. Concrete is less dense than lead or iron and therefore would have a lower attenuation coefficient requiring more material for adequate limitation of exposure.
47. b.
Step 1: Use the formula HVL = 0.693/μ
Step 2: 22 mm = 0.693/μ
Step 3 : 22 (μ) = 0.693
Step 4: μ = 0.0315
48. a. Film badges are easily exposed by low doses of scatter radiation possibly in the vault or at the console. Leaving the badge in the car may allow the badge to be exposed to excessive heat or sunlight, which could 'fog' the film contained in the badge.
49. d. During HDR procedures, radioactive sources are outside of protective containers. To maintain compliance with the ALARA principle, HDR procedures should be conducted in shielded areas such as the simulator or linear accelerator vault
50. c. Following nuclear medicine procedures like the iodine swallow, patients cannot be released until radiation levels around the patient reach less than 5 mrem/hour or the activity remaining is less than 30 microCurie.
51. c. Hydrogen^3 is a gas always present in our bodies. Hydrogen 3 carries charge and releases energy in the form of low radiation.
52. c. Radioactive sources should be transported in shielding containers also known as 'pigs'
53. d. Personnel caring for a patient while radioactive sources are implanted should plan to work as efficiently and quickly as possible to limit exposure to any low dose secondary radiation. Standard precautions are always in order.
54. a.
Step 1: Use the dose equivalent formula
Step 2: Sv = Gray × Quality factor.
Step 3: Quality factor for gamma radiation is 1.
Step 4 : 0.5 Sv = x (1)
55. d.

Use the formula $HVL = \frac{.693}{\mu}$

Step 1: $32 \text{ mm} = \frac{.693}{\mu}$

Step 2: 32 (μ) = 0.693
Step 3: μ = 0.0216
56. d. 1 HVL reduces transmission to 50% so use the formula $0.5^x = .02$

Step 1:	$\log 0.5^x = \log 0.02$
Step 2:	$-0.301x = -1.699$
Step 3:	x = 5.64 HVLs

57. c. One tenth value layer reduces transmission to 10%. $0.1^3 = .001$ or 0.1 %
58. a. Shielding should not allow more than 2 mrem/hour at a distance of 1 meter behind the barrier.
59a.
Answer: 0.063 mm^{-1}

Step 1: $11 \text{ mm} = \frac{.693}{\mu}$

Step 2: μ = 0.063 mm^{-1}
59b. Answer: 55.6 mm lead
Step 1: Use the formulas I/Io = transmission and $I = Io\ e^{-\mu(x)}$

Step 2: $\frac{I}{I_o} = 0.03$

Step 3: $0.03 = e^{-0.063(x)}$

$\ln 0.03 = \ln e^{-0.063(x)}$
$-3.506 = -0.063\ (x)$
$x = 55.6$ mm lead

60a.

Answer: 7.8 cm

Step 1: Use the formula $HVL = \frac{0.693}{\mu}$

Step 2: $\frac{0.693}{HVL} = 0.089 = 7.8$ cm

60b.

Answer: 43.9 cm

Step 1: Use the formulas I/Io = transmission and $I = Io\ e^{-\mu\ (x)}$

Step 2: $\frac{I}{I_o} = 0.02$

Step 3: $0.02 = e^{-0.089(x)}$
$\text{Ln } 0.02 = \ln e^{-0.089(x)}$
$-3.91 = -0.089\ (x)$
$x = 43.9$ cm

CHAPTER 6

Radiation Therapy Equipment and Quality Assurance

1. **b.** The Cobalt source decays at a rate of about 1.09% per month

2. **a.** The protective housing in the gantry of the Cobalt unit should not allow more than 0.1% of beam transmission

3. **b.** The linear accelerator target needs to have a high melting point and high atomic number to accommodate the high-energy electron stream directed toward it

4. **c.** Electrons are burned off the electron gun by thermionic emission

5. **a.** Linear accelerators use transmission targets positioned perpendicular to the stream of electrons, allowing transmission of converted energy on the opposite side of the target. Diagnostic x-ray tubes use reflection targets allowing converted energy to be reflected at an angle away from the target

6. **a.** The large Cobalt source has substantial penumbra. Trimmer bars are the third line of collimators attached to reduce the amount of penumbra reaching the patient

7. Use the penumbra formula

$$P = \frac{2(75 + 5 - 40)}{40} = \frac{80}{40} = 2 \text{ cm}$$

8.

$$P = \frac{3(75 - 5 + 40)}{40} = \frac{120}{40} = 3 \text{ cm}$$

9.

$$P = \frac{2(75 - 5 + 30)}{30} = \frac{100}{30} = 3.33 \text{ cm}$$

10.

$$P = \frac{2(77 + 3 + 40)}{40} = \frac{80}{40} = 2.0 \text{ cm}$$

11. **c.** The Cyclotron accelerates heavy particles like deuterons, neutrons, and protons.

12. **d.** The flattening filter evenly distributes the energy of the photon beam. Without the flattening filter, the photon beam has concentrated energy toward the central axis.

13. The ion chamber monitors dose rate and field symmetry.

14. The magnetron and klystron produce microwaves for acceleration of electrons in the linear accelerator. The klystron amplifies microwaves in the higher power accelerators.

15. The Cobalt unit houses a radioactive source. The penetrating gamma radiation coming from the source is what is used for treatment delivery.

16. The interaction of the gamma rays with the trimmer bars cause secondary radiation. 15 cm spacing allows room for secondary radiation to scatter out before contacting the patient

17. **Increases.** Penumbra is directly proportional to the distance from the source.

18. **Decreases.** The size of penumbra and source to diaphragm distance are inversely proportional. As distance from the source and diaphragm increases, the penumbra region decreases.

19. **Decreases.** The size of penumbra and source size are directly proportional. The larger the source, the larger the penumbra region.

20. **Tungsten.** Tungsten has a sufficient atomic number that electrons striking it will cause Bremsstrahlung and characteristic radiation. At the same time, this type of target allows transmission without eliminating the higher energies of the poly-energetic spectrum produced.

21. No high power current or heat generating mechanics are needed in the cobalt unit.

22. Using bolus materials on/in an irregular anatomical surface losing the skin sparing effect of high-energy photon and electron beams. Standard wedges and custom compensators are positioned within the beam at established distances from the patient's skin surface, therefore preserving the skin-sparing feature of the therapy beam while correcting for irregular surface contour.

23. Radium is expensive to harvest from the earth and has a carcinogenic daughter product—radon gas.

24. **d.** Strontium^{89} is available as an unsealed source and is injectable for diffuse metastatic disease

25. **c.** Phosphorus^{32} emits beta radiation strictly. Cesium, cobalt, and iodine emit gamma radiation

26. **a.** The field light represents the area of radiation

27. **d.** The beam stopper on the cobalt unit serves as a counterbalance for the heavy gantry head and as a primary beam barrier.

28. **b.** The scattering foil is inserted in the path of electrons when the accelerator is operating in the electron mode. The foil scatters electrons across a broad area

29. a. The klystron or magnetron is a source of microwaves in the linear accelerator
30. c. The cyclotron can produce heavy particles like protons, neutrons, and deuterons
31. b. Positioning devices help to achieve the desired patient position for accurate treatment delivery
32. a. Superficial therapy machines operated in the range 50–150 kV
33. a. Long cylinders loaded with isotopes may be positioned in the vagina to deliver dose to the vaginal cavity. Applicators such as Heyman's capsules or tandem and ovoids would deliver dose to endometrium and pelvis side wall. Therapy to the vulva could be deliver using teletherapy beams
34. b. Acceleration of electrons occurs along a linear path in the linear accelerator.
35. b. Cobalt decays at a rate of about 1.09% per month. Output and treatment time calculations would have to be adjusted to reflect decay
36. d. The size of penumbra is influenced by the source size, distance from source and diaphragm or collimator device distance from the source. Refer to penumbra formula
37. f
38. b
39. e
40. d

a. 74.2 days
b. 60 days
c. 30 days
d. 2.7 days
e. 30 years
f. 1622 years
g. 1622 days

41. b. Heyman's capsule looks like a small tampon and is inserted into the uterine cavity delivery dose to the endometrium
42. b. Fletcher's suite consists of tandem and ovoids loaded with low output sources into the female pelvis. This is an example of intra-cavitary brachytherapy. Dose is delivered over a few days.
43. d. The BAT system is a bedside ultrasound unit used for daily target localization
44. a and c. The light field indicates the field size and is relied upon as an indicator of where the radiation field is projected
45. b and c. The performance of the linear accelerator relies on current which is not static and may fluctuate periodically. As equipment wears, the auxiliary and primary power sources can wear down and fluctuate in output therefore affecting the output of the accelerator
46. c. The optical distance indicator (ODI) gives the distance from the source to the patient's skin
47. b. The collimator, gantry, and couch of a conventional simulator must rotate around the isocenter. Tolerance for deviation is 2 mm in diameter
48. b. Lasers should agree with the ODI within 2 mm at isocenter
49. a. Constancy of output should be verified daily for both photon and electron beams on the linear accelerator
50. b. Output values taken during commissioning and acceptance testing should be within 3% of benchmark values supplied by the manufacturer and/or identical systems
51. a and b. Symmetry and flatness may be checked using film or beam profilers. Densitometers need to be used to evaluate the film exposed if this method is chosen
52. b. Field flatness for the photon beam in the linac is recommended to be within 2% across 80% of the beam
53. b. Indicated scan and couch position in the vertical aspect, especially, are recommended to be within 2 mm of actual
54. a and b. radiation room monitors and door interlocks are recommended for daily checks. Beam output should be checked monthly and timer error, yearly
55. c. as a decaying source with a long half-life, output is recommended to be checked monthly; expected change is a decrease of 1.09% per month
56. d. Total overhaul, that is, a review of all technical aspects, should be performed each year
57. a. All sources should be checked for leaks at minimum at the time of receipt. then periodically depending on the half life of the source
58. c. The exact position of sources should be checked using radiographic imaging
59. c and d. Sources should be calibrated before use and then these measurements must be documented and traceable to an accredited calibration laboratory
60. d. In the brachytherapy room, a survey meter must be available for before and after the procedure, a temporary storage container for any unused sources and cutter and long-handled tongs in case sources need to be handled manually
61. a. light and radiation field coincidence should be within 2mm or within 1% on a side.
62. b. Lasers should be within 2 mm of isocenter on simulators
63. K
64. C
65. L, M
66. A
67. B
68. D
69. E
70. F
71. G
72. H
73. H, F, G
74. L
75. B
76. C, M
77. c. Split field testing for longitudinal displacement can be achieved by exposing film allowing one half of the field set at a set collimator angle and then

rotating 180 degrees and exposing the other half of the field

78. b. A spirit level can be used to check the accuracy of gantry digital read-outs. It's acceptable to check readouts at 45-degree increments

79. a. Light field and radiation coincidence can be checked using radiographic film with metallic markers at the field borders to verify against radiation exposed area on the film

80. c. Linear scales may be used for daily treatment set up and translation of patient positions between simulation and treatment

81. d. Recommendation is that the door interlock be checked daily

82. a. The back-up timer, radiation off switch, door interlock, and emergency off switch all put the operator in control of dose delivery. Over-ride switches help avoid unnecessary exposure and indicate the potential exceeding of previously set parameters. Collision rings help prevent patient injury or damage to equipment

83. b. During megavoltage therapy, patients should be monitored using closed circuit intercommunication systems

84. b. Acceptance testing is performed to assure that the manufacturer's specifications on machine performed is actual

85. b. Dose rate constancy should be verified daily and also monthly. The other quality checks are recommended to be performed monthly

86. **1 degree**. AAPM recommends that gantry and collimator indicators are accurate within 1 degree.

87. +3%. Field flatness across the central 80% of the beam should not vary outside of 3%

88. c. Flatness of the beam is influenced by correct position of the flattening filter or target and fluctuations in current. Mirror angulation influences light field and radiation agreement

89. b. Limit switches protect mechanical gears and bearings in the gantry and collimators. If the gantry rotates beyond the end point, the limit switch for the gantry is not fully functional.

90. d. The mechanical distance indicator or pointer is used to verify the accuracy of the ODI and to verify the correct alignment and agreement of lasers

91. b. The mirror and bulb assembly must be in perfect geometrical relationship to accurately represent the radiation beam. Any adjustments or repairs to the system requires quality checking of congruence

92. b. Gold has a half-life of 2.7 days, cesium 30 years, iridium 74 days, and radon 3.8 days

93. b. As cobalt 60 decays, beta particles and gamma rays of energies 1.33 and 1.17 are emitted. The average energy then is 1.25 MV

94. d. The shorter distances in early therapy equipment were used due to rapid percentage depth dose fall off. Secondary radiation augments skin dose at short distance, however, this is a great advantage of longer treatment distance equipment

95. c. Low energy x-ray machines would use filters to harden the beam, filtering out low energy radiation. Increasing the filtration would sift out more soft radiation thereby increasing the overall quality and penetrating power of the beam

96. F. The effective energy of the photon beam is not influenced by how long the beam is on, or by the current (amount of electrons coming across the tube). The effective energy is influenced by increasing the potential across the tube (voltage and supplemental energy boosts from alternating frequency waves).

97. F. The effective energy of the photon beam is not influenced by how long the beam is on, or by the current (amount of electrons coming across the tube). The effective energy is influenced by increasing the potential across the tube (voltage and supplemental energy boosts from alternating frequency waves).

98. T. The effective energy of the photon beam is not influenced by how long the beam is on, or by the current (amount of electrons coming across the tube). The effective energy is influenced by increasing the potential across the tube (voltage and supplemental energy boosts from alternating frequency waves).

99. a. OBI is an acronym for on board imaging devices. OBI devices can take on many forms from simple detectors and video cameras to complexed Cone beam CT attachments

100. a. The cyclotron uses two D-shaped cavities across which, heavy particles are accelerated

101. d. The Klystron is located in the drive stand or in the modulator cabinet

CHAPTER 7

Radiation Therapy Treatment Planning

1. b. Several terms are used for the removable grids that show the crosshairs on a port film. They include BB tray, fiduciary tray, graticule, and reticule

2. **focal spot, point**. SAD is measured from the source to a reference point in space around which the gantry and PSA rotates.

3. c. The cost commonly used database used for treatment planning is CT.

4. d. MRI, PET, CT, and US can be fused and used for therapy treatment planning. PET and CT fusion studies are used often

5. T. xyz coordinates work well for target localization. The patient can be moved and tracked in any direction to a specific distance.

6. Thinner CT slices increase DRR resolution because of additional detail to reconstruct from.

7.

1. Photos
2. Detailed description of set up

3. Good marks on the patient
4. Well made immobilization devices
5. Appropriate, well-fitting positioning aids

8. a. The CT simulator top should be flat so that the patient's anatomy responds the same when on the flat PSA in the treatment room

9. b. Ballpoint pen is not an appropriate tool to use for patient skin markings.

10. F. Unlike conventional radiation therapy, each IMRT port or gantry stop contains a number of beamlets. In most cases, the beamlets are so numerous that filming each one would not be feasible. Instead, QA is chosen to compare output and fluence from a phantom onto which the plan is ran to the output and fluence provided by the treatment planning computer. Usually, orthogonal films are taken to verify isocenter placement.

11. **knee support/sponge.** A support that slightly elevates the knees takes pressure off the lower back and decreases the lordotic curve in the lumbar spine.

12. d. Allowing the breast to find its natural position offers excellent reproducibility and treatment planning conformality.

13. d. Percent depth dose is used for nonisocentric or SSD treatment techniques and represents the fraction of dose at depth

14. b. When beam-shaping devices are used, the effective square should be used to find the percent depth dose, TMR or TAR

15. F. Mayneord's formula is used to change a standard %DD at a standard SSD to a %DD that can be used at a non standard SSD. The formula is based on the inverse square principle.

16. Answers: Pros—More clearance between the gantry and patient
Larger field size can be achieved
Less collimator scatter to the patient
Cons—Patient must be moved between each gantry position
Rotational therapy, IMRT, and conformal therapy would not be feasible

17. Answers:
Patient does not have to be moved between gantry angles
Set up errors are minimized

18. d. Multileaf collimators made intensity modulated radiation therapy a possibility

19. b. Sterling's formula is used to determine the equivalent square

20. a, b, c. Extended SSD technique requires the use of Mayneord's factor (factor goes in the denominator or may convert the old %DD for the new field size) and inverse square.

21. The therapist places radiopaque wires on the patient's skin

22. b. Multiple fields increase the integral dose. An increase in dose is not an advantage to the patient

23.
Lung tumor __6______
Nasopharynx __6_____
Prostate _______18____
Cervix _______18__
Pancreas ________18____
Breast ________6__
Upper arm sarcoma _6__

Thinner anatomical areas or where low-density tissues such as lung tissue are optimally treated with lower energy beams. Whereas, thicker areas with deeply positioned targets require the use of a higher energy beam.

24. **dosimetrically.** Field sizes around a target area should be large enough to give ±5% of the prescribed dose to the target.

25. b. Expediting treatment time should not be a primary consideration for determining gantry positions.

26. **c and d.** Dmax is the point of peak dose in tissue. Peak dose occurs where electronic equilibrium occurs.

27.
PTV
GTV
CTV

28. **false.** Wedges filter out weak photons from polyenergetic beams. The average energy of a polyenergetic beam increases (hardens) after passing through a wedge.

29.
1. Brings Dmax closer to the surface
2. Fills in deficits so that the dose distribution is more homogenous

30. d. TD 5/5 is the dose that will likely cause complications in 5% of the population exposed after 5 years

31. **b and c.** Using the SSD technique, less dose is absorbed as the depth increases. Therefore, any tissues before the target will receive more dose and tissues beyond the target will receive less dose. Refer to an isodose chart.

32. **a and d.** If the beam energy was increased, the same phenomenon would be true. However, comparing low energy to high energy, the high-energy beam spares more tissues near the surface and deposits more at depth.

33. b. A high-energy x-ray beam such as the energies used in therapy will have maximum dose deposit below the surface. The higher the energy, the deeper the point of electronic equilibrium.

34. 6; 18; 18. Higher energy beams have greater penetration and deposit more dose at depth.

35. Direct proportion: 200: 0.65 as x: 0.85, x = 262 cGy
OR
Applied dose = TD/%DD; 200/.65 = 307.6 cGy then....
Applied dose x %DD = TD; 307.6 cGy x 0.85 = 262 cGy

36. Use the formula:
D_{max} dose = TD/%DD
150 cGy/.60 = 250 cGy

37. 2. An electron beam loses about 2 MeV of energy per centimeter of tissue.

38. c. An advantage of electron arc therapy is that Dmax is moved further away from the surface.

39.
1. Safe containment of the isotope
2. Filters out alpha, beta, and lower energy gamma radiation

40. **interstitial.** Seeds are placed within the prostate tissue.

41. **intraluminal.** Source is placed within the lumen created by a balloon.

42. **interstitial.** Ribbons are threaded and secured into the tissues of the tongue.

43. **d.** When more than 2 planes are used, the planes created a 3-dimensional shape conducive to a volume as opposed to an area as a 1 or 2 plane implant provides.

44.

$$\text{Answer: } \frac{\text{Activity(decay constant)}}{\text{Distance}^2}$$

45.

_D__**Patterson–Parker/Manchester**	A) sources of uniform strength spaced 1.0 cm apart.
_B__**Quimby**	B) uniform source distribution with nonuniform dose distribution.
_A__**Memorial**	C) often used for calculating line sources.
_C__**Paris**	D) nonuniform source distribution with uniform dose distribution.

46. **b.** Reference points used in gynecologic brachytherapy are points A and B. Though points B, rectum and bladder doses are evaluated, point A determines the implant duration. Point A is located 2 cm superior and 2 cm lateral of the cervical os.

47. **helium; positive**

48. **negatron**

49. **beta**

50. A magnet could be used. Gamma particles would not react but the charged alpha and beta particles would. The alpha particle has a positive charge but is heavier than the beta particle. The beta particle would be most reactive to the magnet.

51.
1. Cobalt
2. Cesium
3. Palladium
4. Gold
5. Iridium
6. Iodine
7. Phosphorus
8. Ytterbium
9. Strontium
10. Samarium

52. c. Ultrasound is most often used for prostate implant treatment planning because of the ease of visualizing the prostate slice by slice during the procedure.

53. 20

54. 0.5; 2.0

55. b. A change in the field size will change the output. The change should be documented and submitted for recalculation of MU

56. a. Too many fractions to the preliminary field has changed the absorbed dose to all other tissues besides the GTV. Actual dose to other tissues needs to be considered before proceeding to the next phase of the patient's treatment plan.

57. c. Patient measurements must be considered before any dose is administered. Monitor units cannot be calculated without knowing the location of isocenter at minimum.

58. c. Likely during the three week break the patient has lost marks. Changes in weight and anatomical dimensions may have also changed. The three-week break has allowed some tissue healing and possibly regrowth of cancerous cells. BED calculations should be performed so that adjustments to fractions or total dose can be performed.

59. **a and b.** The wedge angle is determined by the tilt of the 50% isodose line in low energy beams such as Cobalt. The dose line at a depth of 10 cm is used to name the wedge angle for higher energy beams used most commonly in therapy today.

60. **d.** The thoracic spine is positioned near the posterior aspect of the body. In patients of normal body habitus, the depth for the upper thoracic vertebral bodies is about 5-6 cm deep. A single posterior low energy beam is sufficient.

61. a. Whole breast irradiation is best delivered using tangential fields. The N1 staging classification likely indicates positive disease in the axillary region which is easily covered using tangential fields. A boost to the tumor bed may be elected to decrease the likelihood of recurrent disease.

62. c. A right temporal tumor is a challenge to treat due to the proximity to the lens. A right sided wedged pair will spare normal brain. Using the vertex field instead of an anterior field will eliminate concern for exceeding tolerance of the lens.

63. b. Wedges are used to compensate for missing tissue and/or to shift dose lines. The aspect of the pelvis through which beams would enter for treatment of the rectum is irregular in contour (rounded) and will likely require the use of wedges positioned appropriately for compensation for missing tissue—heels up toward the posterior aspect.

64. d. Manual contouring can be achieved by using solder wire, calipers, plaster of Paris, or a pantograph. A bite block is a positioning/immobilization device
65. d. Treating the neck often requires lateral beams. Shoulder retractors push the shoulders down out of the potential path of those lateral ports to the neck.
66. d. Optimal hinge angle may be found by using the formula: Hinge = 180 – 2(wedge).
67. b. The separation angle between two beams is known as the hinge angle.
68. b. A good starting point for figuring appropriate wedge size is to first consider the hinge angle between beams and then apply the formula: Hinge = 180 – 2(wedge)
69. b. Using Sterling's formula, the equivalent square for a 15 × 6 cm area is 8.6 cm
70. a. Two adjacent spine fields would have dimensions showing the longest sides as lengths. The two fields would be matched along these lengths. Apply the skin gap formula to compute the skin surface space between the two fields that would allow field overlap at the specified depth: ½ Length #1 (d/SSD) + ½ Length #2 (d/SSD).
71. b. The plan data sheet indicates the use of asymmetric jaws. The field width would be the sum of X1 and X2 jaws and the field length would be the sum of the Y1 and Y2 jaws.
72. a. The gantry angle for the LPO treatment field is shown as 100.0 degrees
73. a. Using the x, y, z coordinate system referenced on an axial view, the data sheet indicates a shift to the patient's right of 1.0 cm. See data labeled Isocenter X on the sheet. On axial image, the patient's right is on the negative side of the x plane.
74. d. Using the x, y, z coordinate system referenced on a sagittal view, the data sheet indicates a shift to posterior to the original isocenter. See data labeled Isocenter Z on the sheet. On sagittal image, the patient's posterior surface is on the negative side of the z plane.
75. c. Using the rules of thumb E/2 = range, E/3 = depth of 80% dose line, E/4 = depth of the 90% dose line. We can calculate that the 20 MeV beam would show the 90% dose line at a depth of 5 cm.

CHAPTER 8

Oncology Patient Care

1. d. In order for infections to spread a germ must be present, the germ must have a place to live and multiply, and a susceptible host must be present with a way for the germ to enter the host. Removing any one of these components breaks the chain of infection
2. d. The normal platelet count in an adult ranges from 140,000–400,000/cc
3. **20 breaths/minute**
4. **medical asepsis**
5. c. Direct contact involves touch, sexual contact, and kissing
6. **epilation**
7.
- **a.** avoid raw vegetable
- **b.** avoid food high in roughage
- **c.** avoid greasy foods
- **d.** increase fluid intake
- **e.** eliminate caffeine products

8.
- **a.** touch
- **b.** sexual contact
- **c.** kissing
- **d.** contaminated food

9.
- **a.** Asepsis—**absence of disease producing microorganism called pathogens**
- **b.** Medical asepsis—**also called (clean technique) practice that helps to reduce the number and hinder the transfer of disease-producing microorganism**
- **c.** Surgical asepsis—**also called (sterile technique) practice which render and keep objects and areas free from all microorganism**
- **d.** Contamination—**process by which something is rendered unclean or unsterile**
- **e.** Disinfection—**process by which pathogenic organism, but generally spores, are destroyed**
- **f.** Antiseptic—**inhibits the growth of bacteria**
- **g.** Sterilization—**process by which all microorganism are destroyed**

10.

COLUMN A	COLUMN B
___E__diarrhea	A. regular diet
___B__nausea	B. clear fluids
___B__vomiting	C. liquids only
___C__mucositis	D. soft liquids
___B, D__dysphagia	E. low residue

11. 98.6 degrees
12. airway; breathing; circulating
13. brachial
14. F. Recapping the needle after use increases risk for needle stick injury
15. F. The normal pulse is about 60–80 beats per minute. Tachycardia means rapid heartbeat
16. Match the following terms with the correct definition

_C___	bluish discoloration of skin	A. syncope
_B___	stroke	B. CVA
_A___	fainting	C. cyanosis
_D___	profuse sweating	D. diaphoresis
_H___	tube used to pass fluids, gases into/out of body	E. tachypnea
_F___	an aggregation of blood	F. thrombus
		G. parenteral
		H. cannula

17. b. Anaphylactic shock occurs when a patient has an allergic response to the iodinated contrast. The contrast triggers a quick and massive release of histamines leading to systemic vasodilation

18. c. Due to constriction of the airway, wheezing, and labored, noisy breathing occurs

19. c. Side effects of radiation therapy depend on the area treated and will occur only in the area being treated

20. d. Radiation recall is defined as the recalling by the skin of previous radiation exposure in response to the administration of certain response-inducing drugs

21. b. Superior vena cava syndrome is caused by the blockage or narrowing of the superior vena cava, often by a tumor in the apex of the lung, decreasing blood flow back to the heart

22. c. Narcotic medications given around the clock have the tendency to cause constipation. Administering mild laxatives helps to maintain normal bowel motility.

23. b. Pressure on the spinal cord can cause compression of nerves that pass through the spaces between the back bone or the bundle of nerves that extend downward from the spinal cord. Compressions secondary to cancers in the lumbar spine may cause tingling in the lower extremities, trouble walking, and incontinence.

24. a. Neutropenia is a blood disorder which is characterize with an abnormally low number of neutrophils. Neutrophils serve as the primary defense against infection

25.

___B___	**low volume of circulating blood**	A. Anaphylactic
___D___	**systemic infection and bacteremia**	B. Hypovolemic
___E___	**injury or emotional trauma**	C. Cardiogenic
___F___	**hypoglycemia**	D. Septic
___C___	**heart failure**	E. Neurogenic
___A___	**severe allergic reaction**	F. Diabetic

26.

___A___	**allergies**	A. Benadryl
___D___	**heart arrhythmia**	B. Lidocaine
___C___	**hypertension**	C. Inderal
___B___	**cardiogenic shock**	D. Lanoxin

27. a. Surgical asepsis dictates the environment is free from all biological contaminants

28. a. Patient safety is first and foremost, after assisting the patient then call for help

29. b. Parenteral routes for medication involves injection into a vein, muscle, artery, abdominal cavity, heart, or fatty tissue. If biological pathogens enter then infection may occur

30. c. Respiration in the adult ranges from 10–20 breaths per minute

31. 37

32. surgical asepsis

33. handwashing

34. F. A nosocomial infection is one acquired in the healthcare facility

35. a. Anaphylactic or allergic reaction is a severe reaction to asparaginase.

36. c. Asepsis is the absence of disease producing microorganisms called pathogens

37. b. Hand washing is instrumental and easiest to achieve in breaking the chain of infection thereby preventing the spread of infection

38. d. The Patient's Bill of Rights says that patients have the right to refuse treatment, know the qualifications of personnel, and trust that records will be secure

39. a. Medical terminology—*Dys-* means lack of or difficulty; *-pnea* refers to breathing

40. b. The definition of epilation is removal of or loss of hair

41. c. Medical terminology—*Anti-* means against; -*emesis* refers to vomiting

42.
- **a.** right patient
- **b.** right drug
- **c.** right route of administration
- **d.** right frequency
- **e.** right dose

43.
- **a.** intravenous
- **b.** oral
- **c.** rectal

44.
- **a.** do not use around flames
- **b.** do not stand oxygen cylinder upright unless it is secured
- **c.** do not carry oxygen cylinder by regulator or valve

45.
- **a.** keep area dry
- **b.** no deodorant in treatment area
- **c.** avoid tight fitting clothes
- **d.** no lotions or creams except those provided by nurse or physician
- **e.** do not scratch skin

46.–55.

	Dose	Intervention
Skin reaction	3000–4000cGy	Keep area dry Loose-fitting clothes No creams or lotions unless prescribed
Diarrhea	2000–5000cGy	Low-residue diet Increase fluid intake No raw vegetables
Fatigue	Variable	Relax Bed rest Increase nutritional supplements

	Dose	Intervention
Pain	Variable depending on source of pain	Take prescribed pain meds Assess weekly with physician
Nausea	1000–3000cGy	Prophylactic antiemetics Liquid diet
Weight loss	Variable	Small frequent meals Increase nutritional supplement Liquid nutrition
Mucositis	3000- 4000cGy	No hot/spicy foods Increase liquid intake Mouth hygiene program
Alopecia	2000cGy	Wear cap No shaving
Cystitis	3000cGy	Urine test monitor Increase liquid intake Antibiotic
Esophagitis	2000cGy	Small, frequent meals Increase liquid intake Antacids

56.–65.

Emergency	Symptoms	Likely cause	Response
Anaphylactic shock	Difficulty breathing Swollen lips Drop in blood pressure Metallic taste Hives	Allergic reaction to medicine Allergic reaction to contrast	Epinephrine
Cardiogenic shock	Weak, rapid pulse Cold hands and feet Fatigue Profuse sweating	Heart attack	Oxygenation Intubation Ventilation
Hypovolemic shock	Rapid breathing Anxiety Clammy skin	Severe blood loss Internal bleeding	Replace blood Replace fluids
Pulmonary embolism	Unexplained shortness of breath Swelling of the ankles Chest pain	Surgery Lying in bed for extended period of time	Anticoagulant Heparin Warfarin
Hypoglycemia	Anxiety Sweating Tremors Confusion	Low blood sugar	Glucose injection
Hyperglycemia	Excessive urine Excessive thirst Dehydration	Diabetes	Fluid correction for dehydration Normalized blood glucose
Respiratory distress	Difficulty breathing Tachypnea Abnormal breath sounds Cyanosis	Blockage of airway Allergic reaction	Provide oxygen Elevate head
Cardiac distress	Cold, clammy skin Irregular pulse Cyanosis	Drug therapy Pre-existing conditions	Check airway Check breathing Check circulation Administer CPR
Seizure	Convulsion Inability to speak Visual hallucinations	Head injury Heat stroke Infection Epilepsy	Protect person from falling Loosen clothes around the neck Place pillow under head Administer phenytoin
Syncope	Loss of consciousness	Low blood pressure Hypoglycemia Circulating disorder	Help patient to the ground Check vitals

66.

1. Beneficence—**acts in the best interest of the patient**
2. Nonmalfeasance—**assumes responsibility for professional decisions**
3. Autonomy—**provides services to humanity with full respect for the dignity of mankind**
4. Justice—**delivers care unrestricted by concerns of personal attributes. . .and without discrimination**
5. Veracity—**advances the principles of the profession**
6. Role fidelity—**adheres to tenets and domains of scope of practice**
7. Confidentiality—**exercises care, discretion and judgment**

67. Make sure that you practice within your scope, take responsibility for continuing education so that you are fully aware of standards of practice, and follow the seven ethical principles.

68. Developing a code of ethics and making it available to the public ensures that both the professional and general public are aware of what we have advocated as the expected, professional code of conduct

69. Protect your patient's privacy by discussing case details discretely among those professionals needing to know. Have consulting room doors closed when interviewing patients. Keep medical records secure and do not peruse through patient information when not warranted. Cover patient's anatomy whenever possible.

70. The ethical principles veracity and role fidelity should govern your response. You should only discuss with the patient the true facts of the error with caution. If you are not fully aware of the details and have any uncertainties, acknowledge the patient's concerns and arrange for them to speak with someone who has the authority to discuss. Follow up to make sure that the patient received the answers he/she was looking for.

71. The ethical principle that should be considered here is confidentiality. Sharing the news with your family is a violation of patient privacy and HIPAA policy. Legal issues may arise, especially if the news you deliver is not true. In the case of mistaken identity as you review a medical record of an individual with the same name, and not that of your family friend, you could find yourself guilty of slander and defamation of character.

72. The patient treated for metastatic brain disease will likely have treatment to the entire brain to a total dose of 30–35 Gy. Treating this volume to this dose, the expected acute effects will likely be epilation, erythema, and slight dry desquamation. You should advise your patient to protect their head from the sun, refrain from scratching and razor shaving. Patient should refrain from any chemical treatments to the scalp. Washing the head with mild soap and lukewarm water is advised. Wigs, turbans, and fun hats are a great filler for thinning hair.

73. d. Tachycardia means rapid pulse. The normal heart rate is 60–80 beats/minute.

74. b. A diuretic helps eliminate excess fluid. Urination is the means by which excess fluid is eliminated.

75. b. Our professional code of ethics commits us to caring for individuals unrestricted of personal attributes, race, or religion. However, other clinicians who may be asked to perform a procedure that is against their personal beliefs (such as abortion) may refer a patient requesting this certain procedure to another qualified professional.

76. a. Professional ethics are a set of principles that have been agreed upon and meant to reflect consensus regarding conduct among a body of professionals in certain work-related situations.

77. b. The ethical principle of confidentiality commits us to holding all patient information in confidence.

78. c. Operating and performing duties outside of your scope of practice puts you and your employer at risk for liability if any harm comes to the patient as a result.

79. c. HIV and HBV are blood borne, therefore needle stick injuries pose the greatest risk for communication of disease.

80. d. Sources of infection are many. Living hosts with pathogens easily transmissible by the airborne, contact or droplet modes may lead to communication of disease.

81. b. Universal precautions were instituted to minimize the transmission of blood-borne disease. It includes the use of protective equipment, aseptic procedures, as well as various types of isolation.

82. b. The scope of practice for radiation therapists describe, in detail, the job responsibilities of the therapist

83. d. *Fide* has a Latin origin and means to be faithful.

84. d. Local radiation therapy locally may cause hyperpigmentation in the area and fatigue if high volumes of bone marrow reserves are treated. Certain chemotherapy drugs cause hyperpigmentation, bone and joint pain, and fatigue follows myelosuppression.

85. a. A patient who is experiencing constipation should increase fiber intake and hydrating by eating fresh fruit and vegetables and drinking plenty of non-carbonated, non-alcoholic liquids.

86. d. Oral mucositis may begin as erythematous patches in the mouth and progress to ulcerations and bleeding. Ulcerating and bleeding sores compromise the patient's ability to speak, eat, drink and take medications.

87. c. Since radiation is a local therapy, nausea and vomiting are likely a side effect of treatment to the upper abdomen or total body where the stomach and small intestine are exposed to radiation.

88. c. Nausea and vomiting may be holistically managed by imagery, relaxation, exercise, ginger root, acupuncture, or hypnosis. Greasy foods should be avoided.

89. c. Cancer cachexia is a progressive, involuntary weight loss caused by a physiological condition such as cancer, hindering the absorption of nutrients or preventing proper intake of food.

90. a. Pelvic irradiation may lead to proctitis, enteritis, cystitis.

CHAPTER 9

Clinical Applications in Radiation Therapy

Head and Neck

1.

- **a.** Oral cavity—swelling or an ulcer that fails to heal
- **b.** Oropharynx—painful swallowing and referred otalgia
- **c.** Hypopharynx—dysphagia, painful neck nodes
- **d.** Nasopharynx—bloody discharge, difficulty hearing
- **e.** Larynx—hoarseness and stridor
- **f.** Maxillary sinus—long-standing sinusitis, nasal obstruction, bloody discharge

2. *See figure, next page.*

3.

F Superior orbital margin (SOM)
N Inferior orbital margin (IOM)
P External occipital protuberance (EOP)
R Mastoid process
I Zygomatic arch
J Glabella
C Nasion
O Inner canthus (IC)
A Outer canthus (OC)
Q Tragus
K Commissure of the mouth
B C1

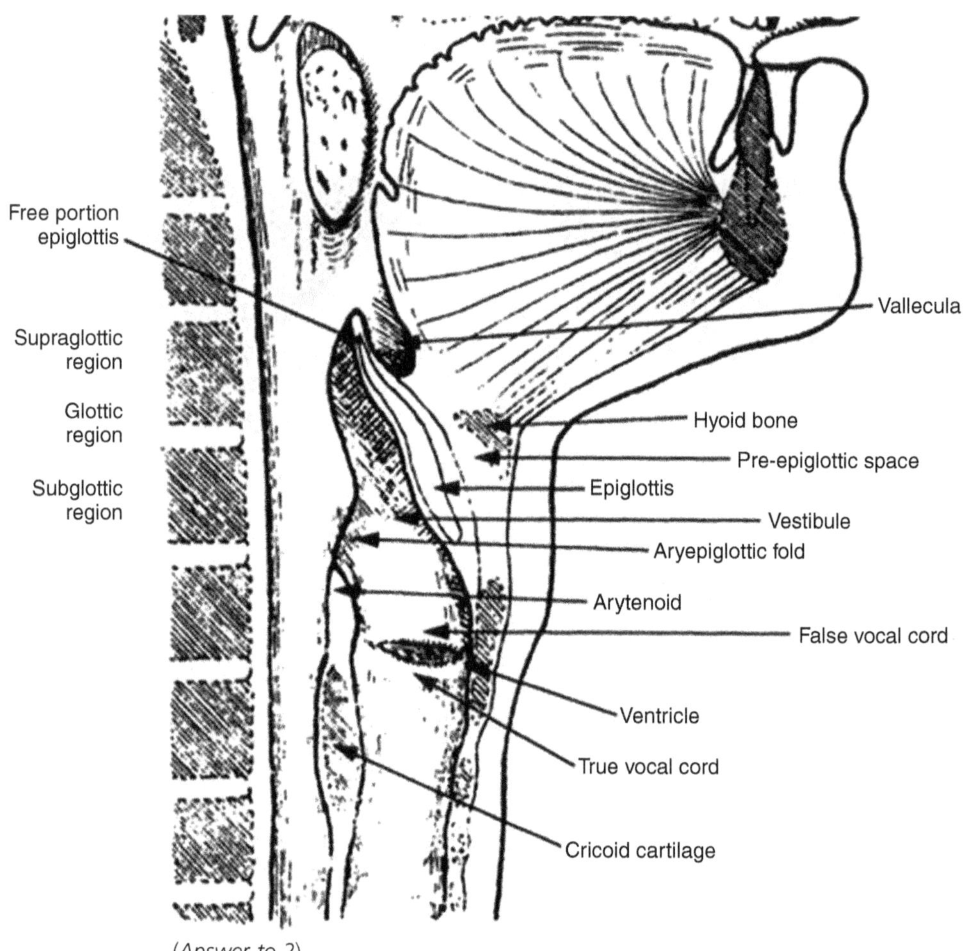

(Answer to 2)

E C2
M C3
H C4
L C6
D C7
G Sternocleidomastoid muscle

4.

U A G S P H S O E	E S O P H A **(G)** U S
N A Y R L X	**(L)** A R Y N X
I O C C D I R	C R I C **(O)** I D
Y R I T O D H	**(T)** H Y R O I D
T C E A A R H	**(T)** R A C H E A
P I E G T O L T S I	E P **(I)** G L O T T I S
V A S L A I Y R	**(S)** A L I V A R Y

5. GLOTTIS
6. Fill in the function of each of the cranial nerves:

Olfactory	I	**Smell**
Optic	II	**Sight**
Oculomotor	III	**Eye movement (up and down)**
Trochlear	IV	**Eye movement (rotation)**
Trigeminal	V	**Sensory (facial) and motor (jaw)**
Abducens	VI	**Eye movement (laterally)**
Facial (masticator)	VII	**Expressions, muscle contractions, and mouthing**
Acoustic	VIII	**Hearing**
Glossopharyngeal	IX	**Tongue and throat movement**
Vagus	X	**Talking and sounds**
Spinal accessory	XI	**Movement of shoulder and head**
Hypoglossal	XII	**Movement of tongue and chewing**

7. b. One-third of the body's lymph nodes are located in the neck divided by convention into six regions labeled by Roman numerals.
8. c. Nine cartilages make up the three regions of the larynx-supraglottis, glottis and subglottis.
9. d. The sternocleidomastoid muscle divides the neck into anterior and posterior triangular regions.
10. c. The jugulodigastric nodes, located in the upper region of cervical node triangle, are commonly enlarged in the presence of cancers in the neck.
11. a. The hyoid bone is an attachment site for muscles needed for swallowing.
12. b. The internal jugular vein is the largest vascular structure in the neck.
13. b. The upper cervical jugulodigastric node may also be referred to as the subdigastric node.
14. b. The hypopharynx includes the posterior and lateral pharyngeal walls below the base of the tongue, the pyriform sinuses, and the post-cricoid region.

15. d. The soft palate is part of the oropharynx, not the oral cavity. The oral cavity ends posteriorly at the hard palate.
16. b. The tonsils are the most common location for cancer in the oropharynx.
17. d. The tonsils are part of the oropharynx and cannot be avoided when treating the oropharynx.
18. d. The upper aerodigestive tract can be easily examined by palpation, direct inspection, and biopsy.
19. b. Rouvière's node is in close proximity to the carotid artery and inaccessible for surgery and should be included in the treatment volume for the nasopharynx.

Define the following symptoms often indicated in specific areas of head and neck cancers. List of the specific areas where they often occur

20. Otalgia—**referred pain to ear, due to tumor in the oropharynx region**
21. Dysphagia—**difficulty swallowing**
22. Stridor—**harsh, raspy breath**
23. Diplopia—**double vision**
24. Erythroplasia—**red, velvety patches on the mucous membrane of the mouth**
25. Leukoplakia—**small, white, raised patches on the mucous membrane**
26. Keratosis—**a lesion on the epidermis marked by the presence of circumcised overgrowth of the horny layer**
27. Dysplasia—**abnormal tissue development**
28. Odynophagia—**painful swallowing**
29. At the site where the tobacco quid rests against the oral mucosa. With constant irritation and possible carcinogenetic link, these areas will eventually develop pre-malignant lesions such as leukoplakia.
30. HPV has been found in oral papillomas, in leukoplakia lesions and oral carcinomas. Cell studies show that high-risk HPVs can transform epithelial cells from cervix, foreskin, and the oral cavity to produce a malignancy. Some studies are indicating these malignancies show no history of smoking and alcohol.
31. Epstein-Barr virus (one of the eight herpes viruses that infect human tissue) and viral DNA have been identified in nasopharyngeal tissue in this type of cancer
32. b. The majority of head and neck cancers are squamous cell carcinomas.
33. b. Smoking and alcohol use are common etiological factors for the development of head/neck cancers.
34. d. When managing head and neck cancers, the main goals are to eradicate disease, maintain function and preserve cosmesis.
35. a. Plummer-Vinson syndrome is an etiological factor for cancers of the oral cavity.
36. c. If the supraclavicular area is treated for the management of head/neck cancer, the typical total dose is 5000 cGy.
37. b. The vallecula is located at the base of the tongue.
38. a. Special care should be taken to make sure that the spinal cord is kept under tolerance while treating the hypopharynx and cervical lymphatics, including Rouvière's node.

Define each of the following areas of the pharynx:

39. Nasopharynx: **This region includes the posterior and lateral pharyngeal walls above the soft plated and the superior surface of the soft palate extending to the posterior choana.**
40. Oropharynx: **This region includes the anterior tonsillar pillar, soft palate, uvula, tonsillar fossa and tonsil, base of tongue and pharyngeal walls.**
41. Hypopharynx: **This region includes the posterior and lateral pharyngeal walls below the base of the tongue, the pyriform sinuses, and post-cricoid region.**
42. b. The highest rate of positive lymph nodes occurs in cancers of the hypopharynx.
43. d. Cranial nerve involvement occurs in 15–25% of case of nasopharyngeal cancers.
44. b. A bite block or tongue blade may serve to separate or displace the palate from the oral cavity.
45. b. The eye, especially the lens, is at the most risk of exceeding tolerance when treating the maxillary antrum.
46. c. The lung is the most common site of distant metastasis from primary head/neck cancers.
47. b. Most cancers of the head/neck are squamous cell carcinomas.
48. a. It is not unusual to see a wedged pair, superior-inferior oblique portal orientation, in the treatment of the parotid gland.
49. b. The maxillary sinus has the highest frequency of malignancy among all sinuses.

Lung

1. Define the following:
   Odynophagia—**painful swallowing**
   Feedback: The proximity of the bronchus to the esophagus and the potential for mediastinal lymphadenopathy may cause a patient with diagnosed lung cancer to experience pain when swallowing food
   Hemoptysis—**coughing up of blood**
   Feedback: Bronchial tumors may begin to break up with persistent coughing and produce bloody sputum
   Dyspnea—**difficulty breathing**
   Feedback: Patients with lung tumors and/or positive mediastinal disease may experience difficulty breathing
   Atelectasis—**collapse of the lung**
   Feedback: The location or persistence of a lung tumor or chronic obstructive conditions of the lung may lead to collapse of the lung

2. List all mediastinal lymph nodes.
   Para-tracheal, para-esophageal, hilar, subcarinal, peri-aortic, interlobar, lobar, segmental, subsegmental
   Feedback: Involvement of mediastinal lymph nodes is common in primary lung cancers
3. Using the cross sectional images below (need posterior lung lesion):
   a. Outline the gross tumor volume
      On image A, mass is located in the left upper lobe, apex region
      On image B, axial cross-section, mass is located in the left lung near the posterior
      On image C, axial image circular nodules in the left mediastinum are enlarged lymph nodes
   b. Outline the critical structures and list tolerance doses for each
      On all images, normal left lung, opposite lung, heart, and spinal cord should be outlined.
      TD 5/5 1/3 of lung 45 Gy; 3/3 of lung 17.5 Gy
      1/3 of heart 60 Gy; 3/3 of heart 40 Gy
      5 cm of cord 50 Gy; 20 cm of cord 47 Gy
   c. Diagram possible directions for off-cord and boost treatment fields
      Off-cord fields would include gross tumor and mediastinal nodes in right anterior and left posterior oblique fields avoiding the spinal cord. Boost fields may be a 90-degree pair including a posterior and left lateral OR a single posterior boost field could deliver high dose to the primary tumor while sparing all normal lung tissue.
4. List four etiologic factors for lung cancer.
   Smoking, asbestos, atmospheric pollution, arsenic, nickel exposure, previous thorax radiation, exposure to ether, chronic obstructive pulmonary disease
   Feedback: The strongest risk factor for the development of lung cancer continues to be cigarette smoking.
5. Note common anatomical locations and physical characteristics for the manifestations of the following lung tumors:
   Adenocarcinoma: **Tend to be located near the periphery of the lung.**
   Squamous cell carcinoma: **Tend to be proximal and involve the hilum. Will likely grow into the bronchial lumen and cause associated pneumonitis.**
   Pancoast tumor: **Located in the apex of the lung.**
   Mesothelioma: **Manifests in the lung pleura.**
   Large cell carcinoma: **Shows up similar to adenocarcinoma.**
6. Briefly explain the situations in which high-dose rate (HDR) brachytherapy would be an appropriate management for lung cancer.

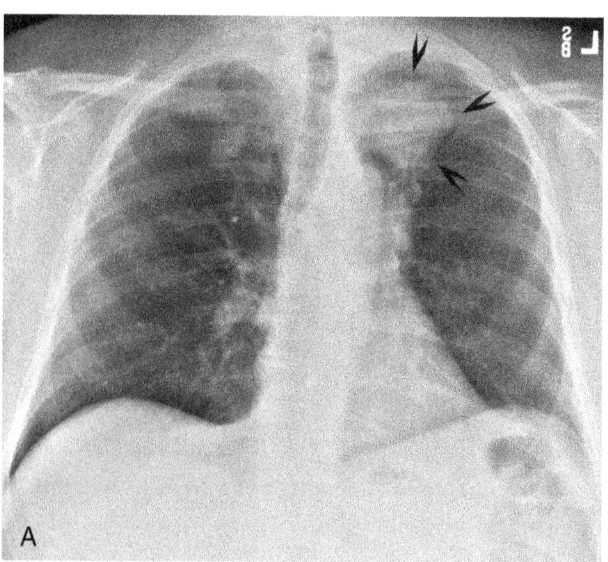

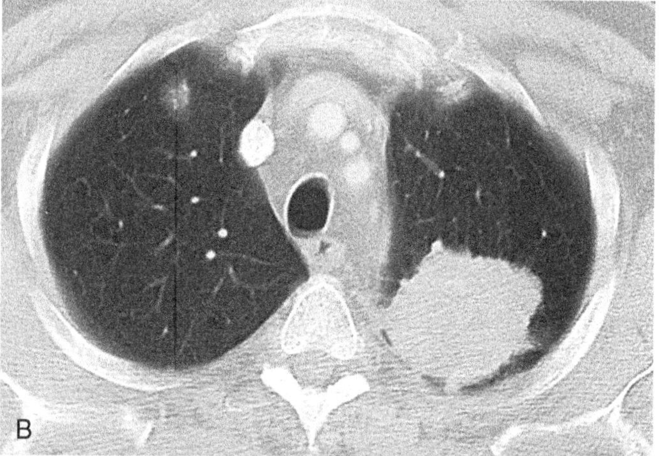

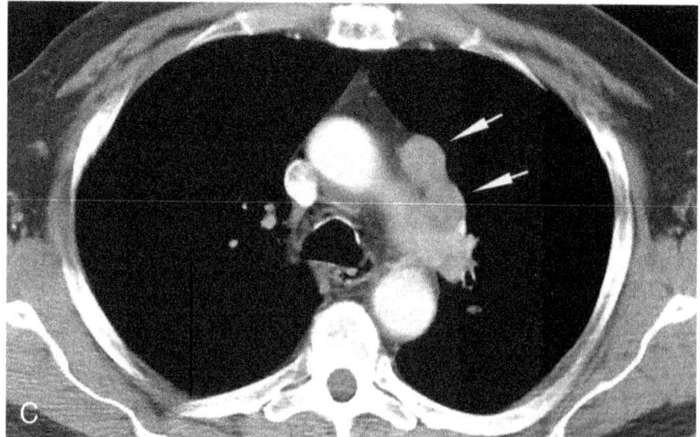

HDR brachytherapy for the management of lung cancer is delivered endobronchial. Patients who have tumors located in or near the main stem bronchus might benefit from endobronchial HDR brachytherapy.

7. **a.** Adenocarcinomas of the lung are commonly seen in patients with no history of smoking.
8. **a.** Clubbing of the fingers is a symptom of COPD or other diseases of the heart or lungs where there is a decreased blood oxygen level.
9. **a.** Oat cell carcinoma, also called small cell carcinoma, is a very aggressive malignancy and is assumed to have begun metastatic spread at the time of diagnosis.
10. **c.** Posteriorly located lung tumor may be easily treated during the boost portion of radiation therapy by using a single posterior field or posterior oblique fields.
11. **a.** The upper thorax has a natural superior slope. The use of a custom compensator or wedge during anterior treatment portal will allow for more even dose distribution within the treatment volume.
12. Using the anatomical diagram draw the likely emergency treatment field for the patient diagnosed with Superior Vena Cava syndrome caused by right Pancoast tumor.

    The appropriate treatment field for the emergency field should be a simple field covering the tumor and moderate margin of about 3 cm on all sides. No lymphatics are included in the initial emergency fields for SVC syndrome.
13. Using the anatomical diagram, draw the likely initial treatment field for the above patient following work-up diagnosed with T2, N0, M0 squamous cell lung carcinoma.

    The appropriate treatment field following work-up for non-small cell lung tumor as described would include the tumor, mediastinal lymph nodes, and bilateral supraclavicular lymph nodes.
14. **c.** Dose for prophylactic radiation to the brain is typically 36–40 Gy.
15. **b.** The CT scan is helpful in establishing the presence and location of a mass and involvement of neighboring tissues but would not supply the clinician with a definite histological type.
16. **b.** The right lobe has 3 lobes while the left lobe has 2
17. **c.** Due to cardiac and respiratory motion, lung tumors move as the heartbeats and also on inspiration and expiration. To decrease the risk of target miss, cardiac or respiratory gating procedures may be utilized.
18. **b.** Mesothelioma has the closest association with asbestos exposure
19. **b.** The slope of the chest causes uneven dose distribution leading to higher dose regions in the upper mediastinum where the anatomy is thinner. Custom compensators, standard wedges, or dynamic wedges may be used to produce more even dose distribution.
20. **a.** Upper lobe tumors of the right lung would require initial fields to include bilateral supraclavicular fossa, mediastinal lymphatics, and margin on the tumor. Opposite lung may be shielded using beam shaping multileaf collimators or custom blocks

Alimentary

1. **posterior.** Review anatomy, esophagus is situated posterior to the trachea, closest to the spine.
2. **splenic flexure.** Anatomy review, junction of transverse and descending colon is in the left upper quadrant of the abdomen anterior to the spleen.
3. **a.** Diverticula are a result of debris causing out pouching and weakening of the intestinal wall
4. **duodenum.** Anatomy review, the duodenum is the first section of the small bowel.
5. **small bowel.** Anatomy review, the small bowel makes up 90% of the alimentary tract
6. Using the diagram below, draw typical AP/PA fields for upper 1/3 esophagus squamous cell carcinoma.

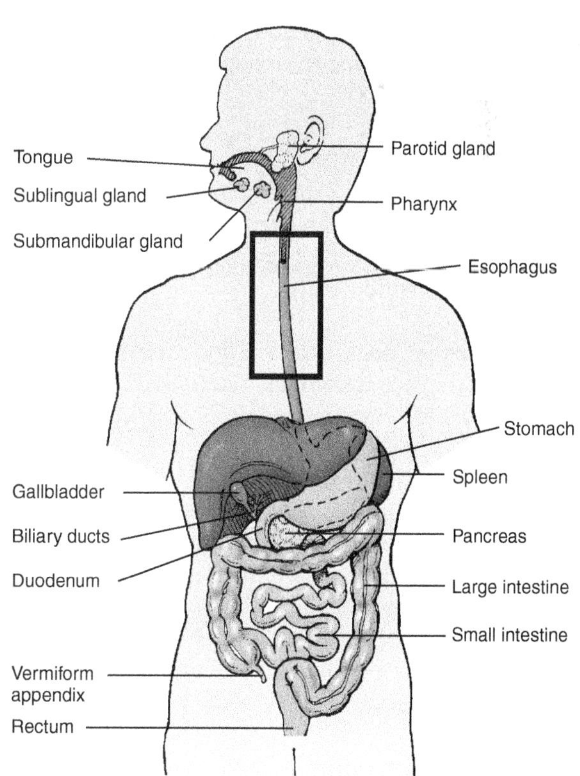

7.

Treatment site	Anatomy included in Typical treatment fields	Critical tissues in the area	Optimal position/ immobilization
Rectum	From L5 to margin on tumor, out beyond pelvic inlet; some small bowel, bladder, common iliac, internal and external iliac nodes and pelvic bones are in the field	Small bowel, bladder, bone marrow	Prone with or without belly board; immobilize lower extremities and pelvis
Anus	From S1 to margin on tumor, wide enough to cover the inguinal lymph nodes in the lower portion of the field; some small bowel, rectum, internal and external iliac and superficial inguinal nodes, bladder and pelvic bones in field	Small bowel, bladder, bone marrow	Supine for inguinal node boost; frog-leg decreases inguinal folds Prone if no inguinal node boost Prone or lithotomy for electron boost to tumor

8. c. Histological types for small bowel cancer include adenocarcinoma, sarcomas, lymphomas, and carcinoid

9. b. Adenocarcinomas comprise about 95 % of stomach cancers

10. c. Surgery has the most promise for cure for stomach cancers. They show slow response to chemotherapy and radiation.

11. c. Most stomach cancer cases are diagnosed late. At the time of presentation, the most common report is a persistent vague discomfort in the area of the stomach

12. Cachexia—**Weight loss caused by physiological malabsorption of nutrients**

Hematemesis—**vomiting blood**
Dysphagia—**difficulty swallowing**

True/False

13. T

14. F. Esophageal tumors of the upper 1/3 of the esophagus are not surgically removed as there's no proximal end to re-connect. They are managed with radiation and chemotherapy.

15. T

16. F. The procedure described is called an exploratory laparotomy. An abdominal perineal resection (APR) resects the rectum and anus and installs an anterior colostomy

17. d. Colon cancers metastasize to the liver, lung and out into the peritoneal cavity

18. d. Studies have shown that gastric cancers are associated with low fiber diets and frequent consumption of salted and smoked foods.

19. b. Primary lymphatic drainage for the anus is to the internal iliac and inguinal lymph nodes. The inguinal nodes should be included in treatment fields

20. c. When unequal weights, add all weights together: $2 + 1 + 1 = 4$. Then divide the total dose by the weights - 50 Gy/4 = 12.5 Gy. This represents 1 weight. Now multiple this by the weight assigned to the point of interest: 12.5(2) = 25 Gy. Check your math.

21. d. In areas where the skin is broken down, it is best to decrease friction and cause more tissue injury. Patting dry instead of wiping is best.

22. c. Having a history of colon polyps increases the risk of developing a malignant colon tumor

23. d. Lower esophagus tumor fields will likely include a section of the stomach. Irradiation to the sensitive lining of the stomach will cause acute nausea.

24. b. Radiation for upper esophagus tumors will cause esophagitis realized by the patient as a difficulty swallowing.

25. c. The layers of the intestinal wall from the inside out are the mucosa, submucosa, muscularis, then serosa

26. c. Prescribed dose for electron fields is often to the 80 or 90% depth dose lines. Rules of thumb: Energy/3 = depth of 80% dose line, Energy/4 = depth of 90% dose line
Energy/3 = 5cm
Energy = 15MeV

27. b. Positioning the patient in the prone position will push some small bowel up and out of the pelvis.

28. a. The 3-field technique with AP/RT/LT are commonly employed when treating the pancreas to decrease dose to the posteriorly located kidneys

29. d. Carcinoid tumors are slow growing and show longer survival rates.

30. a. The Modified Astler-Coller stage A describes a carcinoma in situ with no nodes and distant metastasis. This correlates with Stage 0 using the TNM system

Digestive

1.

Stomach__**inferior and posterior**_______
Duodenum__**tucked in, to the left**____
Liver___**inferior**______

Spleen___**head is medial, tail is in splenic hilum**_____

2. **Secretion of digestive enzymes and sodium bicarbonate to help neutralize acid in the stomach and duodenum. Islets of Langerhans secrete glucagon to regulate sugar levels, insulin for the metabolism of carbohydrates, proteins and fats, and somatostatin which controls the metabolic process.**
3. Stomach__**to the right**___________
   Gallbladder_**superior**_____________
   Aorta_**anterior**_________________
   Inferior vena cava_____**anterior**_____________
   Diaphragm___**inferior**______________
4. **Storage and filtration of blood, secretion of bile, conversion of sugars to glycogen, synthesis and breakdown of fats and temporary storage of fatty acids; helps regulate blood volume, fibrinogen and prothrombin.**
5. **liver**
6. **Stores bile**
7. **d.** The celiac axis from the aorta supplies blood to the spleen, pancreas, stomach and liver
8. **d.** High consumption of alcohol causes cirrhosis of the liver
9. **c.** Jaundice is characterized by yellowish discoloration of the skin and eyes.
10. **c.** Anatomy review; the fundus is the highest portion of the stomach
11. **c.** The biliary ducts carry bile and other digestive juices into the duodenum (beginning of the small intestine)
12. **a.** The gallbladder is in the right abdomen and found tucked under the larger right lobe of the liver
13. **c.** The head of the pancreas is nestled in the curve of the duodenum.
14. **c.** The presence of fats in the stomach triggers the release of bile
15. **c.** The hepatic flexure of the colon is just under the right lobe of the liver.
16. **c.** Excessive radiation of the liver can lead to a severe complication knows as acute hepatitis
17. **c.** Primary liver cancers spread to the lung and brain.
18. **d.** Pancreatic tumors are most often adenocarcinomas.
19.
   Cholelithiasis—**stones in the gallbladder**
   Barrett's esophagus—**a condition where columnar epithelium extends more than 3 cm into the distal esophagus instead of normal squamous epithelium**
   Crohn's disease—**a form of inflammatory bowel disease often at the terminal end of the ileum**
20.
   Abdominal pain
   Dark urine
   Jaundice
   Clay-colored stools
   Newly diagnosed diabetes
21. Complete the table:

Cancer site	2 Signs/ symptoms	3 Methods of detection
Liver	Right abdomen pain Abdominal mass Weight loss, fatigue	Liver function, coagulation studies CA 19-9, CEA markers Ultrasound Computed tomography
Stomach	Vague epigastric discomfort Nausea, vomiting Hematemesis Weight loss, fatigue	Barium swallow Endoscopy Computed tomography Stool examination for blood in stools
Esophagus	Dysphagia Hematemesis Weight loss, fatigue	Barium swallow Ultrasound Computed tomography Esophagoscopy
Colon	Pencil stools Rectal bleeding Constipation Diarrhea	CEA Digital rectal exam Colonoscopy Barium enema Computed tomography

22. **c.** Chemoembolization is the local administration of chemotherapy using proximal venous or arterial access
23. **b.** Hepatocellular carcinoma has a strong association with hepatitis C infection
24. **a.** The Whipple procedure removes a section of the pancreas and small intestine and re-establishes the communication between remaining pancreas, small intestine and biliary tree
25. **c.** Pancreatic carcinomas have proven to be very aggressive and have shown limited response to radiation and chemotherapy. The best chance for cure is surgical removal of the tumor with clear margins.

Breast

1. **c.** The apical nodes are also known as level 3 axillary nodes are the deepest and are most adequately treated using a posterior field (PAB) or midline opposing fields
2. **d.** Lymphatic drainage for the breast includes all three levels of axillary nodes, supraclavicular nodes and internal mammary nodes

3. Using the diagram shown, draw the location of all lymphatic drainage for the breast.

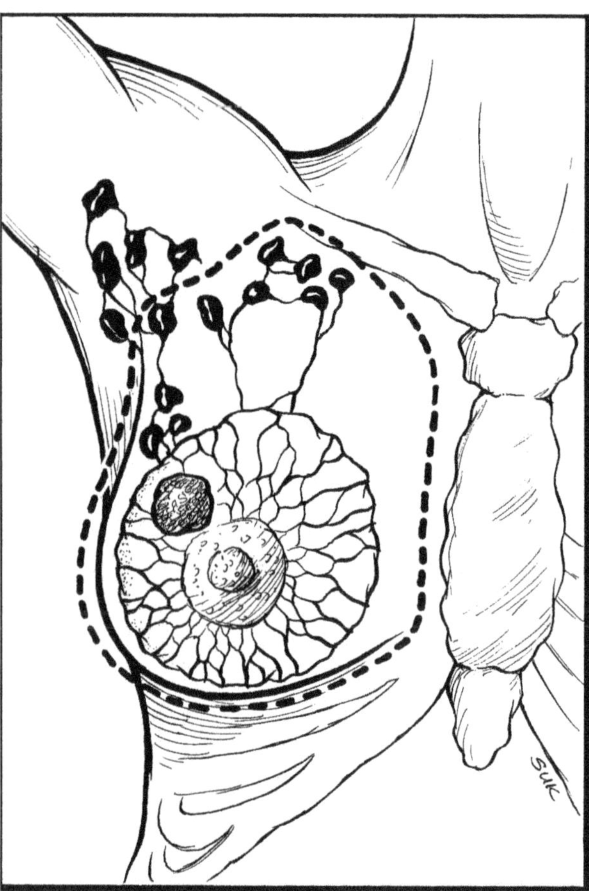

4. b. Tamoxifen is an anti-estrogen administered to counteract the nurturing effects of estrogen on breast cancers.

5.

	Drug Name	Drug Class	Toxicities
C	Cyclophosphamide	Alkylating agent	Myelosuppression, alopecia, nausea vomiting, diarrhea
M	Methotrexate	Anti-metabolite	Mucositis, myelosuppression, mild alopecia,
F	5-flourouracil	Anti-metabolite	Oral and intestinal ulcers, nausea/ vomiting, mild alopecia, radiation recall
C	Cyclophosphamide	Alkylating agent	Myelosuppression, alopecia, nausea vomiting, diarrhea
A	Adriamycin (doxorubicin)	Anti-tumor antibiotic	Myelosuppression, cardiotoxicity, alopecia, nausea/ vomiting
F	5-fluouroracil	Anti-metabolite	Oral and intestinal ulcers, nausea/ vomiting, mild alopecia, radiation recall

Think About It

6. **A unique toxicity associated with adriamycin is cardiac toxicity. Radiation dose should be limited so as not to compound the potential latent injury to the heart.**
7. **Clinical staging includes physical examination taking survey of the skin of the breast, and the status of palpable lymph nodes. Imaging studies may also be used for clinical staging. Pathological staging would include everything necessary for clinical staging but adds surgical exploration and resection with pathological evaluation of tissue sample.**
8.
   $E/4 =$ depth of the 90% dose line
   $E/4 = 5$ cm
   $E = 20$ MeV
9. The objective should be to have the horizontal plane of the electron beam be parallel to the patient's tumor bed area.
   1. The patient may be positioned in left lateral oblique position and slightly inclined to flatten the area
   2. The patient may continue in the same arm up position and the couch and gantry to could be rotated to bring the horizontal axis parallel to the skin (challenge is to clear the patient's arm with this technique)
10.
   a) Tan^{-1} (A/ 2 SSD)
   Tan^{-1} (24/182)
   Tan^{-1} (0.1319) =
   b) **The couch should be angled during treatment of the medial and lateral tangents.**
11.

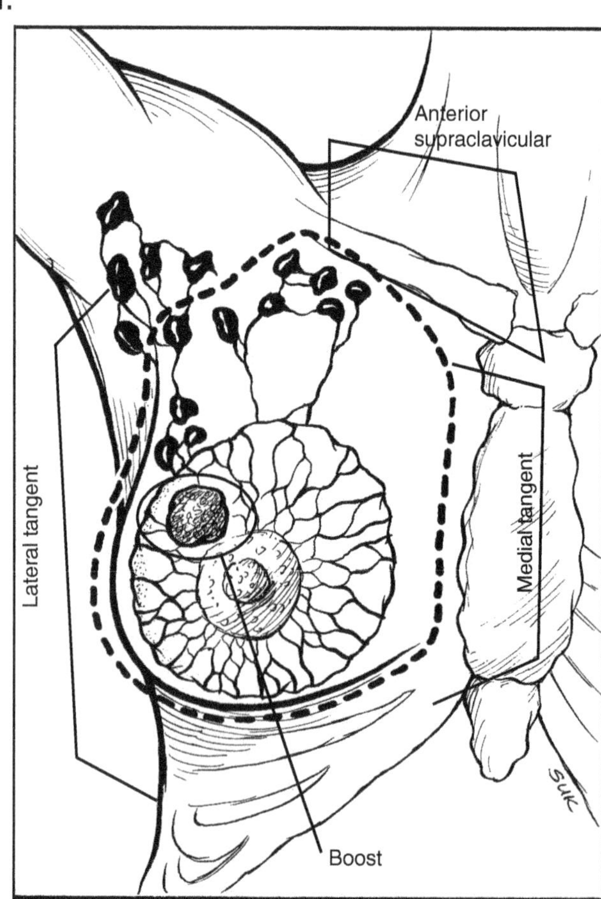

12. Using the information given, calculate the monitor units required for each treatment field per fraction
Prescription:
* 5040 cGy to right breast 180 cGy per fraction-6 MV photons
* 4500 cGy to right supraclavicular fossa 180 cGy per fraction-6 MV photons
* 1000 cGy boost lumpectomy scar 200 cGy per fraction-12 MeV en face electrons
6 MV beam output = 1 cGy/MU 12 MeV beam output = 1 cGy/MU
Medial and lateral tangents
Field size = 8 × 24
SSD = 91 cm
Field size factor = 1.034
TAR @ 9 cm = 0.892
AP Supraclavicular field
Field size = 12 × 10
Field size factor = 1.003
TAR@ 3 cm = 1.002
En face electron boost field
Cone factor = 1.02
Dose to 90% dose line
Answer
Medial and lateral tangents

$$\frac{90\text{ cGy}}{1\text{ cGy/MU} \times 1.034 \times 0.892} = 98\text{ MU}$$

AP Supraclavicular

$$\frac{180}{1\text{ cGy/MU} \times 1.003 \times 1.002} = 179\text{ MU}$$

Electron boost

$$\frac{200\text{ cGy}}{1\text{ cGy/MU} \times 1.02 \times .90} = 218\text{ MU}$$

13. a. A painless lump is the most common sign of breast cancer.
14. Define the following:
Radical mastectomy—**resection of the breast, pectoralis muscles and regional lymph nodes**
HER2neu—**an oncogene expression seen in certain breast cancer patients; an epidermal growth factor**
BRCA1—**a tumor suppressor gene whose failed type is associated with elevated risk for breast cancers**
Peau d'orange—**an orange coloring of the skin of the breast indicating infiltration of cancerous cells into the dermal layers of the breast; skin feels thick and leathery**
15. c. The breast board should be inclined to decrease the slope of the patient's chest to optimize the sparing of lung tissue while covering breast tissue
16. d. The supraclavicular field is best treated using half field technique to prevent overlap into the upper aspect of the tangential fields
17. c. The entire breast following lumpectomy is typically 50 Gy. Then the lumpectomy scar is boosted 10-20 Gy
18. a. Most diagnosed cases of breast cancer are infiltrating ductal carcinoma
19. b. Volume of lung included in the tangential breast fields should be kept at minimum to prevent lung fibrosis. Although some signs of lung pneumonitis may be observed in the small amount of lung irradiated following breast irradiation.
20. d. The change in distance would render an output correct factor of 0.907. Indicating an approximate 10% change. Since distance is increased, dose would be decreased.

$$(100/105)^2 = 0.907$$

21. a. In situ is cancer confined to the lumen of the ducts. This type of tumor has limited capacity for spread and is classified as Stage 0.
22. d. Positive supraclavicular nodes upstage the breast cancer case to Stage IV
23. b. Technetium 99 ad blue dye are injected into the breast tumor area and observed as it flows to lymphatic drainage sites. The node(s) collecting the most Technetium are identified as 'hot' by a gamma camera and resected during a sentinel node biopsy.
24. c. 310 degrees is 40 degrees positive from 270-degree position on the gantry. The opposite angle would be 40 degrees positive from 90-degree position on the gantry. OR 310 degrees is also 50 degrees negative from the 0-degree position. The opposite angle would be 50 degrees negative from the 180-degree position.

Gynecologic

19. Low dose rate and high dose rate are intracavitary treatments to deliver high doses to a direct small area limiting the volume and dose to the bladder, colorectal tissues and small intestines.
Point A—**A prescription point defined as 2 cm superior to the cervical os and 2 cm lateral to the endocervical canal**
Point B—**is 3 cm lateral to point *A***
20. d. The point tolerance dose for the bladder and rectum during gynecologic planning is 7500 cGy.
21. c. There is recent research of increased incidence of endometrial cancer in women taking tamoxifen.
22. b. The outermost portion of the gynecologic tract is the vulva.
23. a. The parametrium is immediately lateral to the uterine cervix.
24. c. Ovarian cancers often involve the abdominal cavity even in the early stage of disease.
25. c. The symptoms of ovarian cancer may include abdominal pain and distention, nausea, heartburn and other non-specific gastrointestinal symptoms.
26. d. CA 125 is a tumor marker helpful in the detection of ovarian cancer.

Gynecologic Tumors

1 ANEMIA
2 TELANGIECTASIS
3 OVARIAN
4 PELVIC INLET
5 CERVIX
6 TANDEM
7 BIOPSY
8 PAPANICOLAOU
9 OVARIES
10 S3
11 FROGLEG
12 DYSURIA
13 ENDOMETRIAL
14 MIDLINE
15 TMRT
16 SQUAMOUS CELL
17 OVOIDS
18 EPITHELIAL

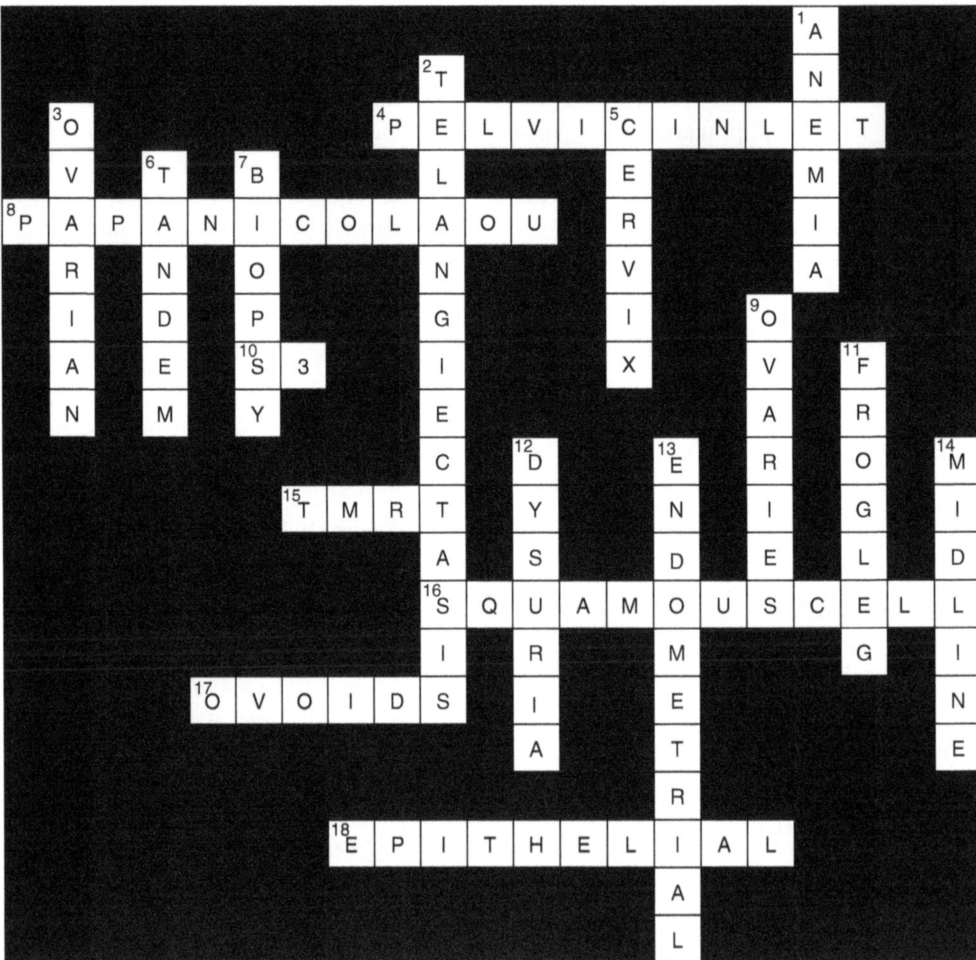

Across

4 The opening into the pelvis into which the baby's head enters

8 Name of the early screening techinque for cervial cancer

10 The posterior border of a lateral pelvic field

15 A treatment technique which would allow a lower dose to the femoral head and neck

16 Pathlolgy for vulva, vagina and cervix cancers

17 Two golf-club-shaped hollow tubes placed laterally to the cervical os into the vaginal fornices

18 Pathlolgy for ovarian cancer

Down

1 The most common side effect from the radiation when treating cervix cancer

2 Fine superficial blood vessels caused from radiation in the areas of the vagina and cervix

3 Most lethal of all gynecologic tumors

5 A slow progressive disease, with the earliest phase (in situ) occurring approximately ten years earlier than invasive cancer

6 A small, hollow, curved cylinder that fits through the cervical os and into the uterus

7 Used to establish a precise diagnosis for cancer

9 The most radiosensitive gynecologic structure

11 Patient position for which a vulva field may be treated

12 Painful or difficulty urination

13 The most prevalent gynecologic malignancy

14 Shielding block used to eliminate dose to the bladder and rectum

27. a. Cervical cancers are seen in younger women stemming from intraepithelial neoplasia.
28. b. The fornices are lateral spaces in the vaginal apex.
29. d. Ovarian cancers are fifth on the list of cancer killers in women according to 2010 statistics.
30. a. Women whose mothers used DES before their birth, show an increased risk of clear cell adenocarcinoma of the cervix and vagina.
31. b. Risk factors for endometrial cancers include; diabetes, hypertension, obesity and use of synthetic hormones.
32. a. The tolerance dose (TD 5/5) for the kidney is 18–23 Gy.
33. b. The normal level of hemoglobin is about 12–16 grams/deciliter.
34. b. Lomotil can be prescribed to manage diarrhea.
35. d. Intracavitary (peritoneal) P32 can be used in the treatment of ovarian cancer.
36. c. Barium sulfate may be used in localizing the rectum during conventional simulation.
37. a. Ovarian cancers are in many instances, detected late and most deadly due to few symptoms and wide dissemination.
38. b. If a patient has paraaortic involvement with a primary cervical cancer, there is an increased risk of spread to the supraclavicular nodes.
39. a. Patient receiving radiation to the pelvis should follow a low-residue diet which would not include whole grain breads.
40. d. An early stage vaginal cancer can be treated with low dose brachytherapy to a dose of 6000 cGy.
41. b. Abdominal distention and hyperactive bowel sounds could indicate bowel obstruction.
42. a. The most radiotolerant structure among the gynecological organs listed is the uterine canal.
43. d. The patient receiving concurrent radiation and chemotherapy should be advised to get plenty of rest and speak to the appropriate professional regarding psychosocial support.
44. d. Inguinal nodes are primary lymphatic drainage for the vagina and should be included in the treatment field.
45. If a patient is having a four-field pelvis treatment, calculate the diameter of the AP to PA, and lateral, using the following:
    AP SSD readout is 85, PA SSD readout is 87.5, right lateral 81; left lateral 79.5
    a. AP/PA diameter = ____27.5____
    b. Rt/Lt lateral = ____39.5____
    AP 100 − 85 = 15 PA 100 − 87.5 = 12.5
    15 + 12.5 = 27.5 cm
    RL 100 − 81 = 19 LL 100 − 79.5 = 20.5
    19 + 20.5 = 39.5 cm

Male Genital

1. c. Seminoma is the most common germ cell cancer of the testis.
2. b. Testicular cancers show up in young men between the ages of 15 and 35.
3. a. Tumor markers for testicular cancer would include alpha-feto-protein (AFP) and beta human chorionic gonadotropin (BHCG).
4. **inferior, anterior.** The prostate gland lies at the base of the bladder and anterior to the rectum.
5. **Gleason's grading system uses 5 different degrees of differentiation.**
6. **superior, anterior.** The seminal vesicles attached to the upper lobes of the prostate gland.
7. Briefly define the following:
   TURP—**transurethral resection of the prostate.** Transurethral resection of the prostate (TURP) can be curative for early stage prostate cancer
   LDH—**lactate dehydrogenase.** Lactate dehydrogenase (LDH) elevated, can be an indicator of tissue destruction and is not only specified in the diagnosis of cancer.
   HCG—**human chorionic gonadotropin.** Human chorionic gonadotropin (HCG) is a blood serum marker helpful in the diagnosis of germ cell tumors such as seminoma.
8. b. Typical radiation doses for the prostate, penis and breast range from 50–78 Gy. Typical doses in the management of seminoma are around 30 Gy.
9. a. Typical doses in the management of breast, penis and testis range from 30–60 Gy. Curative doses in the management of prostate can be as high as 78 Gy.
10. a. For early-stage seminoma, treatment fields should include abdominal paraaortic nodes and ipsilateral pelvic iliac nodes.
11. a. Approximately 98% of prostate cancers are adenocarcinoma.
12. b. Due to the anatomy, size, and location of the prostate gland, low dose rate permanent interstitial seed placement is feasible to deliver high dose to the small gland and spare neighboring tissues such as the bladder and rectum.
13. a. Lupron, a luteinizing hormone inhibitor, is appropriate in the management of prostate cancer since prostate cancers are nurtured by the presence of male hormones.
14.

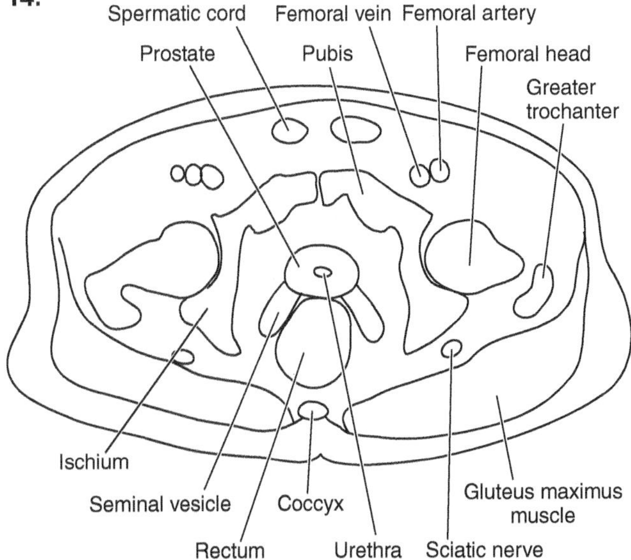

15. c. Patients with diarrhea should be counseled to begin a low-residue or low-fiber diet.

16. a. The hockey-stick field will be treated using AP and PA fields. The upper border would be at the level of thoracic vertebrae 10 and the lower border at the top of the ischium. The patient should be positioned supine with arms up or high on the chest so as not to be included in the upper region of the treatment field.

17. c. Severe wet desquamation should be managed with special dressings to promote healing.

18. d. Seminomas metastasize to the mediastinum and lung.

19. b. Inguinal lymph nodes are included in primary lymphatic drainage for the penis.

20. a. Due to the location of the prostate gland and pelvic lymphatics, the four-field box technique would be appropriate for dose delivery.

21. a. The upper border of the inverted Y for seminoma should be at the level of thoracic vertebrae 10 to include the abdominal paraaortic and renal hilar lymph nodes.

22. b. The lower border of the inverted Y field for seminoma should be at the top of the symphysis pubis to include adequate margin on the external iliac pelvic lymph nodes.

23. d. Following total prostatectomy, radiation dose to the tumor bed would be in the range of 66–75 Gy.

24. d. Using the 80% rule: E/3 = depth of the 80% dose line. The appropriate electron energy would be 15 MeV.

Think About It

25.

40 : 100
45 : x
x = 112.5
A direct proportion is needed since the relationship between distance and field size is direct.

26.

D max for 10 MV = 2.0 cm
ISF = $(100/114.5)^2$ = .763
The inverse square factor is as follows: (SAD/Tx distance + dmax)^2
D max for 10 MV = 2.0 cm.

27.

91.2 %
The answer is determined using Mayneord's correction formula:
(new distance + dmax/old distance + dmax) ^{2} × (old distance + depth/new distance + depth)^2 = F factor
The 'F' factor is 1.203
1.203(.76) = .912

28.

2.8 cm
Use the skin gap formula. L 1/2 (d/SSD) + L 2/ 2 (d/SSD).

29.

280 MU/270 degrees = 1.04 MU/degree
Monitor unit per degree is mathematically expressed by dividing the monitor units by the degree of rotation.

30.

135 degrees
Draw the typical gantry dial with 90 degrees at the right, 270 at the left, and 0 degrees superior. From 225 in the clockwise direction, 270-degree rotation will finish at 135 degrees.

Urinary

1. a. Kidney cancers typically arise in the cortex. Cancers in the medulla and renal pelvis are rare

2. a. Wilms' tumor is another name for nephroblastomas seen in children.

3. d. Renal cell carcinomas metastasize to the lung, liver, bone and brain

4. a. Cancers found in the pelvis of the kidney are commonly transitional cell histology.

5. b. Adenocarcinoma histology is found in kidney cancers arising in the cortex.

6. a. For the detection and confirmation of bladder malignancy, urine cytology, cystoscopy, and/or transurethral resection of the bladder are valuable

7. a, b, and c. Bladder tumors are often found in the posterior-lateral walls and trigone area

8.

Dye working
Chronic bladder infections
Smoking
Exposure to cadmium
Previous pelvic irradiation

9.

Transitional cell
Squamous cell
Adenocarcinoma
Sarcoma
Lymphoma

10. b. If radiation is given preoperatively, a pelvis field including the obturator, external and internal iliac (hypogastric and presacral) nodes is accepted.

11.

Cystectomy—**surgical removal of the bladder**
Intravesical therapy—**chemotherapy drugs inserted directly into the bladder through a urinary catheter. Given weekly for 6–8 weeks with a holding time of about 2 hours.**
TURB—**transurethral resection of the bladder**
IVP—**intravenous pyelogram**

12. b. Anatomy review; the ureters attach to the bladder's posterior lateral surface

13. c. Anatomy review; the kidneys received blood supply from the IVC and abdominal aorta via the renal vein and arteries.

14. c. Anatomy review; the large liver on the right makes the right kidney slightly lower than the left.

15. anterior/inferior; posterior

16. superior; medial/inferior

17. b. Common symptom of bladder cancer is blood in the urine (hematuria).

18. c. Cadmium is a metal found in some kinds of Cerrobend used for custom blocks. Cadmium is a known carcinogen linked to kidney and bladder cancer. Cadmium-free Cerrobend is now available.

19. a. Anatomy review; the ureters are located at the renal pelvis.

20. b. Anatomy review; urine passes to the outside of the body via the urethra.

21.

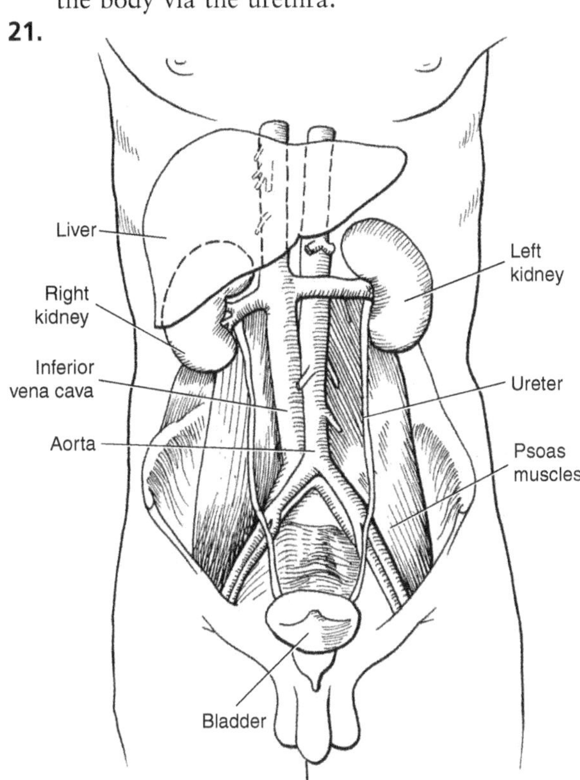

22.

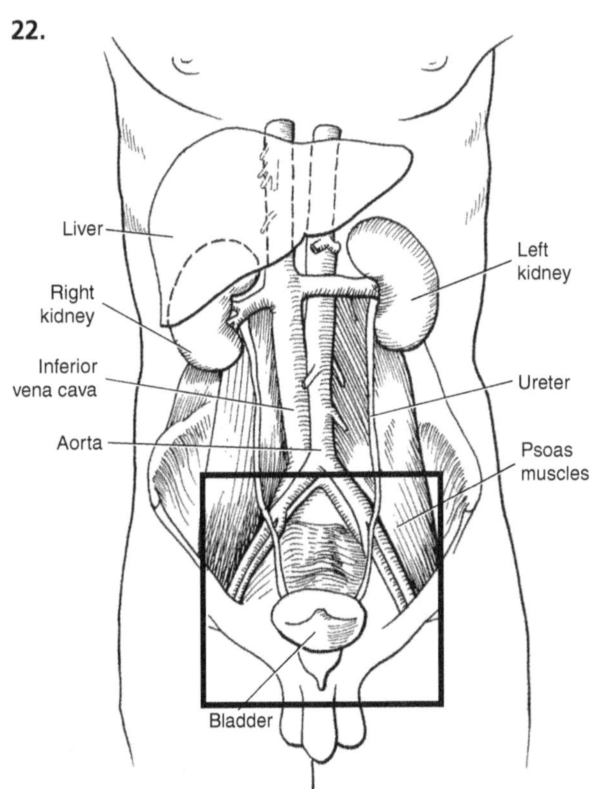

Think About it

23. Calculate the effective equivalent square by using areas. Calculate the area of the open field, then subtract out the area(s) of blocks. Convert the area to an equivalent square by using the square root.

1. $15 \times 20 = 300$
2. $4 \times 5 = 20$
3. $300 - 40 = 260$
4. $\sqrt{260} = 16.1$

24. When the patient is treated, the bladder should be empty so that localization and targeting is consistent. After the patient voids, the bladder is expected to begin filling during set up and treatment.

25. The pediatric patient has greater sensitivity due to dividing immature cells. TD 5/5s we study most often are based mainly on tissue sensitivities in the adult (unless otherwise stated) using standard fractionation. Variables such as patient's age, revised fractionation schedules, irradiated tissue volume, and type of radiation used change the tolerance of tissues. In addition, the pediatric patient is hoped to have a longer life expectancy and therefore the focus has to remain on keeping the possibility of long-term effects at the bare minimum.

Central Nervous System

1. a. The lateral ventricles are located within the cerebral hemispheres
2. b. Sensory and association are controlled in the parietal area.
3. a. The sense of smell is conveyed by the olfactory nerve-cranial nerve I
4. a. Primary brain tumors spread by local invasion; gliomas tend to remain localized
5. c. Medulloblastoma, ependymomas, pineal gland tumors have high potential to spread throughout the CSF
6. d. The majority of primary brain tumors in adults are gliomas
7. c. SRS is reserved for small solitary primary tumors, small solitary metastatic tumors or small solitary recurrent tumors

Think About It

8. One theory is since the central nervous system is central station for all bodily functions it is self-contained for protection from systemic, pathogenic disability. It therefore sets strict limits regarding what comes in and goes out. Permeation is uniquely controlled in either direction. Non-CNS primaries more readily make their way to the CNS (especially the brain) via the blood route than CNS tumors through common vasculature.
9. Noncoplanar beam arrangements allow for smaller doses from each field with more conforming dose distribution than with traditional fields traversing

a single plane and exposing normal tissues to higher total dose

10. Metastatic brain disease is usually multi-focal. Even if not demonstrated as multi-focal at the time of detection, it is accepted that there is likely microscopic disease throughout the brain. Primary tumors are usually solitary and tend to grow radially from the primary location.
11. From the 225-degree gantry position, 270 degrees in the clockwise direction will end at 135 degrees
12. 280 MU/270 degrees = 1.04 MU/degree
13. **field size**
    output
    field size factor
    attenuating factors (if any)
    average TAR/TMR
    prescribed dose to the tumor
14. d. Symptoms of intracranial tumors would not include nocturia (frequent urination during the night)
15. a. Whenever possible, total resection is the primary mode of management for primary brain tumors.
16. e. Pituitary adenomas may show symptoms associated with hormonal imbalance as in diabetes or visual disturbance or sinus pressure due to anatomical location and extension of tumor
17.

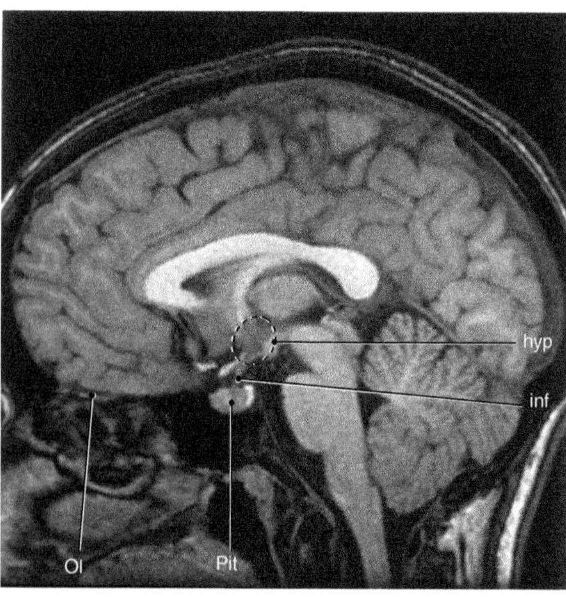

18. e. A tumor compressing the lumbosacral region of the spine could cause incontinence, impotence, and pain down the legs.
19. c. Cranial nerve VII controls movement and sensory of the face
20. a. The TD 5/5 for the lens is 5–10 Gy according to Silverman and Emami
21. a. The TD 5/5 for the optic nerve or chiasm is 50 Gy according to Silverman and Emami
22. a. Injury to the scalp from radiation exposure should be managed by little friction, avoidance of chemicals and perfumes found in shampoos and commercial ointments, and avoidance of extreme temperatures
23. a. Patients with CNS malignancies should always be accompanied and assisted to minimize risk for falling and injury
24. a. Cranial nerve IX controls swallowing and secretion of saliva
25. c. The TD 5/5 for normal brain tissue is 60 Gy; however if only 25% of the brain is included in the treatment volume, tolerance could be pushed to 70 Gy according to Rubin

Skin Cancer

1. F. Melanomas are the most deadly type of skin cancers.
2. T
3. T
4. F. Ulcerating and rolled borders are more characteristic of late stage basal cell or squamous cell skin cancers.
5. T
6. a. Basal cell carcinomas are very curable. In early stages, control rates are 90% or greater.
7. b. Clark's method is based on the depth of invasion through skin layers.
8.
    1. **Pay attention to any changes in the size, color, or status of any existing skin markings**
    2. **Avoid excessive exposure to ultraviolet radiation and use sunscreen of at least 15 SPF**
    3. **People with darkly pigmented skin are not immune to developing skin cancers and should be diligent about monitoring changes in the skin**
    4. **Early diagnosis and early treatment is important. Consult a dermatologist for any questionable changes in the skin**
9.
    1. **Regulation of body temperature; maintain homeostasis**
    2. **Barrier between the environment and the body**
    3. **Produces vitamin D**
    4. **Provides receptors for stimuli like heat, cold and touch**
10. c. Epstein Barr virus is not a known risk factor for skin cancer.
11. a. Melanocytes are found in the stratum basale of the epidermis.
12. a. The stratum basale is the most sensitive to radiation due to high mitotic activity.
13. c. Intense UVA light radiation from tanning beds are damaging to the skin and are just as carcinogenic as ultraviolet rays from the sun.

14. d. Nonmelanomas occur following repeated, long-term UV exposure. Children have not had long-term exposure.
15. c. Lentigo maligna is similar to superficial spreading in that it grows radially to begin with then vertical growth begins. They are usually tan or black and superficial spreading have a variety of reddish tones.

Think About It

16. Immunotherapy is used since melanomas have been noted to regress. Regression is understood to be the body's immune response to disease. Immunotherapy attempts to take advantage of this response and gives the immune system a boost to help fight disease.
17. Using typical fractionation of 40–50 Gy total dose in 2-Gy fractions
    Erythema at 20 Gy
    Dry desquamation at 30 Gy
    Wet desquamation at 40 Gy
18. Use electron beam therapy rule of thumb: $E/4 = \text{depth of } 90\% \text{ dose line}$
    $E/4 = 4\,\text{cm}$
    $E = 16\,\text{MeV}$
19. A lesion in this location would be best treated by electron therapy with careful protection of the lens. A full internal eye shield could be inserted and field shaping by thin lead cut-out placed directly on the skin. Likely, the lesion is small enough to be covered by an extendable, round Lucite cone. Combination of couch and gantry angle to achieve parallel relationship between the surface and horizontal axis of the beam.
20. The lead shield protects the underlying mucosa from residual radiation. Wax behind the shield will further protect the mucosa closest to the septum from secondary radiation from electron/lead interaction.

Leukemia

Define the following terms:

1. Thrombocytopenia—decrease in thrombocytes, also known as platelets
2. Leukapheresis—the sifting out of white cells; selective removal of leukocytes from withdrawn blood that can then be re-transfused
3. Splenomegaly—enlargement of the spleen
4. Leukopenia—decrease in white blood cells
5. Anorexia—weight loss usually associated with a conscious decision to decrease food intake
6. Teratogenic—causing physical defects in the developing embryo; teratogenous- developed from fetal remains
7. Neutropenia—decrease in the number of neutrophils in the blood; neutrophils are granular leukocytes
8. Toxicity—being poisonous; degree of being poisonous or harmful
9. Benzene—a chemical solvent from coal tar; can be used as an insecticide
10. Bone marrow depression—decrease in function of blood forming tissues
11. Auer rods—rod-shaped structures, present in the cytoplasm of myeloblasts, myelocytes, and monoblasts, found in leukemia
12. Nadir—The word nadir means the lowest point. This word is often used in reference to blood counts, particularly white blood cells and platelets. Nadir time can occur within 10-14 days following high doses of chemotherapy. Suppression of blood cell production depends on the drugs administered.
13. Pruritus—Itching that may be caused by inflammation
14. Ecchymoses—A hemorrhagic spot in the skin; looks round or irregular, blue or purplish.

15.–19.

	Drug	Type	Disease	Effect
	Prednisone	Hormonal agent	ALL, CLL	GI-Ulcers/pancreatitis
15.	Chlorambucil	Alkylating agent	CLL	Bone marrow depression (BMD)
16.	Doxorubicin Daunorubicin	Anti-tumor; Anthracycline-antibiotic	ALL, AML	BMD, toxicity of heart and GI
17.	Vinicristine	Plant Alkaloid	ALL	Anorexia, toxicities, myleosuppression, flu-like symptoms
18.	Interferon	Immunotherapeutic drug	CML	Anorexia; weight loss
19.	Hydroxuria	Antimetabolite	ALL	Nausea, vomiting, oral ulcers

20. c. Alfred Velpeau was the first to document a case of leukemia.
21. b. In the case of leukemia, immature white cells accumulate and impair the body's ability to produce adequate red blood cells.
22. a. Wisses blut means white blood.

List the normal values for the following blood values:

23. White blood count **3.90–10.80 thousand/mm³**
24. Red blood count **3.90–5.40 million/mm³**
25. Platelets **150–424 thousand/mm³**
26.

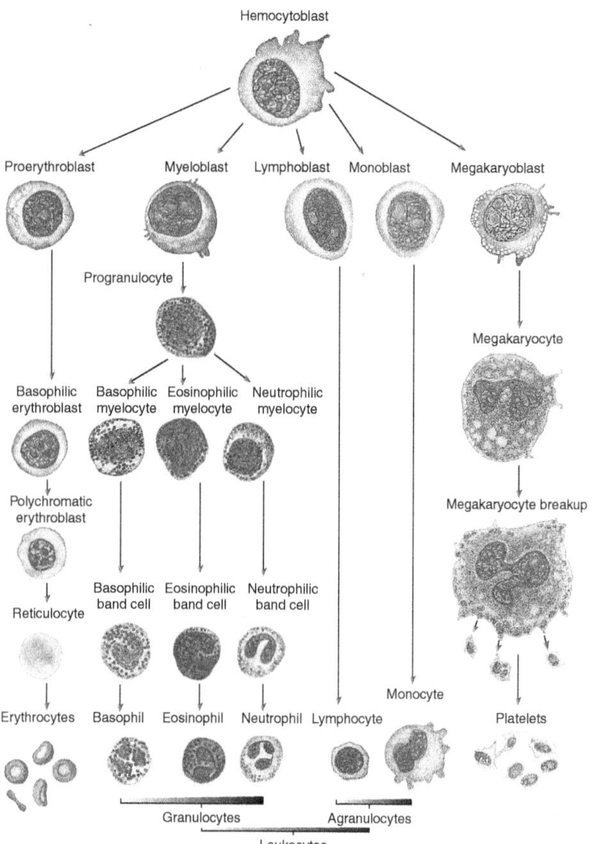

27. List the differential white blood cells:

Basophils	Eosinophils
Neutrophils	Lymphocytes
Monocytes	Platelets

28. a. The type of leukemia seen mostly in children is acute lymphocytic leukemia (ALL).
29. c. Chronic lymphocytic leukemia is not associated with previous radiation exposure.
30. b. Location of the Philadelphia chromosome is a diagnostic factor for detecting CML.
31. **TBI—Total body irradiation may be used in the management of leukemia by having the patient positioned sitting in fetal position at an extended distance from the treatment machine or lying supine or standing. Small children may be treated lying supine as their bodies are small enough to be contained in the collimator area opening. Low dose TBI can be 10 cGy/day to total 4.5 Gy. Special care has to be taken to protect the lungs and lens by varying position or using shields.**
32. Helmet—**This technique is a modification of the whole brain fields. The lower border should be to cervical spine #2 to make sure the fourth ventricle has proper coverage. Lateral fields are appropriate with daily dose of about 1.5 Gy to a total of 25–35 Gy.**
33. CNS—**The total CNS is treated with two lateral brain fields as per the helmet technique and carefully matching a field covering the entire spine from cervical spine #2-3 junction to sacral bone #2 to give margin on the cauda equine. Daily dose is about 1.5 Gy to total 35 Gy to each field.**
34. Bone marrow transplant—**The infusion of bone marrow into a recipient. Donors must be compatible. There are three types: (1) Autologous transplant-donor is also the recipient after marrow has been purged, (2) syngeneic transplant-donor is an identical twin, and (3) allogenic transplant-donor is compatible but unrelated.**
35. **To avoid hot spot where 2 fields may overlap**
36. **Feathering requires the relocation of match points or gaps during treatment of adjacent fields. Movement of match points is suggested to occur every 3–5 treatments.**
37. d. Bone marrow transplants may fail when the recipient experiences graft versus host reaction, the recipient's donated cells are not thoroughly purged or there is recurrence.
38. c. Nadir can occur within 10–14 days in patients who have received methotrexate.
39. d. The integumentary system does not include the blood cells.
40. d. Side effects seen in the skin such as inflammation, change in pigment and hair loss are integumentary side effects from chemotherapy.
41. a. When the spleen in irradiated, a 1-cm margin is recommended.
42. c. Lymphocytosis, or an increase in lymphocytes, is exhibited in patients with CLL.
43. d. Among the four types of leukemia, CML has the worst prognosis.
44. 0.44. Use the gap formula: $L1/2(d/SSD) + L2/2\,(d/SSD)$ $10/2(4/100) + 12/2(4/100) = 0.44$.
45. a. Thermoluminescent dosimeters can be used to verify absorbed dose at specific areas during total body irradiation.
46. c. The subarachnoid mater is not one of the layers of the meninges. They are the dura mater, arachnoid, and pia mater.

47. c. CLL seems to have a hereditary component.
48. b. For a definite diagnosis of ALL, a bone marrow biopsy is imperative.
49. a. The spleen is located in the left upper quadrant of the abdomen.
50. a. In AML, cellular division phases S and M may show a decreased proportion of blastic cells.

Lymphomas

1. Components include lymphatic vessels and nodes and lymphatic organs such as: tonsils, spleen, thymus, and bone marrow. Responsible for immune defenses and circulation of lymph fluid. Filtration of foreign particles and production of lymphocytes.
2. Red blood cells transport oxygen and carbon dioxide. White blood cells are critical to immunity as neutrophils and monocytes carry out phagocytosis and lymphocytes produce antibodies and heparin is produced by basophils and eosinophils help detoxify. Platelets initiate blood clotting and hemostasis.
3. T and B lymphocytes. B cells secrete antibodies. T cells kill cells bearing specific antigens.
4. Lymphatic capillaries merge to form the lymphatic vessels.
5. The lymph vessels lead to collecting ducts that unite with the veins in the thorax. After leaving the lymph nodes, the lymph vessels merge to form larger lymphatic trunks. The trunks drain the lymph from large regions of the body. The trunks join one of two collecting ducts known as the thoracic or right lymph duct.
6. The thoracic duct receives lymph from the cistern chyli and the right lymphatic duct empties into the cisterna.
7. Foreign substances that enter a lymph node are removed or filtered out by phagocytes.
8. Lymph flows into the node through afferent vessels and flow out by way of efferent vessels.
9. The spleen is responsible for hemopoiesis, red blood cell and platelet destruction, and serves as a reservoir for blood.
10. Without a spleen, the other blood forming tissues can take over.
11. Lymphatic vessels have the capacity for repair and regeneration.
12. The thymus traps immature stem cells and pre-processes them so that they become sensitized and capable of maturing into types of lymphocytes essential to developing immunity. This happens in fetal life and typically reaches its maximum performance by puberty.
13. b. The largest lymphatic organ is the spleen.
14. d. The vallecula is not a tonsil.
15. a. The thymus gland atrophies after puberty.
16. b. The B lymphocyte develops from a stem cell in the hematopoietic tissues.
17. c. The lymphatic system consists of lymph fluid, vessels, organs, and nodes.
18. c. Lymph nodes are about 1–25 mm in diameter.
19. b. The thymus gland produces T cells.
20. d. NHL can occur in many sites including nodes, lymph tissue or gastrointestinal tract. Unlike HL, NHL may spread randomly.
21. b. The thoracic duct begins at the cistern chyli.
22. c. Most Hodgkin's disease cases will present as nodular sclerosis type.
23. c. The most common presenting symptom for Hodgkin's disease is a painless cervical node.
24. b. The Reed-Sternberg cell is present in cases of Hodgkin's disease.
25. b. The staging system for lymphomas is traditionally the Ann Arbor staging system.
    Staging of lymphomas may also include the following letters denoting organ. (MATCH)
26. d
27. c
28. b
29. a
30. g
31. e
32. f
33. **True and False.** This is debatable today. Traditionally, radiation therapy has been the primary treatment for early stage Hodgkin's disease. Due to realization of late effects, treatment schemes are being reconsidered putting chemotherapy as the primary and radiation as an adjunct to involved fields
34. c. Although this patient has three lymph node areas involved, they are all above the diaphragm. This is classified as stage II according to Ann Arbor staging.
35. d. Although pruritus can be an associated symptom of Hodgkin's disease, it is not a classic B symptom.
36. d. Both sides of the diaphragm positive with an extralymphatic site would be considered stage IIIE.
37. d. As Waldeyer's ring includes the tonsillar tissues, the treatment field is in close proximity for a treatment field in the management of nasopharynx cancer.
38. c. The traditional mantle field would include the cervical, mediastinal and axillary lymph nodes.
39. d. Treatment to the abdomen may cause the patient to experience nausea, vomiting and fatigue.
40. T. NHL occurs primarily in older persons whereas HD is seen mostly in adolescents and young adults.
41. T. HD tends to spread in an orderly fashion through lymph stations contiguously.
42. b. Lower neck and mediastinal nodes without classic symptoms would be classified as stage IIA.

43. b. Nodular sclerosis carries the most favorable histology. Although, recent studies suggest that histological variation have little influence on prognosis.
44. d. NHL may arise in nodes, gastrointestinal tract or lymphatic tissues such as Waldeyer's ring.
45. c. Non Hodgkin's lymphocytes may arrange themselves in follicular or nodular patterns.
46. c. The optimal dose to the upper mantle is 35-44 Gy.
47. c. The nodes included in the inverted Y field in the management of Hodgkin's lymphoma are the retroperitoneal, common iliac, external and internal iliac and inguinal nodes (superficial inguinal nodes are not included).
48. b. Carditis is inflammation of the heart and can be a chronic side effect of mantle irradiation.
49. b. Dysphagia may be an early effect of mantle irradiation. Dysphagia is difficulty swallowing.
50. b. The appropriate separation between upper and lower fields is known as the skin gap.

Pediatric

1. a. If the entire width of the spine is not included in the radiation field, one portion of the spine will grow normally while the other portion would be stunted, resulting in spinal scoliosis.
2. a. Parasites are not a known risk factor for solid tumors in children.
3. c. Wilms' tumors, or nephroblastomas, are often found by parents feeling a mass in the abdomen of the child.
4. b. Nephroblastomas, or Wilms' tumors, metastasize to the lung
5. a. Neuroblastomas originate in neural crest cells
6. a. Medulloblastomas, ependymomas and pineal gland tumors have high incidence of CSF spread.
7. c. Ewing's sarcoma, or osteogenic cancer, has a common symptom of pain in the bone.
8. a. Although rare, retinoblastoma is the most common malignancy found in the orbit of children
9. b. Wilms' tumors originate in immature kidney cells known as nephroblasts.
10. d. ALL is associated with prophylactic irradiation of the brain or entire CNS to maintain remission.
11.

Allogeneic donor __B__	A. self
Autologous donor __A__	B. compatible match
Syngeneic donor __C__	C. Identical two

12. a and c. Late toxicities of therapy are of great concern when treating children. Delayed bone growth, secondary cancers, and mental deficits (brain) are a few adverse consequences of radiation therapy.
13. c. An enucleation is the removal of the entire orbit
14. c. Preschool aged children are just beginning to communicate and show some independence. Keep instructions honest and simple.
15. d. The adolescent patient is concerned about privacy and personal appearance and can make independent decisions.
16. c. This 17 year old is concerned with physical appearance so assuring her that there are some alternatives is promising.

Think About It

17. Table kick = 6.1 degrees

Use the divergence formula:

1. $\tan^{-1}$ (A/2 SSD)
2. $\tan^{-1}$ (20/186)
3. $\tan^{-1}$ (0.1075)

18. Daily dose will be 1.5 Gy equally weighted; convert to cGy

Equivalent square using Sterling's formula
$= 2(15 \times 20)/35 = 17.1$
Treatment depth = 7 cm as per SSD given

$$\frac{75\,\text{cGy}}{0.996 \times 1.028 \times 0.794} = 92\ \text{MU/per field}$$

19.

b. Using direct proportion

$$\frac{40 : 100\,\text{cm}}{48 : \text{x}} \times = 120\,\text{cm}$$

20.

c. Collimator setting indicates the size of the field area at isocenter. Using direct proportion with the above extended distance of 120 cm. Already know the length from the previous equation, so

$$\frac{8 : 120}{\text{x} : 100} \times = 6.7\,\text{cm}$$

Soft Tissue Sarcoma

1. b. Soft tissue sarcomas spread along the longitudinal axis of the muscle in which it originated
2. c. Treating the entire circumference of the limb should be avoided and a strip of tissue should be spared during high dose radiation treatment of extremities to prevent chronic obstruction of lymphatic fluid flow.
3. a. Lower extremities are almost always treated with the patient reversed on the couch due to equipment limitations; except for young children
4. b. Sarcomas originate in the mesoderm
5. c. Rhabdo- is the prefix for striated. Rhabdomyosarcomas arise from striated muscle
6. d. Lipo- is the prefix for fat. Liposarcomas originate in fatty tissues
7. d. Primary tumors originating in the compact bone metastasize to the lung through the blood route
8. d. Limb salvaging surgery is to preserve functioning of the limb. This may entail performing a biopsy

only through the lesions or taking a section of the bone out and replacing it with tissue grafts or mechanical fixation.

9. b. A lytic lesion would appear moth-eaten with decreased density on x-ray.
10. c. Weight loss and fever are rare symptoms of primary bone cancer except for Ewing's sarcoma and multiple myeloma due to hypercalcemia
11. c.18-23 Gy is the TD 5/5 for the kidney according to Emami
12. a. The periosteum is the outer layer of the bone and acts as a natural barrier for metastasis outside of the bone compartment.
13. c. Haversian systems are the concentric patterns in compact bone.
14. b. The epiphysis is at the end of the bone and is made up of spongy bone.
15. a. A plasmacytoma is another name for a solitary multiple myeloma
16. b. Ewing's sarcoma has a layered onion-skin appearance on x-ray.
17. c. Soft tissue tumors often manifest as painless, fast growing masses (those in the abdomen or near nerves may be painful)
18. d. Ewing's sarcoma is the most common bone tumor in children younger than 10 years old.
19. c. Across all age groups, osteosarcoma is the most common bone primary
20. d. Kaposi's sarcoma has a high incidence in people with AIDS
21. a. Soft tissue sarcomas are primarily controlled by total excision.
22. d. Soft tissue sarcoma grading takes into account the tumor, lymph nodes, metastasis, and grading is very important.
23. T. Soft tissue sarcomas have low incidence in the United States, approximately 6000 cases per year.
24. T. Although rhabdomyosarcomas are not commonly found in the orbit, it is the most common primary orbital malignancy in children
25. F. No lymph nodes are included in primary bone treatment fields because the potential for spread is along the bone and through the vessels in the layers of the bone.

Think About It

26.

- **a.** The patient could be supine with the affected leg elevated and opposite leg positioned flat on the PSA reversed head in toward gantry.
- **b.** The patient could be in lateral position with affected leg bent and resting on the PSA reversed head toward gantry
- **c.** The patient could be in prone position with the affected leg slightly elevated. However, this would likely require the use of collimator angles if lateral fields were used. Reversed on PSA

27.

- **a.** The patient could be positioned supine with arms raised and fields directed toward the right outer abdomen. Immobilize the arms and upper thorax.
- **b.** The patient could be positioned in left lateral decubitus position with arms up toward head and knees bent with field focused on the right outer abdomen. Immobilize the upper torso to minimize rotation. This position may spare more bowel from parallel opposed flank fields.

28.

Ewing's affects mainly adolescents. It originates in the bone marrow versus compact bone. Ewing's has small, round, blue cells versus spindle-type cells found in osteosarcoma. Ewing's tend to show up in the mid-shaft of the bone rather than the ends

29.

Bone metastasis is treated with total doses of about 30 Gy with fractions of 3 Gy. Primary bone tumors are treated with total doses ranging from 50–80 Gy using fraction of 1.8–2 Gy.

30.

Although both may be treated using parallel opposed ports, special care is taken to spare normal tissue during treatment of primary bone tumors to preserve lymphatic flow. Primary bone fields will likely begin with wide margins and then shrink to finally conform to the region of tumor. Metastatic bone fields may begin with wide margins but field sizes remain unchanged throughout the course.

Palliative Care

1. a. Vision problems are symptoms of abnormality in the parietal or occipital lobes of the brain
2. c. Average survival for patients with brain metastasis is between 6 weeks to 6 months
3. The lytic lesion would appear moth-eating and the blastic lesion would appear as dense, abnormal overgrowth of bone on x-ray.
4. Palliative doses for brain metastasis are typically 300 cGy per fraction to a total dose of 30–45 Gy. Doses for primary brain malignancy are typically 180–200 cGy per fraction to total of 60 GY.
   SRS for small, isolated, metastatic lesions may be given to total dose of 20–30 Gy.
   SRT for small, isolated primary lesions may be given to total dose of >60 GY
5. Superior vena cava syndrome—**a compression of the vena cava by tumors in the apex of the lung or mediastinum**

Laminectomy—**removal of a portion of the lamina to decrease or prevent compression of the spinal cord**
Partial hepatectomy—**removal of a portion of the liver**

6. d. Steroids are anti-inflammatory substances
7. d. Brain metastasis may be characterized by many symptoms according to the location of malignancy
8. c. Cauda equine compression may cause incontinence; decreases urethral, vaginal, and rectal sensation
9. c. Strontium, samarium, phosphorus, and rhenium are commonly used radionuclides for bone metastasis
10. a. In the management of SVC syndrome and spinal cord compression, a more immediate response may be prompted by high doses such as 300–400 cGy the first few fractions, then tapering to lower doses depending on the confirmed diagnosis.
11. d. Radiation pneumonitis is not managed by radiation therapy
12. a. Bone metastasis can occur anywhere in the bone; however, the long bones, pelvis, and spine are the most common areas for metastasis
13. a. Metastatic brain malignancy is usually identifiable by its multifocal lesions. Primary brain cancers are usually solitary
14. d. The cervical spine may be treated with the patient supine in neutral head position or prone with neutral head position so as not to put added stress on the cervical region.
15. d. In the thoracic spine region, each thoracic vertebra is about 2.5 cm in length and about 6 centimeters in width, including the transverse processes.
16. b. When treating spinal cord compression, the affected vertebra and one vertebra above and below should be included. A lower lumbar spine compression would require treatment of the sacrum, which is about 12 cm in width. To spare bowel, treatment of the lower lumbar spine and sacrum would be suitable for an upside down T-shaped treatment field
17. a. Since the lumbar spine has concave curvature, it is most appropriate to use opposing anterior-posterior fields for even dose distribution
18. d. A patient having a major seizure should be assisted to a safe place to limit the risk of injury. Therapist should be available to monitor the patient once the event has ended.
19. b. Fainting is a common symptom of SVC syndrome. Therapist should assess patient's breathing and circulation and notify the physician. Patient may resume consciousness without any intervention.
20. a. A malignancy in the liver may prevent the normal flowing out of bile into the small intestine, leading to jaundice.
21. Using the diagram below, draw typical radiation treatment field(s) for confirmed boney metastasis to T6.

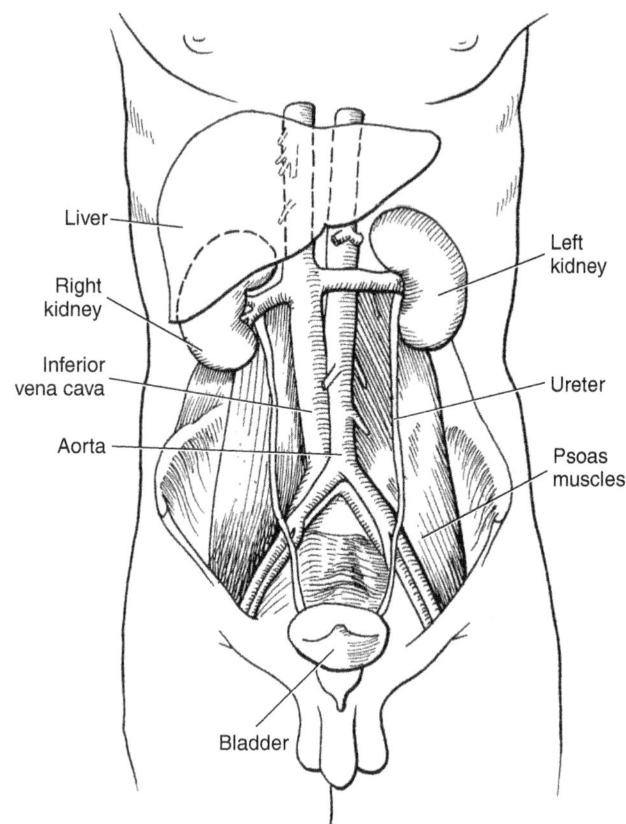

22. Using the diagram below, draw the typical whole brain radiation treatment field(s).

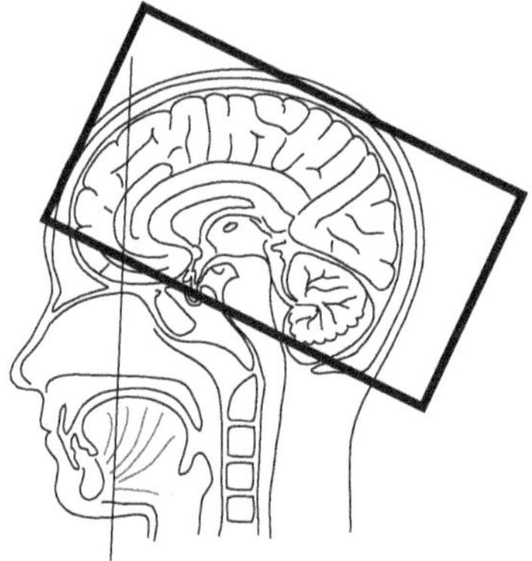

23. a. Primary adenocarcinoma of the lung
24. a. Lymph nodes are not usually a concern when the goal of treatment is palliation since the disease has already metastasized
25. a. A simple daily treatment charge is appropriate for single fields with no beam shaping or modifiers
26. b. The opposing collimator angle to 30 degrees is 330 degrees. Draw the collimator dial to confirm.
27. a. For midline treatment through an area with an interfield distance of 15 cm, isocenter should be placed and calculations done for a depth ½ of the total separation. ½(15) = 7.5cm.

Illustration Credits

Applegate E: *The sectional anatomy learning system: concepts*, ed 3, St. Louis, 2010, Saunders/Elsevier. **Figs. 1-12, 7-2**

Blackburn B, Shahabi, S: *Blackburn's introduction to clinical radiation therapy physics*, ed 1, Madison, 1989, Medical Physics Publishing. **Fig. 7-5**

Bomford CK, Kunkler IH: *Walter and Miller's textbook of radiotherapy*, ed 6, London, 2003, Churchill Livingstone. **Figs. 6-2, 6-4, 7-10**

Bushong, SC: *Radiologic science for technologists*, ed 9, St. Louis, 2008, Mosby. **Figs. 3-4, 3-8**

Christian PE, Waterstram-Rich KM: *Nuclear medicine and PET/CT*, ed 6, St. Louis, 2007, Mosby. **Fig. 3-1**

Cox JD: *Moss' radiation oncology: rationale, techniques, results*, ed 7, St. Louis, 1994, Mosby. **Figs. 9-17, 9-26**

Frank ED, Long BW, Smith BJ: *Merrill's atlas of radiographic positioning and procedures*, ed 11, 2007, Mosby. **Figs. 9-9, 9-19**

Gates R, Fink R: *Oncology nursing secrets*, ed 3, St. Louis, 2008, Mosby. **Fig. 2-3**

Gunderson LL, Tepper JE: *Clinical radiation oncology*, ed 2, Philadelphia, 2007, Churchill Livingstone. **Figs. 2-5, 3-5, 4-2, 7-9, 9-18**

Kahn FM: *The physics of radiation therapy*, ed 3, Philadelphia, 2003, Lippincott Williams & Wilkins. **Fig. 6-3**

Kelley LL, Petersen CM: *Sectional anatomy for imaging professionals*, ed 2, 2007, Mosby. **Figs. 9-5, 9-6, 9-20, 9-21, 9-22, 9-31, 9-32**

Leibel SA, Phillip TL: *Textbook of radiation oncology*, ed 2, Philadelphia, 2004, Saunders. **Figs. 9-1, 9-2, 9-4, 9-7, 9-10**

Mountain CF, Dresler CM: *Regional lymph node classification for staging lung cancer.* Chest 111:1718-1723, 1997. **Fig. 9-3**

Seely R: *Essentials of anatomy and physiology*, St. Louis, 1991, Mosby. **Fig. 9-15**

Seeram E: *Computed tomograhy: physical principles, clinical applications and quality control*, ed 3, St. Louis, 2009, Saunders. **Figs. 6-6, 7-6**

Washington CM, Leaver D: *Principles and practice of radiation therapy*, ed 3, St. Louis, 2010, Mosby. **Figs. 7-1A, 9-8, 9-13, 9-14, 9-16, 9-23, 9-24**

Courtesies

Louis Clark. **Figs. 9-27, 9-28**

Dennis Strete. **Figs. 9-25 (photograph)**

Oldelft Corporation, Fairfax, VA. **Fig. 7-1B**

TomoTherapy, Inc. **Fig. 6-5**

United States Environmental Protection Agency. **Fig. 5-1**, at http://www.epa.gov/radiation/understand/symbols.html. Accessed 12/31/09.

Varian Medical Systems. **Fig. 6-1**

INDEX

Note: Page numbers followed by *b* indicate boxes, *f* indicate figures and *t* indicate tables.

C

D

F

G

H

J

K

L

M

N

O

P

Q

S

T

U